PERIPHERAL NEUROPATHY – ADVANCES IN DIAGNOSTIC AND THERAPEUTIC APPROACHES

Edited by **Ghazala Hayat**

Peripheral Neuropathy – Advances in Diagnostic and Therapeutic Approaches
Edited by Ghazala Hayat

Published by InTech
Janeza Trdine 9, 51000 Rijeka, Croatia

Publishing Process Manager Silvia Vlase

Technical Editor Teodora Smiljanic

Cover Designer InTech Design Team

Additional hard copies can be obtained from orders@intechopen.com

Peripheral Neuropathy – Advances in Diagnostic and Therapeutic Approaches,
Edited by Ghazala Hayat
p. cm.
ISBN 978-953-51-0066-9

For EU product safety concerns:
IN TECH d.o.o., Prolaz Marije Krucifikse Kozulić 3, 51000 Rijeka, Croatia,
info@intechopen.com or visit our website at intechopen.com.

Meet the editor

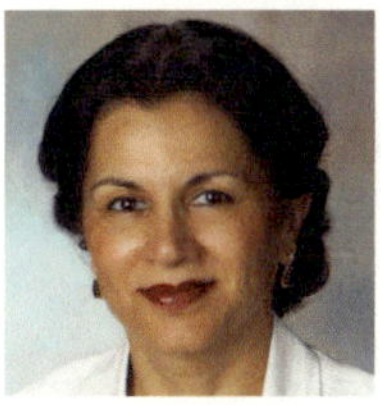

Ghazala Hayat is a professor of Neurology & Psychiatry at the St. Louis University, USA. She is also the director of Neuromuscular, Clinical Neurophysiology services and Clinical Neurophysiology fellowship. After graduating from the King Edward Medical College in Pakistan, prof. Hayat received her training in neurology, neuromuscular disorders and neurophysiology at the Medical College Virginia, USA. Prof. Hayat is board certified in neurology, electrodiagnostic medicine, neuromuscular medicine and clinical neurophysiology. Her interests include peripheral neuropathies, compressive neuropathies, neuromuscular junction disorders and electrodiagnostic studies. She has published on various topics in her area of expertise. Prof. Hayat is a fellow of American Academy of Neurologists, American Association of Neuromuscular disorders & Electrodiagnostic medicine. She was nominated for America's Best Doctors 2007-2012.

Contents

Preface

Over the last two decades we have seen extensive progress within the practice of neurology. We have refined our understanding of the etiology and pathogenesis for both peripheral and central nervous system diseases, and developed new therapeutic approaches towards these diseases.

Peripheral neuropathy is a common disorder seen by many specialists and can pose a diagnostic dilemma. Many etiologies, including drugs that are used to treat other diseases, can cause peripheral neuropathy. However, the most common cause is Diabetes Mellitus, a disease all physicians encounter. Disability due to peripheral neuropathy can be severe, as the patients suffer from symptoms daily.

This book addresses the advances in the diagnosis and therapies of peripheral neuropathy over the last decade. The basics of different peripheral neuropathies is briefly discussed, however, the book focuses on topics that address new approaches to peripheral neuropathies.

The book is divided into four sections: I) Etiology, II) Methods of Investigation, III) Clinical Manifestations and IV) Advances in Therapies of Peripheral Neuropathy. The topics located in the first section address the role of Dynamin in Charcot Marie Tooth, molecular chaperones in diabetic neuropathy and predictors for chemotherapy induced peripheral neuropathy. Section II covers different approaches to investigate peripheral neuropathies. Electrophysiological studies, an integral diagnostic tool, are discussed throughout the book, but a complete chapter was not dedicated to the classical methods of investigation in order to address relatively new methods. MRI scans are increasingly used to diagnose peripheral nerve pathology. A chapter in this section covers the important aspects of this technology and possible indications. Section III consists of clinical manifestations of peripheral neuropathies in children. A chapter is dedicated to the disabling length dependent neuropathies due to compromised balance. Section IV comprises of advances in therapeutic approaches. Gene and cell therapy is the future of many disorders, especially in peripheral nervous system disorders. Cell therapy in diabetic neuropathy and ischemic neuropathies has been discussed in detail. Current therapies for neuropathic pain are also included.

This book will be valuable for specialists in the area and serve as a resource to general neurologists and primary care physicians.

I dedicate this book to our patients who are our inspiration to find the cause and cure for diverse peripheral neuropathies.

I would like to take this opportunity to thank all of the authors for their dedication and effort throughout the editing process. I hope this book will add to our ever expanding knowledge of this common but complex disorder.

Prof. Ghazala Hayat
Department of Neurology & Psychiatry,
Clinical Neurophysiology,
Neuromuscular Diseases,
Saint Louis University,
USA

Part 1

Insights into Etiology of Peripheral Neuropathies

1

Etiological Role of Dynamin in Charcot-Marie-Tooth Disease

Kohji Takei and Kenji Tanabe
Okayama University
Japan

1. Introduction

Charcot–Marie–Tooth disease (CMT) is one of the most common inherited neuropathy, with estimated prevalence of 17 to 40 in 100,000 affected (Patzkó, & Shy, 2011). CMT is characterized by atrophy of muscle tissue and loss of touch sensation of limb, predominantly in the feet and legs, foot drop, and hammer toes. The most frequent initial symptoms include foot drop, claw toe, and muscle wasting in the hands. Symptoms in the advanced cases may include muscle waste in the hands and fore arms, neck and shoulder, vocal cords, which leads to scoliosis and malfunction in chewing, swallowing, or speaking.

The defective neurotransmission stems from either degradation of myelin sheath or breakdown of neuronal axon, which define primary forms of this disease, CMT type 1 and CMT type 2 respectively. CMT type 1 and CMT type 2 can be clinically distinguished based on nerve conduction velocity (NCV). Slow NCV (less than 38 m/s) is characteristic of demyelinating CMT type 1, and the average NCV is slightly below normal, but above 38 m/s in CMT type 2. In addition, dominant intermediate subtypes of CMT (DI-CMT) have been identified, which are characterized by NCVs overlapping both demyelinating and axonal range (25 - 45 m/s).

Number of genes and gene loci has been involved in the pathogenesis of CMT, and despite of diversity of the responsible genes, they are involved in common molecular pathways within Schwann cells and axons that cause these genetic neuropathies (Patzkó & Shy, 2011). CMT Type 1 primarily affects the myelin sheath, and is inherited as dominant, recessive or X-linked. Type 2 primarily affects the axon, and is either dominant or recessive. DI-CMT is classified type A (DI-CMTA), type B (DI-CMTB) type C (DI-CMTC), and type D (DI-CMTD) according to responsible genes and gene loci.

In this review, we focus on dynamin 2 and the mutations, which are responsible for DI-CMTB and axonal CMT type 2. We explain physiological role of dynamin 2 in the regulation of microtubules and propose possible pathogenesis of CMT attributed to dynamin 2 mutants.

2. Dyanmin2 mutation in CMT

As described above, three types of dominantly inherited CMT with intermediate NCV DI-CMT) are known. DI-CMTA was found in a large Italian family and it is linked to chromosome 10q24.1-q25.1 (Rossi et al., 1985; Verhoeven et al., 2001; Villanova et al., 1998), but the responsible gene remains currently unknown. Two unrelated Midwestern-American and Bulgarian families with DI-CMT are linked to chromosome 1p34-p35, and it is classified as DI-CMTC (Jordanova et al., 2003b). In DI-CMTC, a mutation has been identified in tyrosyl-tRNA synthetase (YARS)(Jordanova et al., 2006).

Studies on DI-CMT in unrelated two large pedigrees originating from Australia and North America, has assigned the locus (DI-CMTB) to chromosome 19p12–13.2. (Kennerson et al., 2001; Zhu et al., 2003). Successively, Züchner and coworkers refined the locus of the two DICMTB families and additional Belgian family, and identified mutations in dynamin 2 (Züchner et al., 2005). The North-American family showed a 9-bp deletion of the 3′ end of exon 14 of DNM2, 1652_1659+1delATGAGGAGg which is predicted to result in a shift of the open reading frame leading to a premature stop codon (Lys550fs), and the production of an in-frame mRNA with predicted deletion of three amino acids (Asp551_Glu553del). The Australian family and the Belgian family affect the same amino acid residue of dynamin 2: Lys558. The Australian family carried a missense mutation in exon 15, 1672A→G, resulting in the amino acid substitution Lys558Glu. The Belgian family showed a deletion of a single amino acid, Lys558del (1672_1674delAAG). Dynamin mutations in DI-CMTB identified in the original report were restricted in its PH domain (Züchner et al., 2005, Fig. 2).

Subsequently, Claeys et al., analyzed the three original families and in three additional unrelated Spanish, Belgian and Dutch families with DI-CMTB and found two novel mutations in dynamin 2 (Claeys et al., 2009). They identified the novel missense mutation Gly358Arg (1072G4A) in exon 7 of dynamin 2 in the Spanish family, and the novel Thr855_Ile856del (2564_2569delCCATTA) mutation in exon 19 in the index patient of the Belgian family. These mutations are situated in the middle domain and proline-rich domain of dynamin 2, respectively (Fig. 2). Other mutations of dynamin 2 have been identified in CMT patients who present with symptoms typical of axonal CMT (CMT2)(Fabrizi et al., 2007; Bitoun et al., 2008). The later study identified a heterozygous three base-pair deletion located in exon 15 of dynamin 2 (1675_1677delAAA) which results in the loss of the highly conserved lysine 559 (Lys559del) located in the PH domain (Fig.2).

3. Overview of dynamin

Before mentioning possible pathogenesis of CMT caused by the mutation of dynamin 2, the key molecule will be outlined here. In addition to the biochemical characteristics of the molecule, when and how the protein has been identified and studied, or what has been known so far regarding to its functions, will be described below.

3.1 Identification of dynamin

Long before the discovery of mammalian dynamin, Drosophila melanogaster mutant shibire (shi^{ts}), a temperature-sensitive paralytic mutant, has been known (Grigliatti et al., 1973) Ultrastructural analysis of the neuromuscular junction of shi^{ts} mutant fly revealed depletion of synaptic vesicles and accumulation of endocytic pits at presynaptic plasma membrane of neurons (Kosaka & Ikeda, 1983). Thus, the paralysis of shi^{ts} mutant fly is caused by synaptic dysfunction due to blockage of synaptic vesicle endocytosis.

Mammalian dynamin was originally isolated from bovine brain as a microtubule-binding protein (Shpetner & Vallee, 1989). Purified dynamin bound and interconnected microtubules, and supported microtubule gliding (Shpetner & Vallee, 1989, Fig. 1).

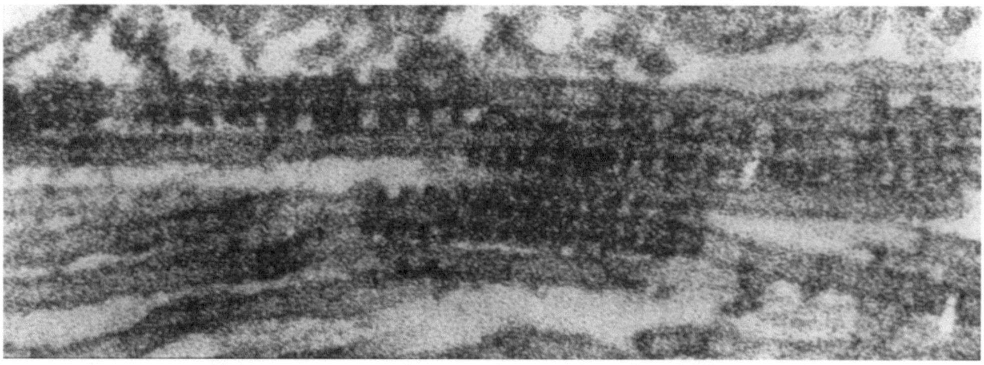

Fig. 1. Electron micrograph of dynamin polymerizing around microtubules.
Bundle of microtubules decorated with dynamin (from Shpetner & Vallee, 1989).

Following the identification, dynamin was cloned and sequenced (Obar et al., 1990). The amino acid sequence contained three consensus elements characteristic of GTP-binding proteins and suggested that it is a GTPase (Obar et al., 1990). As suggested, dynamin was turned out to be a GTPase, which was highly stimulated by the presence of microtubules (Shpetner & Vallee, 1992). Later on, Drosophila shibire gene was cloned and sequenced (Obar et al., 1990; van der Bliek et al., 1991), which revealed considerably high homology of mammalian dynamin and shibire gene product (66% identity, 78% similarity). This revelation immediately put dynamin in the central stage of endocytosis research. In a short while, endocytosis was examined in COS and HeLa cells overexpressing mutant dynamin, and it was found that an endocytosis is blocked at an intermediate stage (Herskovits et al., 1993; van der Bliek et al., 1993).

3.2 Dynamin Isoforms and their expression

The mammalian brain dynamin was exclusively expressed in neurons (Scaife & Margolis, 1990), preferentially after postnatal day 7 (Nakata et al., 1991). This neuron-specific isoform is termed dynamin 1 after two other isoforms with different tissue distributions were identified. Dynamin 2 is expressed ubiquitously (Cook et al., 1994), and dynamin 3 is expressed highly in brain, testis, lung and heart (Nakata et al., 1993).

3.3 Domain structure of dynamin

Dynamin isoforms were highly homologous, and all the dynamin isoforms share five characteristic domains (Fig. 2). They include highly conserved N-terminal GTPase domain, middle domain that binds to γ-tubulin (Thompson et al., 2004), pleckstrin homology domain (PH) that serves as binding motif for phophinositide-4, 5-bisphosphate (PIP_2)(Barylko et al., 1998), and GTPase effector domain (GED). C-terminal Proline/arginine -rich domain (PRD) considerably varies between dynamin isoforms, and mediates interaction with various SH3-domains containing molecules, which include endocytic proteins amphiphysin 1 (David et al., 1996; Yoshida et al., 2004), endophilin (Ringstad et al., 1997), intersectin (Zamanian et al., 2003), and sorting nexin 9 (Ramachandran & Schmid, 2008). Actin binding proteins, such as cortactin and Abp1, also contain SH3 domain and bind to dynamin PRD (McNiven et al., 2000; Kessels et al., 2001).

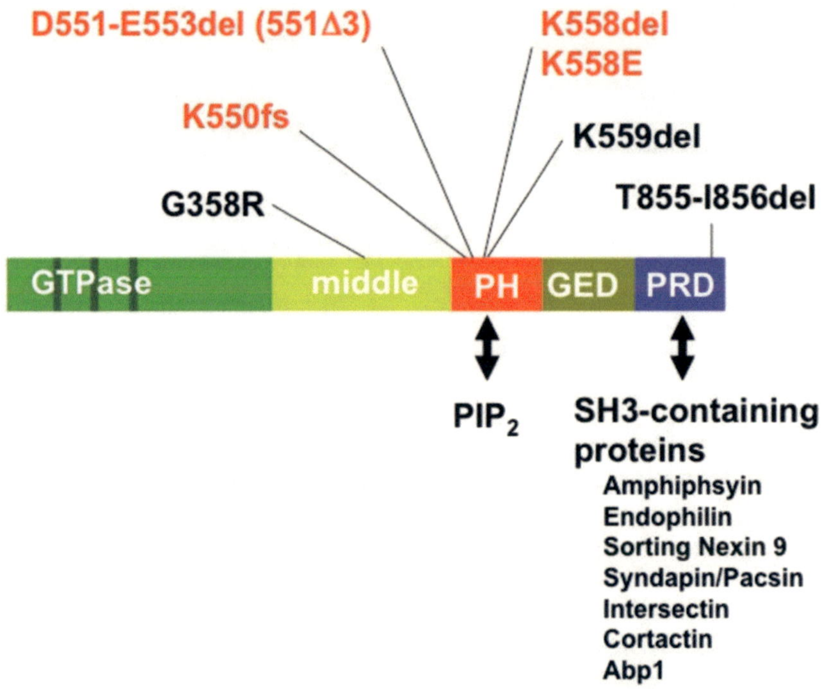

Fig. 2. Domain structure of dynamin and its mutation cites identified in CMT patients
All dynamin isoforms contains five functional domains. Reported mutations found in CMT patients are shown. Among these, four mutations indicated in red are reported in the first study on dynamin mutation in CMT (Züchner et al., 2005). Counterparts of dynamin's binding motifs, PH and PRD, are also shown. GTPase: GTPase domain, middle: middle domain, PH: pleckstrin homology domain, GED: GTPase effector domain, PRD: Proline/arginine -rich domain, PIP_2: phophinositide-4, 5-bisphosphate.

3.4 Function of dynamin in endocytosis

Dynamin self-assembles, or assembles with a binding partner molecule into rings and spirals *in vitro* (Hinshaw & Schmid, 1995; Takei et al., 1999). Furthermore, in presence of lipodsomes, dynamin polymerizes on the lipid membranes and deform them into narrow tubules, and constricts the lipid tubules to fragments upon GTP-hydrolysis (Sweitzer & Hinshaw, 1998; Takei et al., 1998; Stowell et al., 1999). This biophysical property of dynamin seems to support its role in the fission of endocytic pits in endocytosis.

Physiologically, dynamin assembles into rings and spirals at the neck of deeply invaginated endocytic pits formed on the plasma membrane (Takei et al., 1995), and conformation of the polymerized dynamin is changed upon GTP hydrolysis providing a driving force to squeeze the neck to membrane fission (Sweitzer & Hinshaw, 1998; Takei et al., 1998; Marks et al., 2001; Roux et al., 2006; Ramachandran & Schmid, 2008)(Fig.3). This mechanism of action of dynamin in endocytosis is referred as pinchase model (McNiven, 1998). Another model, in which conformational change of dynamin cause the extension of the dynamin spirals to pop off of the endocytic pit, is also proposed as popase model (Stowell et al., 1999). In either case, dynamin functions as a GTPase-driven mechanoenzyme in endocytosis.

Dynamin GTPase activity is stimulated by self-assembly (Warnock et al., 1996), by PH domain-mediated interaction with membrane lipids such as PIP_2 (Lin et al., 1997), or by PRD-mediated interaction with subset of SH3 domain-containing proteins (Yoshida et al., 2004). This enzymatic characteristic of dynamin would be favorable for its function as a mechanochemical enzyme in endocytosis.

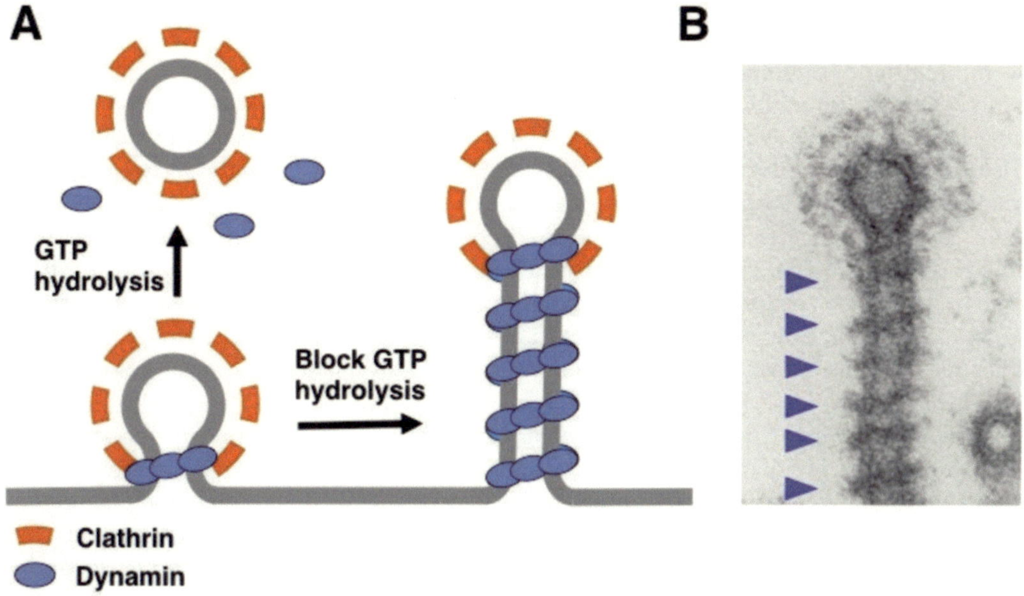

Fig. 3. Function of domain in endocytosis A: Dynamin assembles into rings at the neck of deeply invaginated endocytic pits formed on the plasma membrane. Conformational change of the polymerized dynamin upon GTP hydrolysis provides a driving force to squeeze the endocytic pit to membrane fission (left). Experimentally inhibiting the GTP hydrolysis results in overpolymerization of dynamin around elongated endocytic pit (middle).
B: Electron micrograph of elongated endocytic pit decorated with dynamin (arrowheads, from Takei et al., 1995)

Dynamin PRD interacts with various SH3 domain-containing endocytic proteins enriched in the synapse, including amphiphysin 1 (David et al., 1996; Takei et al., 1999; Yoshida et al., 2004), endophilin (Farsad et al., 2001), sorting nexin 9 (Ramachandran & Schmid, 2008; Shin et al., 2008), syndapin (Kessels et al., 2004), and intersectin (Yamabhai et al., 1998). Such interactions may be utilized to incorporate various functional molecules synchronously required for endocytosis. For example, by interacting with amphiphysin or endophilin, BAR domain–containing endocytic proteins, BAR domain's function of sensing or inducing membrane curvature would be synchronized with dynamin's fission activity (Yoshida et al., 2004; Itoh et al., 2005). By interacting with Abp1 or cortactin, actin dynamics would take place at the site of endocytosis (Kessels et al., 2001). Treatment with Latrunculin B, actin monomer-sequestering agent that blocks fast actin polymerization, results in the inhibition of fission reaction, supporting an implication of actin dynamics in endocytosis (Itoh et al., 2005).

Dynamin 1 is phosphorylated by several kinases including PKC and CDK5, and dephosphorylated by carcinerurin. Dynamin-dependent endocytosis is enhanced in presence of Roscovitine, CDK5 inhibitor, indicating that CDK5-dependent phosphorylation of dynamin1 negatively regulates endocytosis. CDK5 phosphorylates not only dynmain1 but also amphiphsyin1, its biding partner in endocytosis, and phosphorylation of these molecules decreases the binding affinity of these endocytic molecules (Tomizawa et al., 2003).

3.5 Implication of dynamin in actin dynamics

Involvement of dynamin in the regulation of actin dynamics is based largely on studies using dynamin 2, a ubiquitous isoform. Dynamin 2 is enriched in variety of actin-rich structures, such as podosomes (Ochoa et al., 2000), invadopodia (Baldassarre et al., 2003), lamellipodia and dorsal membrane ruffles (Cao et al., 1998; Krueger et al., 2003; McNiven et al., 2000), phagocytic cups (Gold et al., 1999), and Listeria actin comets (Lee & De Camilli, 2002; Orth et al., 2002). Several studies suggest functional implication of dynamin GTPase in actin dynamics. Expression of dynamin K44A, a GTPase defective mutant, reduces the formation of actin comets (Lee & De Camilli, 2002; Orth et al., 2002), podosomes (Ochoa et al., 2000; Bruzzaniti et al., 2005), and drastically changes cell shape (Damke et al., 1994).

Consistent with the localization and implication of dynamin in these actin-rich structures, molecular interactions of dynamin 2 with actin (Gu et al., 2010) and actin-regulating proteins such as Abp1 (Kessels et al., 2001), profilin (Witke et al., 1998) and cortactin (Schafer et al., 2002; McNiven et al., 2000) have been reported. Some studies emphasizes that these interactions represent mechanisms to incorporate actin dynamics in dynamin-dependent endocytosis. For example, interaction between dynamin 2 and cortactin, SH3-domain containing actin binding protein that binds also F-actin and actin-regulating Arp2/3 complex (Ammer & Weed, 2008), is associated with clathrin and dynamin-dependent endocytosis (Krueger et al., 2003; Cao et al., 2003; Zhu et al., 2005). On the other hand, however, the same dynamin-cortactin interaction is considered as a mechanism to recruit dynamin to the site of actin dynamics in other studies (McNiven et al., 2000; Schafer et al., 2002; Mooren et al., 2009; Yamada et al., 2009).

Assembly and remodeling of actin filaments by dynamin 2, through an interaction with cortactin, has been investigated by in vitro experiments (Schafer et al., 2002; Mooren et al., 2009). In their recent study, they demonstrated that, in the presence of dynamin, GTP led to remodeling of actin filaments in vitro via the actin-binding protein cortactin (Mooren et al., 2009). As the mechanism of the actin regulation, they suggests that GTP hydrolysis-induced conformational change within dynamin is transduced to cortactin, which in turn alters orientation of the F-actin so that actin's sensitivity to cofilin, an actin depolymerizing factor, is increased (Mooren et al., 2009). However, as interactions between dynamin's PRD and cortactin's SH3 domain does not require GTP binding nor hydrolysis by dynamin, it remains uncertain how GTP hydrolysis dependent conformational change within dynamin might be transmitted to cortactin. More recently, direct interaction between dynamin and actin has been identified, and it was proposed that the interaction leads to release of gelsolin, an actin capping protein, from the actin filament (Gu et al., 2010). However, it remains unclear how dynamin GTPase activity is utilized to alter the affinity of F-actin to the actin regulatory factor.

4. Implication of dynamin in microtubule dynamics

As described above, dynamin 1 was originally identified as a microtubule-binding protein (Shpetner & Vallee, 1989), and its GTPase activity was stimulated by microtubules (Shpetner & Vallee, 1989; Maeda et al., 1992). However, physiological significance of the dynamin-microtubule interaction has not been elucidated yet.

The association between dynamin and microtubules was recently investigated in relation to mitosis, in which tubulin plays a role as in mitotic spindle and centrosome. In mitotic cells, dynamin 2 was concentrated at microtubule bundles at mitotic spindle (Ishida et al., 2011), spindle midzone, and intercellular bridge in cytokinesis (Thompson et al., 2002). The middle domain of dynamin 2 binds to γ-tubulin, and they colocalize at the centrosome, where dynamin 2 is thought to play a role in centrosome cohesion (Thompson et al., 2004). Consistent with such observation, dynamin is enriched in spindle midbody extracts (Thompson et al., 2002).

4.1 Dynamin CMT mutant 551Δ3 impairs microtubule dynamics

Dynamin's role of on microtubules at interphase was incidentally revealed as a result of our recent investigation on dynamin mutations found in CMT patents (Tanabe & Takei 2009).

In order to elucidate molecular pathogenesis of dynamin 2-cused CMT disease, we overexpressed dynamin CMT mutants, 551Δ3 and K558E, in COS-7 cells, and examined the dynamin's role on microtubules. Endocytosis, which was assessed by transferrin uptake, was completely blocked by K558E as reported before (Züchner et al., 2005). Interestingly, 551Δ3 did not block endocytosis, but the transferrin-containing early and recycling endosomes no longer accumulated at the perinuclear region suggesting dysfunction of microtubule-dependent vesicular transport in dynamin 2-caused CMT (Fig.4).

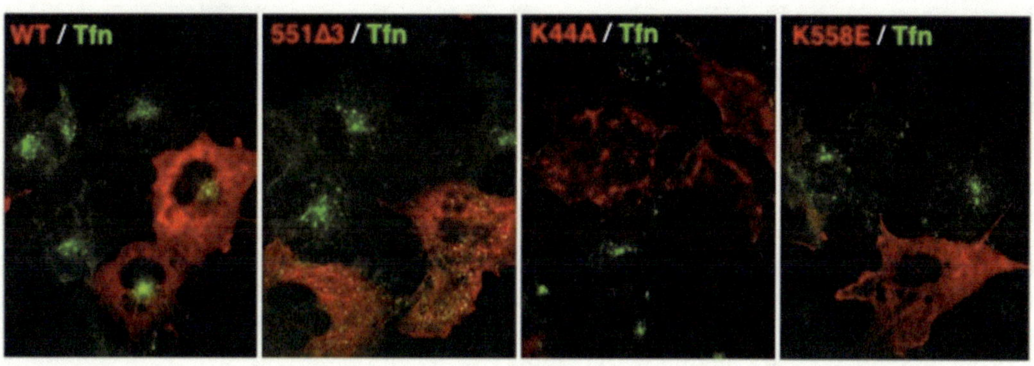

Fig. 4. Endocytosis of transferrin in dynamin 2 mutant expressing cells. COS-7 cells transfected with the indicated constructs were incubated with Alexa Fluor 488-transferrin for 30 min, and exogenous dynamin was stained by immunofluorescence (red). Note that transferrin (green) is internalized in 551Δ3 expressing cells, but the transferrin is not accumulated at perinuclear region (second panel from the left) in contrast to dynamin WT expressing cells (left). Endocytosis is blocked in dynamin K44A and K558E expressing cells (right two panels). (from Tanabe & Takei, 2009)

As mentioned above, dynamin was originally identified as a microtubule-associated protein (Shpetner & Vallee, 1989). Both dynamin 1 and dynamin 2 polymerizes around microtubules, and the interactions lead to the stimulation of dynamin GTPase activity (Maeda et al., 1992; Warnock et al., 1997). Consistently, in cells, subpopulation of dynamin 2 is present at microtubules in addition to the plasma membrane and cytosol. Localization of dynamin at microtubules become more prominent in 551Δ3 expressing cells (Züchner et al., 2005; Tanabe & Takei, 2009), probably because of its increased affinity to microtubules.

Microtubules can be very stable or highly dynamic depending on the cell cycle stage, and on position of the cell within the organism (Schulze & Kirschner, 1987). Microtubule typically comprises 13 protofilaments, which are consisted of α/β tubulin heterodimers. The tubulin dimers can depolymerize as well as polymerize, and microtubules can undergo rapid cycles of assembly and disassembly. GTP-bound tubulin is added onto plus-tips of microtubules and hydrolysis of GTP induces conformational change in tubulin dimer, which induces microtubule depolymerization. This dynamic instability of microtubules is regulated by many factors (Howard & Hyman, 2007).

Stable microtubules are subject to acetylation (Piperno et al., 1987; Westermann & Weber, 2003), thus they can be distinguished from dynamic microtubules by measuring acetylated tubulin. Acetylated tubulin was massively increased in 551Δ3 expressing cells compared to WT dynamin (Fig.5), in spite of the protein expression levels were unchanged, indicating that the 551Δ3 mutation of dynamin 2 impairs dynamic instability of microtubules.

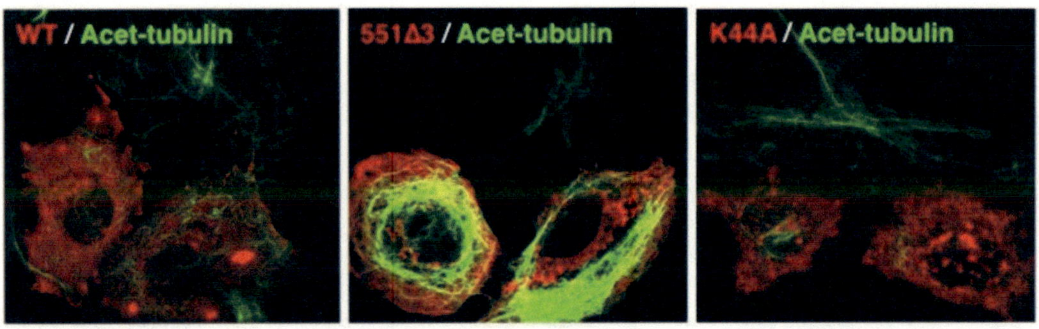

Fig. 5. Expression of 551Δ3 dynamin 2 mutant causes accumulation of acetylated tubulin. COS-7 cells were transfected with the indicated dynamin constructs and visualized by immunofluorescence for exogenous dynamin (red) and acetylated tubulin (green). Note the accumulation of abundant acetylated tubulin in 551Δ3 expressing cells (middle). (from Tanabe & Takei, 2009)

Impaired dynamic instability of microtubules is known to inhibit intracellular trafficking along microtubules (Mimori-Kiyosue & Tsukita, 2003; Vaughan, 2005). Microtubule-dependent traffic can be analyzed by examining the formation of the Golgi apparatus because the biogenesis involves transport process of pre-Golgi compartment from cell periphery to perinuclear region, and this transport is dependent on microtubules (Thyberg & Moskalewski, 1999) (Fig.6).

While mature Golgi apparatus is ribbon-shaped localized at perinuclear region, immature pre-Golgi compartments are scattered throughout the cytoplasm. Golgi apparatus in the 551Δ3 expressing cells were massively fragmented, representing impaired microtubule-dependent vesicular traffic in the cells (Fig.7). This is consistent with impaired dynamic instability of microtubules in 551Δ3 expressing cells.

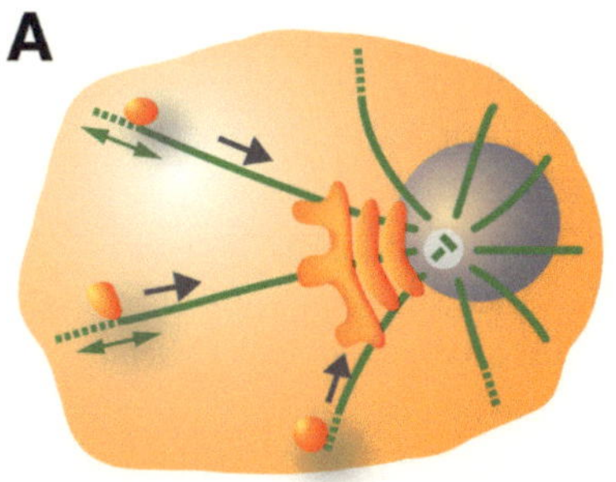

Fig. 6. Formation of mature Golgi apparatus by microtubule-dependent vesicular transport. Scheme showing radially arranged microtubules (green) and the formation of matured Golgi by microtubule dependent vesicular transport of immature pre-Golgi compartments (orange). Plus end of microtubules extends and shrinks dynamically and capture the cargo. (A). Loss of dynamic instability of microtubules impairs the microtubule-dependent transport.

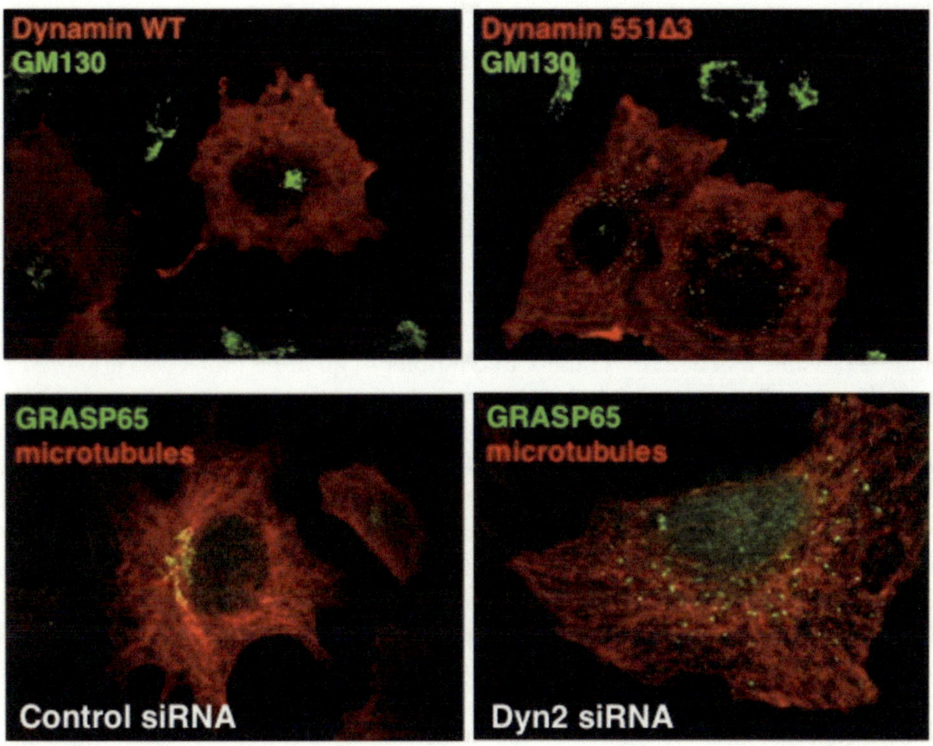

Fig. 7. Dynamin CMT mutant or dynamin 2 RNAi impairs the formation of Golgi apparatus. Upper panels: Expression of 551Δ3 dynamin 2 leads to Golgi fragmentation (right). COS-7 cells transfected with the indicated dynamin constructs were visualized by immunofluorescence for exogenous dynamin (red) and GM130, a Golgi marker (green). Lower panels: Dynamin 2 RNAi causes fragmentation of Golgi apparatus (right). HeLa cells were transfected with the indicated siRNAs and visualized with antibodies a Golgi marker GRASP65 (green) and α-tubulin (red). (from Tanabe & Takei, 2009)

4.2 Depletion of dynamin affects microtubule dynamics

Accumulation of acetylated microtubules and impairment of microtubule-dependent vesicular traffic induced by the 551Δ3 mutation are thought to be due to 'loss of function' of dynamin 2, because depletion of endogenous dynamin 2 in HeLa cells by RNAi resulted in similar phenotypes (Tanabe & Takei, 2009). Golgi apparatus was fragmented in approximately 90 % of dynamin 2 siRNA cells, indicating suppressed microtubule-dependent membrane transport. The dynamin 2 siRNA-treated cells did not show any apparent reorganization of microtubules by immunofluorescence. However, acetylated tubulin in the cells was increased approximately twofold while total tubulin protein level remain unchanged. In addition, EB1, which localizes at the plus-end of dynamic/growing microtubules, was significantly reduced in dynamin 2 siRNA cells, even though the EB1 expression levels were unaffected by the siRNA (Fig.8). This indicates that depletion of endogenous dynamin 2 reduces dynamic, growing microtubules.

5. Possible mechanism of the regulation of microtubule dynamics by dynamin

As described above, dynamin 2 is implicated in the dynamic instability of microtubules, and deletion or mutation of the protein impairs the microtubule dynamics. Then how dynamin regulates the microtubule dynamics?

Microtubule is regulated, both in polymerization and depolymerization, by many factors. While microtubule depolymerizing factors involve MCAK, a member of kinesin-13 family (Hunter ey al., 2003; Walczak, 2003), polymerization factors includes XMAP215, tau and doublecortin (Howard & Hyman, 2007; Kerssemakers et al., 2006). Furthermore, the microtubule plus-end proteins, including EB1, CLASPs and CLIP170, are also essential for dynamic instability of microtubules.

It would be possible that activity of these microtubule-regulating molecules is altered by the presence of dynamin on microtubules. In another words, microtubule-bound dynamin 2 might function as "ratchet" that limits the access of these molecules to microtubules. Physiologically, dynamin transiently interact with microtubules, resulting only small population of dynamin stays at "microtubule-bound" state. On the other hand, dynamin with CMT mutation has higher affinity to microtubules and preferably localizes at microtubules (Tanabe & Takei, 2009). This would lessen the access of microtubule-regulating molecules to microtubules, and as a result, causes to decrease polymerization-depolymerization cycle. It would be also possible that abundant presence of mutant dynamin on microtubules may mechanically obstruct polymerization and depolymerization of microtubules (Fig 9).

It is known that blocking interconversion between stable and dynamic microtubules using Taxol, a microtubule depolymerization inhibitor, results in abnormal rearrangement of microtubules (Green & Goldman, 1983). Consistently, abnormal accumulation of acetylated microtubules is observed in dynamin 551Δ3 expressing cells (Tanabe & Takei, 2009).

Live cell imaging of GFP tubulin stably expressed in HeLa cells revealed that dynamic instability of microtubules in dynamin 2-depleted cells was apparently decreased compared with control cells (Tanabe & Takei, 2009).

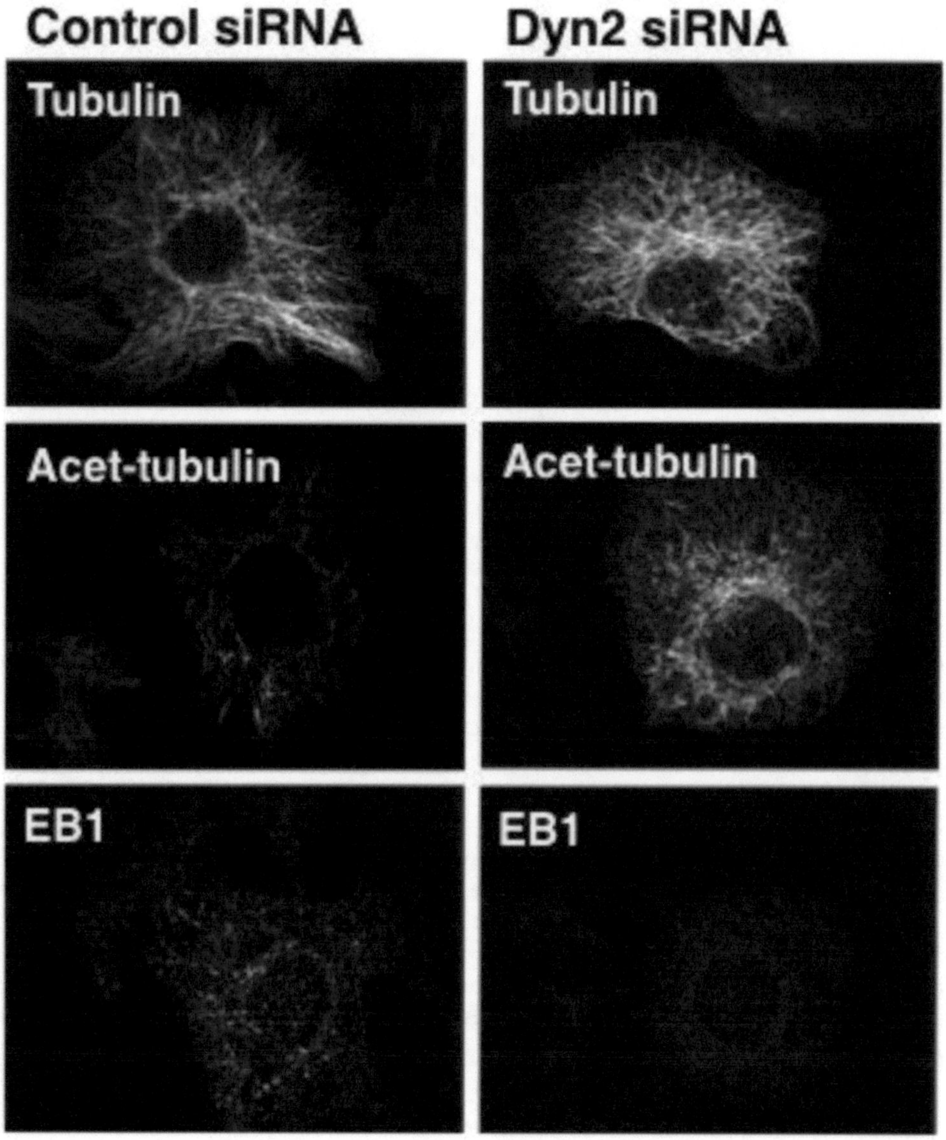

Fig. 8. Depletion of endogenous dynamin 2 by RNAi results in stable microtubule accumulation. HeLa cells cells transfected with control or dynamin 2 siRNA were stained by immunofluorescence as indicated. Note the increase of acetylated tubulin in dynamin 2 knocked-down cells (middle panels) while total tubulin is unchanged (top panels). In the knocked-down cells, punctate staining of EB1, microtubules plus end factor is lost (bottom panels). (from Tanabe & Takei, 2009)

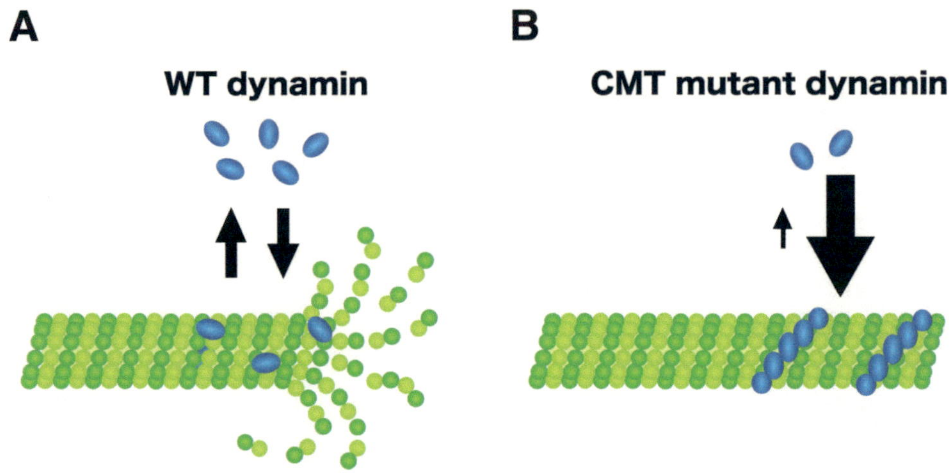

Fig. 9. Possible role of dynamin in the regulation of microtubule dynamics. Transient interaction of dynamin with microtubules would be essential for dynamic instability of microtubules (left). Mutation of dynamin would increase dynamin's affinity of to microtubules, which in turn obstructs polymerization-depolymerization cycle of microtubules either mechanically, or indirectly via microtubule-regulating molecules.

6. Conclusion

Dynamin has been originally identified as a microtubule-binding protein in 1989. However, the most of dynamin studies in the last two decades has been focused on its functions in endocytosis and actin dynamics. Our recent investigation on CMT mutant dynamin revealed impairment of microtubule dynamics and microtubule-dependent transport. Furthermore, this study led to the discovery of a novel role of dynamin, i.e. regulation of dynamic instability of microtubules.

It remains to be clarified which cells are more affected in the dynamin-caused CMT, in a correlation with clinical features of the disease. Since dynamin 2 is a ubiquitously expressed isoform, CMT mutations in dynamin 2 could affect either neurons, Schwan cells, or both. Precise molecular mechanism how dynamin regulates dynamic instability of microtubules would require future studies. Especially, it would be of importance which molecules function with dynamin in the microtubule regulation, or how dynamin-microtubule interaction is regulated.

7. References

Ammer, A.G. & Weed, S.A. (2008). Cortactin branches out: roles in regulating protrusive actin dynamics. *Cell Motil. Cytoskeleton,* 65, pp. 687-707, ISSN 0886-1544

Baldassarre, M., Pompeo, A., Beznoussenko, G., Castaldi, C., Cortellino, S., McNiven, M.A., Luini, A. & Buccione, R. (2003). Dynamin participates in focal extracellular matrix degradation by invasive cells. *Mol. Biol. Cell,* 14, pp. 1074-1084, ISSN 1059-1524

Barylko, B., Binns, D., Lin, K., Atkinson, M., Jameson, D., Yin, H. & Albanesi, J.P. (1998). Synergistic activation of dynamin GTPase by Grb2 and phosphoinositides. *J Biol Chem,* 273(6), pp. 3791-3797, ISSN 0021-9258

Bitoun, M., Stojkovic, T., Prudhon, B., Maurage, C.A., Latour, P., Vermersch, P. & Guicheney, P. (2008). A novel mutation in the dynamin 2 gene in a Charcot-Marie-Tooth type 2 patient: clinical and pathological findings. *Neuromuscul Disord,* 18(4), pp. 334-338, ISSN 1873-2364

Bruzzaniti, A. Neff, L., Sanjay, A., Horne, W.C., De Camilli, P. & Baron R. (2005). Dynamin forms a Src kinase-sensitive complex with Cbl and regulates podosomes and osteoclast activity. *Mol Biol Cell,* 16, pp. 3301-3313, ISSN 1059-1524

Cao, H., Garcia, F. & McNiven, M.A. (1998). Differential distribution of dynamin isoforms in mammalian cells. *Mol Biol Cell,* 9, pp. 2595-2609, ISSN 1059-1524

Cao, H., Orth, J.D., Chen, J., Weller, S.G., Heuser, J.E. & McNiven, M.A. (2003). Cortactin is a component of clathrin-coated pits and participates in receptor-mediated endocytosis. *Mol Biol Cell,* 23, pp. 2162-2170, ISSN 1059-1524

Claeys, K.G., Züchner, S., Kennerson, M., Berciano, J., Garcia, A., Verhoeven, K., Storey, E., Merory, J.R., Bienfait, H.M., Lammens, M., Nelis, E., Baets, J., De Vriendt, E., Berneman, Z.N., De Veuster, I., Vance, J.M., Nicholson, G., Timmerman, V. & De Jonghe, P. (2009). Phenotypic spectrum of dynamin 2 mutations in Charcot-Marie-Tooth neuropathy. *Brain,* 132 (Pt 7), pp. 1741-1752, ISSN 0006-8950

Cook, T.A., Urrutia, R. & McNiven, M.A. (1994). Identification of dynamin 2, an isoform ubiquitously expressed in rat tissues. *Proc Natl Acad Sci USA,* 91(2), pp. 644-648, ISSN 0027-8424

Damke, H., Baba, T., Warnock, D.E. & Schmid, S.L. (1994). Induction of mutant dynamin specifically blocks endocytic coated vesicle formation. *J Cell Biol,* 127, pp. 915-934, ISSN 0021-9525

David, C., McPherson, P., Mundigl, O. & De Camilli, P. (1996). A role of amphiphysin in synaptic vesicle endocytosis suggested by its binding to dynamin in nerve terminals. *Proc Natl Acad Sci USA,* 93(1), pp. 331-335, ISSN 0027-8424

Fabrizi, G.M., Ferrarini, M., Cavallaro, T., Cabrini, I., Cerini, R., Bertolasi, L. & Rizzuto, N. (2007). Two novel mutations in dynamin-2 cause axonal Charcot-Marie-Tooth disease *Neurology,* 69(3), pp. 291-295, ISSN 0028-3878

Farsad, K., Ringstad, N., Takei, K., Floyd, S.R., Rose, K. & De Camilli, P. (2001). Generation of high curvature membranes mediated by direct endophilin bilayer interactions. *J Cell Biol,* 155, pp. 193-200, ISSN 0021-9525

Gold, E.S., Underhill, D.M., Morrissette, N.S., Guo, J., McNiven, M.A. & Aderem, A. (1999). Dynamin 2 is required for phagocytosis in macrophages. *J Exp Med,* 190, pp. 1849-1856, ISSN 0022-1007

Grigliatti, T.A., Hall, L., Rosenbluth, R. & Suzuki, D.T. (1973). Temperature-sensitive mutations in Drosophila melanogaster. XIV. A selection of immobile adults. *Mol Gen Genet,* 120(2), pp. 107-114, ISSN 0026-8925

Gu, C., Yaddanapudi, S., Weins, A., Osborn, T., Reiser, J., Pollak, M., Hartwig, J. & Sever, S. (2010). Direct dynamin-actin interactions regulate the actin cytoskeleton. *EMBO J.* 29, pp. 3593-3606, ISSN 0261-4189

Herskovits, J.S., Burgess, C.C., Obar, R.A. & Vallee, R.B. (1993). Effects of mutant rat dynamin on endocytosis. *J Cell Biol,* 122(3), pp. 565-578, ISSN 0021-9525

Hinshaw, JE, Schmid, SL. (1995). Dynamin, self-assembles into rings suggesting a mechanism for coated vesicle budding. *Nature,* 374(6518), pp. 190-192, ISSN 0028-0836

Howard, J. & Hyman, A.A. (2007). Microtubule polymerases and depolymerases. *Curr Opin Cell Biol,* 19(1), pp. 31-35, ISSN 0955-0674

Hunter, A.W., Caplow, M., Coy, D.L., Hancock, W.O., Diez, S., Wordeman, L. & Howard, J. (2003). The kinesin-related protein MCAK is a microtubule depolymerase that forms an ATP-hydrolyzing complex at microtubule ends. *Mol Cell,* 11(2), pp. 445-457, ISSN 1097-2765

Ishida, N., Nakamura, Y., Tanabe, K, Li, S.A. & Takei, K. (2011). Dynamin 2 associates with microtubules at mitosis and regulates cell cycle progression *Cell Struct Funct,* 6(2), pp.145-154, ISSN 0386-7196

Itoh, T., Erdmann, K.S., Roux, A., Habermann,B., Werner, H. & De Camilli, P. (2005). Dynamin and the actin cytoskeleton cooperatively regulate plasma membrane invagination by BAR and F-BAR proteins. *Dev Cell,* 9(6), pp. 791-804, ISSN 1534-5807

Jordanova, A., Irobi, J., Thomas, F.P., Van Dijck, P., Meerschaert, K., Dewil, M., Dierick, I., Jacobs A., De Vriendt, E., Guergueltcheva, V., Rao, C.V., Tournev, I., Gondim, F.A., D'Hooghe, M., Van Gerwen, V., Callaerts, P, Van Den Bosch, L, Timmermans JP, Robberecht, W., Gettemans, J., Thevelein, J.M., De Jonghe, P., Kremensky, I. & Timmerman, V. (2006). Disrupted function and axonal distribution of mutant tyrosyl-tRNA synthetase in dominant intermediate Charcot-Marie-Tooth neuropathy. *Nat Genet,* 38(2), pp. 197-202, ISSN1061-4036

Jordanova, A., Thomas, F.P., Guergueltcheva, V., Tournev, I., Gondim, F.A., Ishpekova, B., De Vriendt, E., Jacobs, A., Litvinenko, I., Ivanova, N., Buzhov, B., De Jonghe, P., Kremensky, I. & Timmerman, V. (2003). Dominant intermediate Charcot-Marie-Tooth type C maps to chromosome 1p34-p35. *Am J Hum Genet,* 73(6), pp. 1423-1430, ISSN 0002-9297

Kennerson, M.L., Zhu, D., Gardner, R.J., Storey, E., Merory, J., Robertson, S.P. & Nicholson, G.A. (2001). Dominant intermediate Charcot-Marie-Tooth neuropathy maps to chromosome 19p12-p13.2. *Am J Hum Genet,* 69(4), pp. 883-888, ISSN 0002-9297

Kerssemakers, J.W.J., Munteanu, E.L., Laan, L., Noetzel, T.L. & Janson, M.E. (2006). Dogterom M. Assembly dynamics of microtubules at molecular resolution. *Nature,* 442(7103), pp. 709-712, ISSN 0028-0836

Kessels, M., Engqvist-Goldstein, A., Drubin, D. & Qualmann, B. (2001). Mammalian Abp1, a signal-responsive F-actin-binding protein, links the actin cytoskeleton to endocytosis via the GTPase dynamin. *J Cell Biol,* 153(2), pp. 351-366, ISSN 0021-9525

Kessels, M.M. & Qualmann, B. (2004). The syndapin protein family: linking s trafficking with the cytoskeleton. *J Cell Sci,* 117, pp. 3077-3086, ISSN 0021-9533

Kosaka, T. & Ikeda, K. (1983). Reversible blockage of membrane retrieval and endocytosis in the garland cell of the temperature-sensitive mutant of Drosophila melanogaster, shibirets1. *J Cell Biol,* 97(2), pp. 499-507, ISSN 0021-9525

Krueger, E.W., Orth, J.D., Cao, H. & McNiven, M.A. (2003). A dynamin-cortactin-Arp2/3 complex mediates actin reorganization in growth factor-stimulated cells. *Mol. Biol. Cell* 14, pp. 1085-1096, ISSN1059-1524

Lee, E. & De Camilli, P. (2002). Dynamin at actin tails. *Proc. Natl. Acad. Sci. U S A* 99, pp. 161-166, ISSN 0027-8424

Lin, H., Barylko, B., Achiriloaie, M. & Albanesi, J. (1997). Phosphatidylinositol (4,5)-bisphosphate-dependent activation of dynamins I and II lacking the proline/arginine-rich domains. *J Biol Chem,* 272(41), pp. 25999-26004, ISSN 0021-9258

Maeda, K., Nakata, T., Noda, Y., Sato-Yoshitake, R. & Hirokawa, N. (1992). Interaction of dynamin with microtubules: its structure and GTPase activity investigated by using highly purified dynamin. *Mol Biol Cell,* 3(10), pp. 1181-1194, ISSN 1059-1524

Marks, B., Stowell, M.H., Vallis, Y., Mills, I.G., Gibson, A., Hopkins, C.R. & McMahon, H.T. (2001). GTPase activity of dynamin and resulting conformation change are essential for endocytosis. *Nature,* 410, pp. 231-235, ISSN 0028-0836

McNiven, M.A. (1998). Dynamin: a molecular motor with pinchase action. *Cell,* 94(2), pp. 151-154, ISSN 0092-8674

McNiven, M.A., Kim, L., Krueger, E., Orth, J., Cao, H. & Wong, T. (2000). Regulated interactions between dynamin and the actin-binding protein cortactin modulate cell shape. J Cell Biol, 151(1), pp. 187-198, ISSN 0021-9525

McNiven, M.A., Kim, L., Krueger, E.W., Orth, J.D., Cao, H. & Wong, T.W. (2000). Regulated interactions between dynamin and the actin-binding protein cortactin modulate cell shape. *J. Cell Biol.* 151, pp. 187-198, ISSN 0021-9258

Mimori-Kiyosue, Y., Grigoriev, I., Lansbergen, G., Sasaki, H., Matsui, C., Severin, F., Galjart, N., Grosveld, F., Vorobjev, I., Tsukita, S. and Akhmanova, A. (2005). CLASP1 and CLASP2 bind to EB1 and regulate microtubule plus-end dynamics at the cell cortex. *J Cell Biol,* 168, pp. 41-153, ISSN 0021-9525

Mooren, O.L., Kotova, T.I., Moore, A.J. & Schafer, D.A. (2009). Dynamin 2 GTPase and cortactin remodel actin filaments. *J. Biol. Chem,* 284, pp. 23995-24005, ISSN 0021-9258

Nakata, T., Iwamoto, A., Noda, Y., Takemura, R., Yoshikura, H. & Hirokawa, N. (1991). Predominant and developmentally regulated expression of dynamin in neurons. *Neuron,* 7(3), pp. 461-469

Nakata, T., Takemura, R. & Hirokawa, N. (1993). A novel member of the dynamin family of GTP-binding proteins is expressed specifically in the testis. *J Cell Sci,* 105(Pt 1), pp. 1-5, ISSN 0021-9525

Obar, R., Collins, C., Hammarback, J, Shpetner, H.S. & Vallee, R. (1990). Molecular cloning of the microtubule-associated mechanochemical enzyme dynamin reveals homology with a new family of GTP-binding proteins. *Nature,* 347(6290), pp. 256-261, ISSN 0028-0836

Ochoa, G.C., Slepnev, V.I., Neff, L., Ringstad, N., Takei, K., Daniell, L., Kim, W., Cao, H., McNiven, M., Baron, R. & De Camilli, P. (2000). A functional link between dynamin and the actin cytoskeleton at podosomes. *J Cell Biol,* 150, pp. 377-389, ISSN 0021-9525

Orth, J.D., Krueger, E.W., Cao, H. & McNiven, M.A. (2002). The large GTPase dynamin regulates actin comet formation and movement in living cells. *Proc. Natl. Acad. Sci. U S A,* 99, pp. 167-172, ISSN 0027-8424

Patzkó, A. & Shy, M.E. (2011). Update on Charcot-Marie-Tooth disease. *Curr Neurol Neurosci Rep,* 11(1), pp. 78-88, ISSN 1528-4042

Piperno, G., LeDizet, M. & Chang, X.J. (1987). Microtubules containing acetylated alpha-tubulin in mammalian cells in culture. *J Cell Biol,* 104, pp. 289-302, ISSN 0021-9525

Ramachandran, R. & Schmid, S.L. (2008). Real-time detection reveals that effectors couple dynamin's GTP-dependent conformational changes to the membrane. *EMBO J*, 27(1), pp. 27-37, ISSN 0261-4189

Ringstad, N., Nemoto, Y. & De Camilli, P. (1997). The SH3p4/Sh3p8/SH3p13 protein family: binding partners for synaptojanin and dynamin via a Grb2-like Src homology 3 domain. *Proc Natl Acad Sci U S A*, 94(16), pp. 8569-8574, ISSN 0027-8424

Rossi, A., Paradiso, C., Cioni, R., Rizzuto, N. & Guazzi, G. (1985). Charcot-Marie-Tooth disease: study of a large kinship with an intermediate form. *J Neurol*, 232(2), pp. 91-98, ISSN 0340-5354

Roux, A., Uyhazi, K., Frost, A. & De Camilli, P. (2006). GTP-dependent twisting of dynamin implicates constriction and tension in membrane fission. *Nature*, 441, pp. 528-531, ISSN 0028-0836

Scaife, R. & Margolis, R.L. (1990). Biochemical and immunochemical analysis of rat brain dynamin interaction with microtubules and organelles in vivo and in vitro. *J Cell Biol*, 111(6 Pt 2), pp. 3023-3033, ISSN 0021-9525

Schafer, D.A., Weed, S.A., Binns, D., Karginov, A.V., Parsons, J.T. & Cooper, J.A. (2002). Dynamin 2 and cortactin regulate actin assembly and filament organization. *Curr Biol*, 12, pp. 1852-1857, ISSN 0960-9822

Schulze, E. & Kirschner, M. (1987). Dynamic and stable populations of microtubules in cells. *J Cell Biol*, 104, pp. 277-288, ISSN 0021-9525

Shin, N., Ahn, N., Chang-Ileto, B., Park, J., Takei, K., Ahn, S.G., Kim, S.A., Di Paolo, G. & Chang, S. (2008). SNX9 regulates tubular invagination of the plasma membrane through interaction with actin cytoskeleton and dynamin 2. *J Cell Sci*, 121, pp. 1252-1263, ISSN 0021-9533

Shpetner, H.S. & Vallee, R.B. (1989). Identification of dynamin, a novel mechanochemical enzyme that mediates interactions between microtubules. *Cell*, 59(3), pp. 421-432, ISSN 0092-8674

Shpetner, H.S. & Vallee, R.B. (1992). Dynamin is a GTPase stimulated to high levels of activity by microtubules. *Nature*, 355(6362), pp. 733-735, ISSN 0028-0836

Stowell, M.H., Marks, B., Wigge, P. & McMahon, H.T. (1999). Nucleotide-dependent conformational changes in dynamin: evidence for a mechanochemical molecular spring. *Nat Cell Biol*, 1(1), pp. 27-32, ISSN1465-7392

Sweitzer, S.M. & Hinshaw, J.E. (1998). Dynamin undergoes a GTP-dependent conformational change causing vesiculation. *Cell*, 93, pp. 1021-1029, ISSN 0092-8674

Takei, K., Haucke, V., Slepnev, V., Farsad, K., Salazar, M., Chen, H. & De Camilli, P. (1998). Generation of coated intermediates of clathrin-mediated endocytosis on protein-free liposomes. *Cell*, 94(1), pp. 131-141, ISSN 0092-8674

Takei, K., McPherson, P.S., Schmid, S.L. & De Camilli, P. (1995). Tubular membrane invaginations coated by dynamin rings are induced by GTP-γS in nerve terminals *Nature*, 374, pp. 186-190, ISSN 0028-0836

Takei, K., Slepnev, V.I., Haucke, V. & De Camilli, P. (1999). Functional partnership between amphiphysin and dynamin in clathrin-mediated endocytosis. *Nat Cell Biol*, 1, pp. 33-39, ISSN 1465-7392

Tanabe, K. & Takei, K. (2009). Dynamic instability of microtubules requires dynamin 2 and is impaired in a Charcot-Marie-Tooth mutant. *J Cell Biol*, 185(6), pp. 939-948, ISSN 0021-9525

Thompson, H.M., Cao, H., Chen, J., Euteneuer, U. & McNiven, M.A. (2004). Dynamin 2 binds gamma-tubulin and participates in centrosome cohesion. *Nat Cell Biol,* 6(4), pp. 335-342, ISSN 1465-7392

Thompson, H.M., Skop, A.R., Euteneuer, U., Meyer, B.J. & McNiven, M.A. (2002). The large GTPase dynamin associates with the spindle midzone and is required for cytokinesis. *Curr Biol,* 12(24), pp. 2111-2117, ISSN 0960-9822

Thyberg, J. & S. Moskalewski. (1999). Role of microtubules in the organization of the Golgi complex. *Exp Cell Res,* 246, pp. 263-279, ISSN 0014-4827

Tomizawa, K., Sunada, S., Lu, Y-F., Oda, Y., Kinuta, M., Ohshima, T., Saito, T., Wei, F.Y., Matsushita, M, Li S.T., Tsutsui, K., Hisanaga, S., Mikoshiba, K., Takei, K. & Matsui, H. (2003). Cophosphorylation of amphiphysin I and dynamin I by Cdk5 regulates clathrin-mediated endocytosis of synaptic vesicles. *J Cell Biol,* 163(4), pp. 813-824, ISSN 0021-9525

Toyoshima, Y.Y., Miki-Noumura, T., Shimizu, T., Kokubu, T., Ohashi, S., Hisanaga, S. & Toyoshima, C. (1991). Dynamin is a microtubule plus end-directed moter.(Biochemistry)(Proceedings of the Sixty-Second Annual Meeting of the Zoological Society of Japan). *Zoological science,* 8(6), pp. 1138, ISSN 0289-0003

van der Bliek, A. & Meyerowitz, E. (1991). Dynamin-like protein encoded by the Drosophila shibire gene associated with vesicular traffic. *Nature,* 351(6325), pp. 411-414, ISSN 0028-0836

van der Bliek, A.M., Redelmeier, T.E., Damke, H., Tisdale, E.J., Meyerowitz, E.M. & Schmid, S.L. (1993). Mutations in human dynamin block an intermediate stage in coated vesicle formation. *J Cell Biol,* 122(3), pp. 553-563, ISSN 0021-9525

Vaughan, K.T. (2005). Microtubule plus ends, motors, and traffic of Golgi membranes. *Biochim Biophys Acta,* 1744, pp. 316-324, ISSN 0006-3002

Verhoeven, K., Villanova, M., Rossi, A., Malandrini, A., De Jonghe, P. & Timmerman, V. (2001). Localization of the gene for the intermediate form of Charcot-Marie-Tooth to chromosome 10q24.1-q25.1. *Am J Hum Genet,* 69(4), pp. 889-894, ISSN 0002-9297

Villanova, M., Timmerman, V., De Jonghe, P., Malandrini, A., Rizzuto, N., Van Broeckhoven, C., Guazzi, G. & Rossi, A. (1998). Charcot-Marie-Tooth disease: an intermediate form. *Neuromuscul Disord,* 8(6), pp. 392-393, ISSN 0960-8966

Walczak, C.E. (2003). The Kin I kinesins are microtubule end-stimulated ATPases. Mol Cell, 11(2), pp. 286-288, ISSN 1097-2765

Warnock, D.E., Hinshaw, J.E. & Schmid, S.L. (1996). Dynamin self-assembly stimulates its GTPase activity. *J Biol Chem,* 271(37), pp. 22310-22314, ISSN 0021-9258

Westermann, S. & Weber, K. (2003). Post-translational modifications regulate microtubule function. *Nat Rev Mol Cell Biol,* 4, pp. 938-947, ISSN1471-0072

Witke, W., Podtelejnikov, A.V., Di Nardo, A., Sutherland, J.D., Gurniak, C.B., Dotti, C. & Mann, M. (1998). In mouse brain profilin I and profilin II associate with regulators of the endocytic pathway and actin assembly. *EMBO J,* 17, pp. 967-976, ISSN 0261-4189

Yamabhai, M., Hoffman, N.G., Hardison, N.L., McPherson, P.S., Castagnoli, L., Cesareni ,G. & Kay, B.K. (1998). Intersectin, a novel adaptor protein with two Eps15 homology and five Src homology 3 domains. *J Biol. Chem.* 273, pp. 31401-31407, ISSN 0021-9258

Yamada, H., Abe, T., Li, S.A., Masuoka, Y., Isoda, M., Watanabe, M., Nasu, Y., Kumon, H., Asai, A. & Takei, K. (2009). Dynasore, a dynamin inhibitor, suppresses lamellipodia formation and cancer cell invasion by destabilizing actin filaments. *Biochem Biophys Res Commun,* 390, pp. 1142-1148, ISSN 0006-291X

Yoshida, Y., Kinuta, M., Abe, T., Liang, S., Araki, K., Cremona, O., Di Paolo, G., Moriyama, Y., Yasuda, T., De Camilli, P. & Takei, K. (2004). The stimulatory action of amphiphysin on dynamin function is dependent on lipid bilayer curvature. *EMBO J,* 23(17), pp. 3483-3891, ISSN 0261-4189

Zamanian, J.L. & Kelly, R.B. (2003). Intersectin 1L guanine nucleotide exchange activity is regulated by adjacent src homology 3 domains that are also involved in endocytosis. *Mol Biol Cell,* 14(4), pp. 1624-1637, ISSN 1059-1524

Zhu, D., Kennerson, M., Merory, J., Chrast, R., Verheijen, M., Lemke, G. & Nicholson, G. (2003). Refined localization of dominant intermediate Charcot-Marie-Tooth neuropathy and exclusion of seven known candidate genes in the region. *Neurogenetics,* 4(4), pp. 179-183, ISSN 1364-6745

Zhu, J., Zhou, K., Hao, J.J., Liu, J., Smith, N. & Zhan, X. (2005). Regulation of cortactin/dynamin interaction by actin polymerization during the fission of clathrin-coated pits. *J. Cell Sci.* 118, pp. 807-817, ISSN 0021-9533

Züchner, S., Noureddine, M., Kennerson, M., Verhoeven, K., Claeys, K., De Jonghe, P., Merory, J., Oliveira, S.A., Speer, M.C., Stenger, J.E., Walizada, G., Zhu, D., Pericak-Vance, M.A., Nicholson, G., Timmerman, V. & Vance, J.M. (2005). Mutations in the pleckstrin homology domain of dynamin 2 cause dominant intermediate Charcot-Marie-Tooth disease. *Nat Genet,* 37(3), pp. 289-294, ISSN 1061-4036

2

Predictors of Chemotherapy-Induced Peripheral Neuropathy

Yuko Kanbayashi[1,2] and Toyoshi Hosokawa[2,3,4]
[1]*Department of Hospital Pharmacy and*
[2]*Pain Treatment & Palliative Care Unit, University Hospital,*
[3]*Department of Anaesthesiology and*
[4]*Pain Management & Palliative Care Medicine*
Kyoto Prefectural University of Medicine, Graduate School of Medical Science, Kyoto, Japan

1. Introduction

Chemotherapy-induced peripheral neuropathy (CIPN) is a dose-limiting toxicity of chemotherapy that often develops in response to administration of various drugs, including, molecularly targeted therapeutic agents (bortezomib), taxanes (paclitaxel, docetaxel), platinum compounds, platinum-containing drugs (cisplatin, carboplatin, oxaliplatin), vinca alkaloids (vincristine), thalidomide, lenalidomide, and epothilones (ixabepilone) (Kannarkat et al., 2007; Ocean et al., 2004; Park et al.,2008; Walker et al., 2007; Windebank et al., 2008; Wolf et al., 2008). It has been postulated that CIPN may represent the initial stage in the development of neuropathic pain. Although the symptoms of CIPN are diverse, the condition consistently reduces patient quality of life (QOL). Unfortunately, effective strategies for preventing or treating CIPN remain elusive.

To identify significant predictors for CIPN which would contribute to improving QOL among chemotherapy patients, we conducted a study, entitled, "Statistical identification of predictors for peripheral neuropathy associated with administration of bortezomib, taxanes, oxaliplatin or vincristine using ordered logistic regression analysis" (Kanbayashi et al., 2010). In this review, we will discuss the predictors for CIPN and review other studies.

2. Predictors of CIPN

CIPN is a dose-limiting toxicity of chemotherapy that often develops in response to administration of various drugs, in particular, bortezomib, taxanes (paclitaxel, docetaxel), oxaliplatin and vincristine (Kannarkat et al., 2007; Ocean et al., 2004; Park et al.,2008; Walker et al., 2007; Windebank et al., 2008; Wolf et al., 2008). However, effective strategies for preventing or treating CIPN are lacking. Accordingly, we conducted a retrospective study to identify significant predictors for CIPN which would contribute to improving QOL among chemotherapy patients (Kanbayashi et al., 2010). Patients had been administered bortezomib (n=28), taxanes (paclitaxel or docetaxel; n=58), oxaliplatin (n=52) or vincristine (n=52) at our hospital between April 2005 and December 2008.

	Bortezomib (*N*=28)	Taxanes (*N*=58)	Oxaliplatin (*N*=52)	VCR (*N*=52)
Demographic				
Sex (male), *N* (%)	16 (57.1)	36 (62.1)	32 (61.5)	27 (51.9)
Age, Mean (SD)	59.9 (13.9)	65.3 (9.3)	62.2 (12.3)	63.8 (13.0)
Age ≥60 years, *N* (%)	17 (60.7)	40 (67.0)	32 (61.5)	25 (48.1)
Comorbidity				
DM, *N* (%)	3 (10.7)	5 (8.6)	6 (11.5)	4 (7.7)
Concomitant medication				
Opioid, *N* (%)	5 (17.9)	8 (13.7)	10 (19.2)	8 (15.4)
NSAIDs, *N* (%)	8 (28.6)	21 (36.2)	16 (30.8)	12 (23.1)
NSAIDs (COX-2), *N* (%)	-	10 (17.2)	-	-
Analgesic adjuvant (%)	17 (60.7)	-	8 (15.4)	10 (19.2)
Concomitant use of cancer drugs				
DEX, *N* (%)	13 (46.4)	-	-	5 (9.6)
Thalidomide, *N* (%)	1 (3.8)	-	-	-
Cisplatin, *N* (%)	-	14 (24.1)	-	-
TS-1, *N* (%)	-	12 (20.7)	-	-
Number of chemotherapy cycles (1), Mean (range)	11.1±14.5 (3-75)	6.6±7.7 (1-46)	8.2±6.0 (1-25)	3.8±2.9 (1-18)
Number of chemotherapy cycles (2) (<6/6-10/>10)	9/14/5	34/17/7	20/19/13	37/15/0
Type of cancer				
Gastric cancer, *N* (%)		20 (34.5)		
Esophageal cancer, *N* (%)		35 (60.3)		
Cecal cancer, *N* (%)		1 (1.7)		
Cholangiocarcinoma, *N* (%)		1(1.7)		
Malignant mesothelioma, *N* (%)		1(1.7)		
Colorectal cancer, *N* (%)			52 (100)	
MM, *N* (%)	28 (100)			5 (9.6)
NHL, *N* (%)				39 (75.0)
Leukemia, *N* (%)				8 (15.4)

DM, diabetes mellitus; VCR, vincristine; NSAID, non-steroidal anti-inflammatory drug; COX, cyclooxygenase; DEX, dexamethasone; TS-1, tegafur, 5-chloro-2,4-dihydroxypyridine, and oteracil potassium; MM, multiple myeloma; NHL, non-Hodgkin lymphoma

Table 1. Clinical characteristics of patients and factors potentially affecting occurrence of peripheral neuropathy.

Table 1 presents the clinical characteristics of the patients administered bortezomib, taxanes (paclitaxel or docetaxel), oxaliplatin or vincristine, as well as selected predictors (=*X:* independent variable) related to the manifestation of CIPN. The analgesic adjuvants that were co-administered consisted of anti-epileptic agents (gabapentin, clonazepam, and carbamazepine), tricyclic antidepressants (amitriptyline), mexiletine, vitamin B_{12} and

Japanese herbs (Shakuyaku-Kanzo-To and Gosha-Jinki-Gan). Table 2 provides data on the severity of CIPN at the time of chemotherapy completion (=*Y:* dependent variable), graded from 0 to 5 in accordance with the Common Terminology Criteria for Adverse Events (CTCAE) v3.0 (Table 3). We elucidated predictors for CIPN using ordered logistic regression analysis (Table 4). Among patients administered bortezomib, the risk of CIPN was significantly increased among males, but significantly decreased by the co-administration of dexamethasone. The number of drug administration cycles was a significant predictor of CIPN risk among patients administered taxanes, oxaliplatin, or vincristine. The risk of CIPN among patients administered oxaliplatin was decreased by the co-administration of non-steroidal anti-inflammatory drugs (NSAIDs). Finally, the co-administration of an analgesic adjuvant increased CIPN risk among patients administered vincristine. We used a statistical approach to identify predictors for CIPN. CIPN will be alleviated by coadministration of dexamethasone with bortezomib and NSAIDs with oxaliplatin. Our study has limitations in terms of the retrospective nature of the investigation and the relatively small number of patients analyzed, but the statistical identification of predictors for CIPN should contribute to the establishment of evidence-based medicine in the prophylaxis of CIPN and improving QOL for patients undergoing chemotherapy.

	Number of patients			
CTCAE v3.0	Bortezomib (n=28)	Taxanes (n=58)	Oxaliplatin (n=52)	Vincristine (n=52)
0	10	48	26	31
1	5	2	8	3
2	6	4	16	15
3	7	4	2	3
4	0	0	0	0
5	0	0	0	0

Table 2. Results of sensory peripheral neuropathy assessments using CTCAE v3.0.

	Grade					
Adverse event	0	1	2	3	4	5
Neuropathy-sensory	Normal	Asymptomatic; loss of deep tendon reflexes or paresthesia (including tingling) but not interfering with function	Sensory alteration or paresthesia (including tingling), interfering with function but not interfering with ADL	Sensory alteration or paresthesia interfering with ADL	Disabling	Death

ADL, activities of daily living.

Table 3. National Cancer Institute Common Toxicity Criteria - version 3 (2006).

Variable	EV	SE	χ^2 value	P	OR	CI of OR	
						Lower 95%	Upper 95%
Table 4-1: Bortezomib (accuracy=14/28)							
DEX	-0.809	0.389	4.32	0.0376*	0.445	0.208	0.955
Sex (male)	1.110	0.411	7.30	0.0069*	3.035	1.356	6.793
Table 4-2: Taxanes (accuracy=49/58)							
Number of chemotherapy cycles (2)	0.867	0.424	4.17	0.0412*	2.379	1.035	5.466
DM	0.690	0.495	1.94	0.1632	1.993	0.756	5.257
Table 4-3: Oxaliplatin (accuracy=34/52)							
Number of chemotherapy cycles (2)	1.128	0.336	11.25	0.0008*	3.089	1.598	5.972
NSAIDs	-0.934	0.353	7.00	0.0082*	0.393	0.197	0.785
Table 4-4: Vincristine (accuracy=42/52)							
Age	0.795	0.458	3.01	0.0828	2.215	0.902	5.438
Number of chemotherapy cycles (2)	1.794	0.593	9.14	0.0025*	6.015	1.880	19.248
Analgesic adjuvant	1.363	0.530	6.62	0.0101*	3.907	1.383	11.031
NSAIDs	0.842	0.460	3.35	0.0670	2.320	0.943	5.711

* $P < 0.05$

EV, estimated value; SE, standard error; CI, confidence interval; OR, odds ratio; DEX, dexamethasone; DM, diabetes mellitus; NSAIDs, non-steroidal anti-inflammatory drugs

Table 4. Results of logistic regression analysis for variables extracted by forward selection.

2.1 Bortezomib

Bortezomib is a dipeptide boronic acid analogue with antineoplastic activity. Bortezomib reversibly inhibits the 26S proteasome, a large protease complex that degrades ubiquinated proteins. By blocking the targeted proteolysis normally performed by the proteasome, bortezomib disrupts various cell signaling pathways, leading to cell cycle arrest, apoptosis, and inhibition of angiogenesis. Specifically, the agent inhibits nuclear factor (NF)-kappaB, a protein that is constitutively activated in some cancers, thereby interfering with NF-kappaB-mediated cell survival, tumor growth, and angiogenesis. In vivo, bortezomib delays tumor growth and enhances the cytotoxic effects of radiation and chemotherapy (National Cancer Institute., 2011). Mitochondrial and endoplasmic reticulum damage seems to play a key role in bortezomib-induced PN genesis, since bortezomib is able to activate the mitochondrial-based apoptotic pathway (Pei et al., 2004).

Among cases complicated by diabetes mellitus (DM), the administration of thalidomide reportedly increased the risk of bortezomib-induced PN (Badros et al., 2007). Reducing the dosage of bortezomib and/or changing the treatment schedule are also reportedly effective in alleviating bortezomib-induced PN (Argyriou et al., 2008a). However, neither the number of chemotherapy cycles nor the diagnosis of DM predicted bortezomib-induced PN (Kanbayashi et al., 2010). Additionally, since the use of thalidomide is not covered by the health insurance system in Japan, few patients (1 of 28 patients treated with bortezomib) received thalidomide co-administration (Kanbayashi et al., 2010). Thus, we did not include thalidomide in our analysis. However, we found that co-administration of dexamethasone was able to alleviate bortezomib-induced PN. A recent report found that the immune system is involved in bortezomib-induced PN (Ravaglia et al., 2008), and that administration of a steroid may help to mitigate involvement of the immune system. In addition, we found that bortezomib-induced PN was most likely to manifest in male patients. To our knowledge, no reports of sex differences in CIPN have been described. Although Mileshkin et al. studied the occurrence of PN in patients treated with thalidomide, they also found no sex differences (Mileshkin et al., 2006). In terms of cancer pain, however, an earlier study reported that pain was significantly exacerbated when the patient was male (Kanbayashi et al., 2009). This issue of sex-related bortezomib-induced PN warrants further investigation.

Corso et al. concluded that the incidence, severity and outcome of bortezomib-induced PN are similar in untreated and pre-treated multiple myeloma (MM) patients (Corso et al., 2010). The only exception to this finding was a lower incidence and shorter duration of neuropathic pain in untreated patients with less frequent need for bortezomib discontinuation. The authors reported age to be the most relevant risk factor for bortezomib-induced PN, with a 6% PN risk increase for every additional year of age. Dimopoulos et al. demonstrated that bortezomib induced PN is dose-related and cumulative up to a ceiling and is consistently reversible in the majority of patients (Dimopoulos et al., 2011). In multivariate analysis, the authors found prior PN to be the only significant risk factor for bortezomib-induced PN in a newly diagnosed patient population. Importantly, there was no correlation in this study between occurrence of PN and reduced response rate or median time to progression (TTP). Lanzani et al. also indicated that the course of bortezomib-induced peripheral neurotoxicity can be severe in subjects with normal neurological examination at baseline, thereby suggesting careful monitoring during treatment in such patients (Lanzani et al., 2008). Their results confirm that pre-existing neuropathy is a risk factor for the development of more severe bortezomib-induced peripheral neurotoxicity and that severe PN may occur only after a few cycles of treatment. However, from the perspective of daily clinical practice, it is important to note that individual cases of severe bortezomib toxicity (in one case leading to drug treatment withdrawal only after two cycles of treatment) can also occur in naïve first-line patients or in pretreated patients with a normal neurological examination prior to bortezomib administration.

Furthermore, other studies have clarified the relationship between genetic factors and bortezomib-induced PN. Broyl et al. suggested an interaction between myeloma-related factors and the patient's genetic background in the development of CIPN, with different molecular pathways being implicated in bortezomib- and vincristine-induced PN (Broyl et al., 2010). Additionally, Favis et al. reported that genes associated with immune function (CTLA4, CTSS), reflexive coupling within Schwann cells (GJE1), drug binding (PSMB1), and neuron function (TCF4, DYNC1I1) were associated with bortezomib-induced PN (Favis et al., 2011).

2.2 Taxanes (paclitaxel, docetaxel)

The taxanes are intravenously administered microtubule stabilizing agents (MTSA) that interfere with mitotic spindles during cell mitosis. They include paclitaxel, docetaxel, and a new albumin-bound formulation of paclitaxel. This class is widely used in some of the most prevalent solid tumors including lung, breast, and prostate cancer, often in combination with platinum agents or after platinum treatment. Combination of a taxane and platinum is often first-line cancer treatment, and taxane monotherapy is reserved for refractory or metastatic disease settings. CIPN is more common with paclitaxel than docetaxel (Kannarkat G et al., 2007). Paclitaxel is a compound extracted from the Pacific yew tree Taxus brevifolia with antineoplastic activity. Paclitaxel binds to tubulin and inhibits the disassembly of microtubules, thereby resulting in the inhibition of cell division. This agent also induces apoptosis by binding to and blocking the function of the apoptosis inhibitor protein Bcl-2 (B-cell Leukemia 2) (National Cancer Institute., 2011). Docetaxel is a semi-synthetic, second-generation taxane derived from a compound found in the European yew tree Taxus baccata. Docetaxel displays potent and broad antineoplastic properties; it binds to and stabilizes tubulin, thereby inhibiting microtubule disassembly which results in cell-cycle arrest at the G2/M phase and cell death. This agent also inhibits pro-angiogenic factors such as vascular endothelial growth factor (VEGF) and displays immunomodulatory and pro-inflammatory properties by inducing various mediators of the inflammatory response. Docetaxel has been studied for use as a radiation-sensitizing agent (National Cancer Institute., 2011).

The risk of PN due to administration of taxanes increased in concert with the number of cycles of chemotherapy (Kanbayashi et al., 2010). This result agrees with earlier studies which reported PN to be a dose-limiting factor in taxane therapy (Argyriou et al., 2008; Hagiwara & Sunada, 2004; Makino, 2004).

In a recent review paper discussing neuropathy induced by MTSA, neuropathies induced by taxanes were found to be the most extensively studied (Lee & Swain, 2006). This type of neuropathy usually presents as sensory neuropathy (SN) and is more common with paclitaxel than with docetaxel administration. The incidence of MTSA-induced neuropathy seems to depend on the MTSA dose per treatment cycle, the schedule of treatment, and the duration of the infusion. Although there have been several small clinical trials testing neuroprotective agents, early recognition and supportive care remain the best approaches for prevention and management of MTSA-induced neuropathy (Lee & Swain, 2006). In another review, Argyriou et al. found that the incidence of taxane-induced PN is related to possible causal factors, such as, a single dose per course and cumulative dose (Argyriou et al., 2008b; Fountzilas et al., 2004; Nabholtz et al., 1996; Smith et al., 1999). Specifically, Hilkens et al. reported that severe docetaxel neuropathy is most likely to occur following treatment with a cumulative dosage over 600 mg/m^2 (Hilkens et al., 1997). The risk of taxane-induced PN was also found to be related to treatment schedule, prior or concomitant administration of platinum compounds or vinca alcaloids, age and pre-existing PN due to heredity or medical conditions, such as DM, alcohol abuse, paraneoplastic syndromes, and others (Argyriou et al.,2008b; Chaudhry et al., 2003).

Although it has been previously proposed that elderly patients are more prone to higher risk of manifesting taxanes-induced PN (Akerley et al., 2003), our study did not find advanced age to be a predictor for taxane-induced PN. Argyriou et al. also indicated that elderly cancer patients did not have a greater risk of CIPN, nor was advanced age associated with worst severity of CIPN (Argyriou et al., 2006; Argyriou et al., 2008b).

In terms of infusion time, Markman reported that a 3-h infusion of paclitaxel is associated with a lower risk of neutropenia and a greater risk of PN, compared to either 24-h infusion paclitaxel or docetaxel (1-h infusion) (Markman, 2003). On the contrary, Mielke et al. observed a drastic increase in PN risk during the course of weekly paclitaxel administrations without significant differences between 1- and 3-h infusions (Mielke et al., 2003). This later finding is in contrast to pharmacokinetic observations indicating that a shortening of infusion time might enhance neurotoxicity by increasing the area under the curve of Cremophor (Mielke et al., 2003).

Some studies have also investigated the relationship between genetic factors and taxane-induced PN. In their pilot study, Sissung et al. suggested that paclitaxel-induced neuropathy and neutropenia might be linked to inherited variants of ABCB1 through a mechanism that is unrelated to altered plasma pharmacokinetics (Sissung et al., 2006). Specifically, polymorphisms that are associated with ABCB1 expression and function may be linked to treatment efficacy and the development of neutropenia and neurotoxicity in patients with androgen-independent prostate cancer receiving docetaxel. The authors also suggested that docetaxel-induced neuropathy, neutropenia grade, and overall survival could be linked to ABCB1 allelic variants with ensuing negative implications for docetaxel treatment in patients carrying ABCB1 variant genotypes (Sissung et al., 2008). Moreover, Mir et al. found a significant correlation between Glutathione-S-transferases P1 (GSTP1) (105) Ile/ (105) Ile genotype and the development of grade > or = 2 docetaxel -induced PN (Mir et al., 2009). Given that GSTs regulate the cellular response to oxidative stress, this finding strongly suggests a role for oxidative stress in the pathophysiology of docetaxel-induced PN.

2.3 Platinum-containing drugs (cisplatin, carboplatin, and oxaliplatin)

Platinum compounds covalently bind and damage DNA and include cisplatin, carboplatin, and oxaliplatin. These drugs are used in nearly all types of solid tumors. Though all three are known to cause classic symptoms of CIPN, higher incidences are seen with cisplatin and oxaliplatin. CIPN due to cisplatin is more often irreversible than in cases with oxaliplatin. CIPN is a dose-limiting toxicity with both cisplatin and oxaliplatin (Kannarkat G et al., 2007). Oxaliplatin will be primarily focused in this section.

Oxaliplatin is an organoplatinum complex in which the platinum atom is complexed with 1, 2-diaminocyclohexane (DACH) and with an oxalate ligand as a 'leaving group.' A 'leaving group' is an atom or a group of atoms that is displaced as a stable species taking with it the bonding electrons. After displacement of the labile oxalate ligand leaving group, active oxaliplatin derivatives, such as monoaquo and diaquo DACH platinum, alkylate macromolecules, forming both inter- and intra-strand platinum-DNA crosslinks, which result in inhibition of DNA replication and transcription and cell-cycle nonspecific cytotoxicity. The DACH side chain appears to inhibit alkylating-agent resistance (National Cancer Institute., 2011). Oxaliplatin is used for the treatment of colorectal, lung, breast and ovarian cancers. While oxaliplatin does not cause renal or hematologic toxicity, it can induce neuropathic pain which hampers the success of chemotherapy (Meyer et al., 2011). Oxaliplatin-induced PN (OXLIPN) is presented with two distinct syndromes, one of acute neurosensory toxicity and a chronic form that closely resembles the cisplatin-induced PN (Argyriou et al., 2008c). Oxaliplatin causes significant neurotoxicity that is experienced primarily in the hands during therapy and in the feet during follow-up. In a minority of patients the neurotoxicity is long lasting (Land et al., 2007).

The risk of OXLIPN increased as the number of drug administration cycles increased and when no non-steroidal anti-inflammatory drugs (NSAIDs) were co-administered (Kanbayashi et al., 2010). Thus, in agreement with prior reports, PN appears to be a dose-limiting factor in oxaliplatin therapy. As for an influence of NSAIDs, several groups have reported that cyclooxygenase (COX) 2-dependent prostaglandin (PG) E2 may be a causative factor in PN (Broom et al., 2004; Ma & Quirion, 2008; Suyama et al., 2004; Vo et al., 2009). Moreover, there have been reports that COX-2 is involved in diabetic PN, although that pathology is a separate entity to CIPN (Kellogg et al., 2007; Kellogg et al., 2008). Further investigation will be needed to elucidate the prophylactic efficacy of COX2-specific NSAIDs in relation to CIPN.

The incidence of OXLIPN is usually related to various risk factors, including treatment schedule, dosage, cumulative dose, infusion duration, and pre-existing peripheral neuropathy (Argyriou et al, 2008c). High cumulative doses of oxaliplatin are strongly associated with occurrence of chronic peripheral nerve damage, which could be attributed to the oxaliplatin dose accumulation. Indeed, it is documented that at cumulative doses that reach 800 mg/m^2, the occurrence of OXLIPN is highly likely; severe (grade 3) OXLIPN occurs in 15% after cumulative doses of 750–850 mg/m^2 and in 50% after a total dose of 1170 mg/m^2 (Grothey, 2005). Clinical and neurophysiological examinations of such cases show an acute and transient neurotoxicity and a cumulative dose-related sensory neuropathy in nearly all the patients (Pietrangeli et al., 2006). Pasetto et al. also reported that OXLIPN is usually late-onset and correlated with the cumulative-dose of oxaliplatin (Pasetto et al., 2006).

In another study, Brouwers et al. found that the severity of neuropathy secondary cisplatin administration was related to the cumulative dose and sodium thiosulfate use (Brouwers et al., 2009). However, OXLIPN did not appear to be related to the dose within the studied dose range. No relationship was demonstrated between risk of PN and platinum levels, renal function, glutathione transferase genotypes, DM, alcohol use, or co-medication. The authors concluded that since their study was explorative, the issues discussed need to be investigated further. In their retrospective analysis of 1587 cases, Ramanathan et al. indicated that oxaliplatin-based therapy does not influence the incidence, severity, or time to onset of peripheral sensory neuropathy in asymptomatic DM patients with colorectal cancer who meet eligibility criteria for clinical trials (Ramanathan et al., 2010). Attal et al. identified thermal hyperalgesia as a relevant clinical marker of early oxaliplatin neurotoxicity that may predict severe neuropathy (Attal et al., 2009).

Some studies have also investigated the connection between genetic polymorphisms and OXLIPN. Inada et al. suggested that ERCC1, C118T and GSTP1 Ile105Val polymorphisms are more strongly related to the time until onset of neuropathy than to the grade of neuropathy (Inada et al., 2010). This finding suggests that these polymorphisms influence patients' sensitivity to neuropathy. Antonacopoulou et al. reported that although ITGB3 L33P seems to be unrelated to the development of OXLIPN, it appears to be related to its severity (Antonacopoulou et al., 2010). Two independent studies in advanced colorectal cancer patients treated with oxaliplatin looked at the GST genes for patients who experienced grade 3 cumulative neuropathy (McWhinney et al., 2009; Ruzzo et al., 2007; Lecomte et al., 2006). Ruzzo et al. described an association between the GSTP1 105 Val G/G allele and the development of grade 3 neuropathy secondary to oxaliplatin treatment of 166 patients (Ruzzo et al., 2007). Additionally, Lecomte and colleagues reported a significant association between the GSTP1 105 Val G/G allele and risk of developing neurotoxicity in a cohort of 64 patients (Lecomte et al., 2006). Gamelin et al. proposed that key components of the oxalate synthesis pathway could be associated with platinum-drug neurotoxicity (Gamelin et al., 2007). In their study of patients treated with oxaliplatin, a minor haplotype in glyoxylate aminotransferase (AGXT) predicted both acute and chronic neurotoxicity. Although this was the first study to indicate the contribution of AGXT, it warrants further analysis in larger patient cohorts. On the other hand, Argyriou et al. failed to provide evidence to support a causal relationship between the voltage-gated sodium channel gene SCN2A R19K polymorphism and OXLIPN (Argyriou et al., 2009).

2.4 Vinca alkaloids

Vinca alkaloids are plant-derived microtubule assembly inhibitors. This class includes vincristine, vinblastine and vinorelbine. Vincristine, the oldest and most neurotoxic of the class, is still widely used in leukemias, lymphomas, myeloma, and various sarcomas. CIPN is the most common dose-limiting toxicity of vincristine. Symptoms range from peripheral sensorimotor loss to autonomic dysfunction related to paralytic ileus, orthostasis, and sphincter problems. Central nervous system (CNS) involvement is much less common but can manifest as ataxia, cranial nerve palsies, cortical blindness and seizures. Vinblastine and vinorelbine have much lower incidences of neurotoxicity than their predecessor (Kannarkat G et al., 2007).

Vincristine is the sulfate salt of a natural alkaloid isolated from the plant Vinca rosea Linn with antimitotic and antineoplastic activities. Vincristine binds irreversibly to microtubules and spindle proteins in S phase of the cell cycle and interferes with the formation of the mitotic spindle, thereby arresting tumor cells in metaphase. This agent also depolymerizes microtubules and may also interfere with amino acid, cyclic AMP, and glutathione metabolism; calmodulin-dependent Ca++ -transport ATPase activity; cellular respiration; and nucleic acid and lipid biosynthesis (National Cancer Institute., 2011).

The risk of CIPN due to vincristine administration increased as the number of chemotherapy cycles increased (Kanbayashi et al., 2010). This result supports earlier reports that concluded vincristine-induced PN (VIPN) to be a dose-limiting factor of therapy (Ja'afer et al., 2006; Verstappen et al., 2005; Weintraub et al., 1996). Moreover, analgesic adjuvants used to relieve the symptoms of PN during chemotherapy did not show adequate prophylactic efficacy. Thus, in agreement with prior studies (Kannarkat et al., 2007; Ocean et al., 2004; Park et al.,2008; Walker et al., 2007; Windebank et al., 2008; Wolf et al., 2008) it can be concluded that no effective analgesic adjuvants are currently available for CIPN. Verstappen et al. reported that while neuropathic changes were observed in both dose intensity groups, the higher dose intensity group reported significantly more symptoms during therapy, whereas neurologic signs were significantly more prominent after a cumulative dose of 12 mg vincristine (Verstappen et al., 2005). Furthermore, off-therapy exacerbation of symptoms (24%) and signs (30%) occurred unexpectedly in that trial. Weintraub et al. reported that colony-stimulating factors could precipitate a severe atypical neuropathy when given in conjunction with vincristine (Weintraub et al, 1996). The development of this severe atypical neuropathy was most strongly associated with the cumulative dose of vincristine. Conversely, the size of individual doses and the number of doses given in cycle 1 were important only to the extent that they influenced the cumulative dose.

Studies have also attempted to clarify the relationship between genetic factors and VIPN. For example, Egbelakin et al. evaluated the relationship between cytochrome P450 (CYP)

3A5 genotype and VIPN in children with precursor B cell acute lymphoblastic leukemia (preB ALL) (Egbelakin et al., 2011). They concluded that CYP3A5 expressers experience less VIPN, produce more primary metabolite (M1), and have lower metabolic ratios compared to CYP3A5 non-expressers. Broyl et al. reported that early-onset VIPN was characterized by the up-regulation of genes involved in cell cycle and proliferation, including AURKA and MKI67, and also by the presence of single-nucleotide polymorphisms (SNPs) in genes involved in these processes, such as GLI1 (rs2228224 and rs2242578) (Broyl et al., 2010). In this study, late-onset VIPN was associated with the presence of SNPs in genes involved in absorption, distribution, metabolism, and excretion. Graf et al. showed that a 17p11.2-12 duplication predisposed patients to severe neurotoxicity from vincristine, suggesting that this drug should be avoided in patients with CMT1A (Graf et al., 1996). Thus, it is essential to obtain a detailed family history for all oncology patients to screen for possible hereditary neuropathies. In patients with unexplained or preexisting familial neuropathy, testing for 17p11.2-12 duplication should be carried out prior to initiating vincristine therapy. Patients with other hereditary neuropathies may also be at risk for severe neurotoxic reactions.

2.5 Thalidomide

Thalidomide is a synthetic derivative of glutamic acid (alpha-phthalimido-glutarimide) with teratogenic, immunomodulatory, anti-inflammatory and anti-angiogenic properties. Thalidomide acts primarily by inhibiting both the production of tumor necrosis factor alpha (TNF-alpha) in stimulated peripheral monocytes and the activities of interleukins and interferons. This agent also inhibits polymorphonuclear chemotaxis and monocyte phagocytosis. In addition, thalidomide inhibits pro-angiogenic factors such as vascular endothelial growth factor (VEGF) and basic fibroblast growth factor (bFGF), thereby inhibiting angiogenesis (National Cancer Institute., 2011).

Harland et al. concluded that changes in nerve conductivity were a frequent but unpredictable adverse effect of thalidomide (< or = 200 mg/day), and that smoking might protect against such changes (Harland et al., 1995). The authors suggested that nerve conduction studies are required before and during treatment, irrespective of the prescribed dose. Molloy et al. found that thalidomide neuropathy occurred concurrently with a decline in the sensory nerve action potential (SNAP) index (Molloy et al., 2001). Thus, the SNAP index can be used to monitor PN, but not for early detection. Older age and cumulative dose were possible contributing factors for thalidomide-induced PN. Neuropathy may thus be a common complication of thalidomide therapy in older patients. Bastuji-Garin et al. found the risk of thalidomide neuropathy seems to be negligible for doses less than 25 mg per day, regardless of the duration of therapy (Bastuji-Garin et al., 2002). In patients with advanced MM, a thalidomide daily dose of 150 mg was found to minimize PN without jeopardizing response and survival (Offidani et al., 2004). Torsi et al. reported that the severity of neurotoxicity was not related to cumulative or daily thalidomide dose, but only to the duration of the disease prior to thalidomide treatment (Torsi et al., 2005). However, no patients presented with neurological symptoms at study entry. The results of this study suggest that long-term thalidomide therapy in MM may be hampered by the remarkable neurotoxicity of the drug, and that a neurological evaluation should be mandatory prior to thalidomide treatment, in order to identify patients at risk of developing a PN. Others suggest that the majority of patients would develop PN given sufficient length of treatment with thalidomide (Mileshkin et al., 2006). Accordingly, therapy should be limited to less than 6 months in order to minimize the risk of neurotoxicity. These authors also found that electrophysiologic monitoring provides no clear benefit versus careful clinical evaluation for the development of clinically significant neuropathy. On the other hand, Souayah et al. reported that symptom severity was correlated with the time of onset, but not with cumulative dose (Souayah et al., 2010). In this study, five patients partially improved when the thalidomide was withdrawn, and three patients developed tremor with the neuropathy. Since the sensory symptoms occurred shortly after thalidomide was introduced, it is advisable that older patients with macular degeneration be carefully screened for risk factors of PN before thalidomide is used in their treatment.

Finally, a number of studies investigated the relationship between genetic factors and thalidomide-induced PN. Johnson et al. demonstrated that an individual's risk of developing a PN after thalidomide treatment could be mediated by polymorphisms in genes governing repair mechanisms and inflammation in the peripheral nervous system (Johnson et al., 2011). These authors concluded that their findings could contribute to the development of future neuroprotective strategies with thalidomide therapy. Finally, Cibeira et al. found that a polymorphism in GSTT1 (rs4630) was associated with a lower frequency of thalidomide-induced PN (p=0.04) (Cibeira et al., 2011).

3. Conclusion

Although various analgesic adjuvants, including antidepressants and anti-epileptics, have been tested as therapeutic agents for CIPN, none have shown clear efficacy. Our results supported this notion, with CIPN occurring even with co-administration of analgesic adjuvants. Despite previous reports showing an opioid to effectively relieve PN (Gatti et al., 2009; Watson et al., 2003), the lack of co-administration of opioids was not identified as a predictor for CIPN (Kanbayashi et al., 2010). Further research is warranted in regard to the potential prophylactic effects of agents such as steroids, NSAIDs (particularly COX2-specific NSAIDs), gabapentinoids (gabapentin or pregabalin) and opioids on the development of CIPN (Attal et al., 2006; Rao et al., 2007; Tsavaris et al., 2008; Vanotti et al., 2007; Vondracek et al.,2009). Risk factors for CIPN such as gene polymorphism have already been reported, but the interrelationship of CIPN and gene polymorphism in particular will need to be verified at a later date. Further investigation of these issues will be needed to establish evidence-based medicine in the prophylaxis of CIPN and improve QOL for patients undergoing chemotherapy.

4. References

Akerley, W., Herndon, JE., Egorin, MJ., Lyss, AP., Kindler, HL., Savarese, DM., Sherman, CA., Rosen, DM., Hollis, D., Ratain, MJ., & Green, MR. (2003). Weekly, high-dose paclitaxel in advanced lung carcinoma: a phase II study with pharmacokinetics by the Cancer and Leukemia Group B. *Cancer*, Vol.97, No.10, (May 2003), pp. (2480-6), ISSN 0008-543X

Antonacopoulou, AG., Argyriou AA., Scopa CD., Kottorou A., Kominea A., Peroukides, S., & Kalofonos, HP. (2010). Integrin beta-3 L33P: a new insight into the pathogenesis of chronic oxaliplatin-induced peripheral neuropathy? *Eur J Neurol*, Vol.17, No.7, (July 2010), pp. (963-8), ISSN 1351-5101

Attal, N., Cruccu, G., Haanpää, M., Hansson, P., Jensen, TS., Nurmikko, T., Sampaio, C., Sindrup, S., & Wiffen, P., EFNS Task Force. (2006). EFNS guidelines on pharmacological treatment of neuropathic pain. *Eur J Neurol*, Vol.13, No.11, (November 2006), pp. (1153-69), ISSN 1351-5101

Argyriou, AA., Polychronopoulos, P., Koutras, A., Iconomou, G., Gourzis, P., Assimakopoulos, K., Kalofonos, HP., & Chroni, E. (2006). Is advanced age associated with increased incidence and severity of chemotherapy-induced peripheral neuropathy? *Support Care Cancer*, Vol.14, No.3, (March 2006), pp. (223-9), ISSN 0941-4355

Argyriou, AA., Iconomou, G., & Kalofonos, HP. (2008a) Bortezomib-induced peripheral neuropathy in multiple myeloma: a comprehensive review of the literature. *Blood*, Vol.112, No.5, (September 2008), pp. (1593-9), ISSN 0006-4971

Argyriou, AA., Koltzenburg, M., Polychronopoulos, P., Papapetropoulos, S., & Kalofonos, HP. (2008b). Peripheral nerve damage associated with administration of taxanes in patients with cancer. *Crit Rev Oncol Hematol*, Vol.66, No.3, (June 2008), pp. (218-28), ISSN 1040-8428

Argyriou, AA., Polychronopoulos, P., Iconomou, G., Chroni, E. & Kalofonos, HP. (2008c). A review on oxaliplatin-induced peripheral nerve damage. *Cancer Treat Rev*, Vol.34, No.4, (June 2008), pp. 368-77, ISSN 0305-7372

Argyriou, AA., Antonacopoulou, AG., Scopa, CD., Kottorou, A., Kominea, A., Peroukides, S., & Kalofonos, HP. (2009). Liability of the voltage-gated sodium channel gene SCN2A R19K polymorphism to oxaliplatin-induced peripheral neuropathy. *Oncology*, Vol.77, No.3-4, pp. (254-6), ISSN 0030-2414

Attal, N., Bouhassira, D., Gautron, M., Vaillant, JN., Mitry, E., Lepère, C., Rougier, P., & Guirimand, F. (2009). Thermal hyperalgesia as a marker of oxaliplatin neurotoxicity: a prospective quantified sensory assessment study. *Pain*, Vol.144, No.3, (August 2009), pp. (245-52), ISSN 0304-3959

Badros, A., Goloubeva, O., Dalal, JS., Can, I., Thompson, J., Rapoport, AP., Heyman, M., Akpek, G., & Fenton, RG. (2007). Neurotoxicity of bortezomib therapy in multiple myeloma: a single-center experience and review of the literature. *Cancer*, Vol.110, No.5, (September 2007), pp. (1042-9) ISSN 0008-543X

Broom, DC., Samad, TA., Kohno, T., Tegeder, I., Geisslinger, G., & Woolf, CJ. (2004). Cyclooxygenase 2 expression in the spared nerve injury model of neuropathic pain. *Neuroscience*, Vol.124, No.4, (June 2004), pp. (891-900), ISSN 0306-4522

Bastuji-Garin, S., Ochonisky, S., Bouche, P., Gherardi, RK., Duguet, C., Djerradine, Z., Poli, F., & Revuz, J., Thalidomide Neuropathy Study Group.(2002). Incidence and risk factors for thalidomide neuropathy: a prospective study of 135 dermatologic patients. *J Invest Dermatol*, Vol.119, No.5, (November 2002), pp. (1020-6), ISSN 0022-202X

Brouwers, EE., Huitema, AD., Boogerd, W., Beijnen, JH., & Schellens, JH. (2009). Persistent neuropathy after treatment with cisplatin and oxaliplatin. *Acta Oncol*, Vol.48, No.6, pp. (832-41), ISSN 0284-186X

Broyl, A., Corthals, SL., Jongen, JL., van der Holt, B., Kuiper, R., de Knegt, Y., van Duin, M., el Jarari, L., Bertsch, U., Lokhorst, HM., Durie, BG., Goldschmidt, H., & Sonneveld, P. (2010). Mechanisms of peripheral neuropathy associated with bortezomib and vincristine in patients with newly diagnosed multiple myeloma: a prospective analysis of data from the HOVON-65/GMMG-HD4 trial. *Lancet Oncol*, Vol.11, No.11, (November 2010), pp. (1057-65) ISSN 1470-2045

Chaudhry, V., Chaudhry, M., Crawford, TO., Simmons-O'Brien, E., & Griffin, JW. (2003). Toxic neuropathy in patients with pre-existing neuropathy. *Neurology*, Vol.60, No.2, (January 2003), pp. (337-40), ISSN 0028-3878

Cibeira, MT., Fernández de Larrea, C., Navarro, A., Díaz, T., Fuster, D., Tovar, N., Rosiñol, L., Monzó, M., & Bladé, J. (2011). Impact on response and survival of DNA repair single nucleotide polymorphisms in relapsed or refractory multiple myeloma patients treated with thalidomide. *Leuk Res*, ISSN 0145-2126

Corso, A., Mangiacavalli, S., Varettoni, M.; Pascutto, C.; Zappasodi, P., & Lazzarino, M. (2010). Bortezomib-induced peripheral neuropathy in multiple myeloma: a comparison between previously treated and untreated patients. *Leuk Res*, Vol.34, No.4, (April 2010), pp. (471-4), ISSN 0145-2126

Dimopoulos, MA., Mateos, MV., Richardson, PG., Schlag, R., Khuageva, NK., Shpilberg, O., Kropff ,M., Spicka, I., Palumbo, A., Wu, KL., Esseltine, DL., Liu, K., Deraedt, W., Cakana, A., Van De Velde, H., & San Miguel, JF. (2011). Risk factors for, and reversibility of,peripheral neuropathy associated with bortezomib-melphalan-prednisone in newly diagnosed patients with multiple myeloma: subanalysis of the phase 3 VISTA study. *Eur J Haematol,* Vol.86, No.1, (January 2011), pp. (23-31), ISSN 0902-4441

Egbelakin, A., Ferguson, MJ., MacGill, EA., Lehmann, AS., Topletz, AR., Quinney, SK., Li, L., McCammack, KC., Hall, SD., & Renbarger, JL.(2011). Increased risk of vincristine neurotoxicity associated with low CYP3A5 expression genotype in children with acute lymphoblastic leukemia. *Pediatr Blood Cancer,* Vol.56, No.3, (March 2011), pp. (361-7), ISSN 1545-5009

Favis, R., Sun, Y., van de Velde, H., Broderick, E., Levey, L., Meyers, M., Mulligan, G., Harousseau, JL., Richardson, PG., & Ricci, DS. (2011). Genetic variation associated with bortezomib-induced peripheral neuropathy. *Pharmacogenet Genomics*, Vol.21, No.3, (March 2011), pp. (121-9), ISSN 1744-6872

Fountzilas, G., Kalofonos, HP., Dafni, U., Papadimitriou, C., Bafaloukos, D., Papakostas, P., Kalogera-Fountzila, A., Gogas, H., Aravantinos, G., Moulopoulos, LA., Economopoulos, T., Pectasides, D., Maniadakis, N.; Siafaka, V.; Briasoulis, E.; Christodoulou, C.; Tsavdaridis, D.; Makrantonakis, P.; Razis, E.; Kosmidis, P.; Skarlos, D., & Dimopoulos, MA. (2004). Paclitaxel and epirubicin versus paclitaxel and carboplatin as first-line chemotherapy in patients with advanced breast cancer: a phase III study conducted by the Hellenic Cooperative Oncology Group. *Ann Oncol,* Vol.15, No.10, (October 2004), pp. (1517–26), ISSN 0923-7534

Gatti, A.; Sabato, AF.; Occhioni, R.; Colini Baldeschi, G., & Reale, C. (2009). Controlled-release oxycodone and pregabalin in the treatment of neuropathic pain: results of a multicenter Italian study. *Eur Neurol,* Vol.61, No.3, pp. (129-37), ISSN 0014-3022

Gamelin L., Capitain, O., Morel, A., Dumont, A., Traore, S., Anne le, B., Gilles, S., Boisdron-Celle, M., & Gamelin, E. (2007). Predictive factors of oxaliplatin neurotoxicity: the involvement of the oxalate outcome pathway. *Clin Cancer Res*, Vol.13, No.21, (November 2007), pp. (6359-68), ISSN 1078-0432

Graf, WD., Chance, PF., Lensch, MW., Eng, LJ., Lipe, HP., & Bird, TD. (1996). Severe vincristine neuropathy in Charcot-Marie-Tooth disease type 1A. *Cancer,* Vol.77, No.7, (April 1996), pp. (1356-62), ISSN 0008-543X

Grothey, A. (2005). Clinical management of oxaliplatin-associated neurotoxicity. *Clin Colorectal Cancer,* Vol.5, Suppl 1, (April 2005), pp. (S38-46), ISSN 1533-0028

Hagiwara, H., & Sunada, Y. (2004). Mechanism of taxane neurotoxicity. *Breast Cancer,* Vol.11, No.1, pp. (82-5), ISSN 1340-6868

Harland, CC., Steventon, GB., & Marsden, JR. (1995). Thalidomide-induced neuropathy and genetic differences in drug metabolism. *Eur J Clin Pharmacol,* Vol.49, No.1-2, pp. (1-6), ISSN0031-6970Hilkens, PH., Verweij, J., Vecht, CJ., Stoter, G., & van den Bent, MJ. (1997). Clinical characteristics of severe peripheral neuropathy induced by docetaxel (Taxotere). *Ann Oncol,* Vol.8, No.2, (February 1997), pp. (187-90), ISSN 0923-7534

Inada, M., Sato, M., Morita, S., Kitagawa, K., Kawada, K., Mitsuma, A., Sawaki, M., Fujita, K., & Ando, Y. (2010). Associations between oxaliplatin-induced peripheral neuropathy and polymorphisms of the ERCC1 and GSTP1 genes. *Int J Clin Pharmacol Ther,* Vol.48, No.11, (November 2010), pp. (729-34), ISSN 0946-1965

Ja'afer, FM., Hamdan, FB., & Mohammed, FH. (2006).Vincristine-induced neuropathy in rat: electrophysiological and histological study. *Exp Brain Res,* Vol.173, No.2, (August 2006), pp. (334-45), ISSN 0014-4819Johnson, DC., Corthals, SL., Walker, BA., Ross, FM., Gregory, WM., Dickens, NJ., Lokhorst, HM., Goldschmidt, H., Davies, FE., Durie, BG., Van Ness, B., Child, JA., Sonneveld, P., & Morgan, GJ. (2011). Genetic factors underlying the risk of thalidomide-related neuropathy in patients with multiple myeloma. *J Clin Oncol,* Vol.29, No.7, (March 2011), pp. (797-804), ISSN 0732-183X

Kanbayashi, Y., Okamoto, K., Ogaru, T., Hosokawa, T., & Takagi, T. (2009). Statistical validation of the relationships of cancer pain relief with various factors using ordered logistic regression analysis. *Clin J Pain,* Vol.25, No.1, (January 2009), pp. (65-72), ISSN 0749-8047

Kanbayashi, Y., Hosokawa, T., Okamoto, K., Konishi, H., Otsuji, E., Yoshikawa, T., Takagi, T., & Taniwaki ,M. (2010). Statistical identification of predictors for peripheral neuropathy associated with administration of bortezomib, taxanes, oxaliplatin or vincristine using ordered logistic regression analysis. *Anticancer Drugs,* Vol.21, No.9, (October 2010), pp. (877-81), ISSN 0959-4973

Kannarkat, G., Lasher, EE., & Schiff, D. (2007). Neurologic complications of chemotherapy agents. *Curr Opin Neurol,*Vol.20,No.6, (December 2007), pp. (719-25), ISSN 1350-7540

Kellogg, AP., Cheng, HT., & Pop-Busui, R. (2008). Cyclooxygenase-2 pathway as a potential therapeutic target in diabetic peripheral neuropathy. *Curr Drug Targets,* Vol.9, No.1, (January 2008), pp. (68-76), ISSN 1389-4501

Kellogg, AP., Wiggin, TD., Larkin, DD., Hayes, JM., Stevens MJ., & Pop-Busui R. (2007). Protective effects of cyclooxygenase-2 gene inactivation against peripheral nerve dysfunction and intraepidermal nerve fiber loss in experimental diabetes. *Diabetes,* Vol.56, No.12, (December 2007), pp. (2997-3005), ISSN 0012-1797

Land, SR., Kopec, JA., Cecchini, RS., Ganz, PA., Wieand, HS., Colangelo, LH., Murphy, K., Kuebler, JP., Seay, TE., Needles, BM., Bearden, JD 3rd., Colman, LK., Lanier, KS., Pajon, ER Jr., Cella, D., Smith, RE., O'Connell, MJ.; Costantino, JP., & Wolmark, N. (2007). Neurotoxicity from oxaliplatin combined with weekly bolus fluorouracil and leucovorin as surgical adjuvant chemotherapy for stage II and III colon cancer: NSABP C-07. *J Clin Oncol,* Vol.25, No.16, (June 2007), pp. (2205-11), ISSN 0732-183X

Lanzani, F., Mattavelli, L., Frigeni, B., Rossini, F., Cammarota, S., Petrò, D., Jann, S., & Cavaletti, G. (2008). Role of a pre-existing neuropathy on the course of bortezomib-induced peripheral neurotoxicity. *J Peripher Nerv Syst,* Vol.13, No.4, (December 2008), pp. (267-74), ISSN 1085-9489

Lecomte, T., Landi, B., Beaune, P., Laurent-Puig, P., & Loriot, MA. (2006). GlutathioneS-transferase P1 polymorphism (Ile105Val) predicts cumulative neuropathy in patients receiving oxaliplatin-based chemotherapy. *Clin Cancer Res* ,Vol.12,No.10, (May 2006), pp. (3050-6), ISSN 1078-0432Lee, JJ. & Swain, SM. (2006). Peripheral neuropathy induced by microtubule-stabilizing agents. *J Clin Oncol,* Vol.24, No.10, (April 2006), pp. 1633-42, ISSN 0732-183X

Ma, W., & Quirion, R. (2008). Does COX2-dependent PGE2 play a role in neuropathic pain? *Neurosci Lett,* Vol.437, No.3, (June 2008), pp. (165-9), ISSN 0304-3940

Makino, H. (2004). Treatment and care of neurotoxicity from taxane anticancer agents. *Breast Cancer,* Vol.11, No.1, pp. (100-4), ISSN 1340-6868

Markman, M. (2003). Management of toxicities associated with the administration of taxanes. *Expert Opin Drug Saf,* Vol.2, No.2, (March 2003), pp. (141-6), ISSN 1474-0338

McWhinney, SR., Goldberg, RM., & McLeod, HL. (2009).Platinum neurotoxicity pharmacogenetics. Platinum neurotoxicity pharmacogenetics. *Mol Cancer Ther,* Vol.8, No.1, (January 2009), pp. (10-6), ISSN 1535-7163

Meyer, L., Patte-Mensah, C., Taleb, O., & Mensah-Nyagan, AG. (2011). Allopregnanolone prevents and suppresses oxaliplatin-evoked painful neuropathy: multi-parametric assessment and direct evidence. *Pain* ,Vol.152, No.1, (January 2011), pp. (170-81), ISSN 0304-3959

Mielke, S., Mross, K., Gerds, TA., Schmidt, A., Wäsch, R., Berger, DP., Lange, W., & Behringer, D. (2003). Comparative neurotoxicity of weekly non-break paclitaxel infusions over 1 versus 3 h. *Anticancer Drugs,* Vol.14, No.10, (November 2003), pp. (785-92), ISSN 0959-4973

Mileshkin, L., Stark, R., Day, B., Seymour, JF., Zeldis, JB., & Prince, HM. (2006). Development of neuropathy in patients with myeloma treated with thalidomide: patterns of occurrence and the role of electrophysiologic monitoring. *J Clin Oncol,* Vol.24, No.27, (September 2006), pp. (4507-14), ISSN 0732-183X

Mir, O., Alexandre, J., Tran, A., Durand, JP., Pons, G., Treluyer, JM., & Goldwasser, F. (2009). Relationship between GSTP1 Ile (105) Val polymorphism and docetaxel-induced peripheral neuropathy: clinical evidence of a role of oxidative stress in taxane toxicity. *Ann Oncol,* Vol.20, No.4, (April 2009), pp. (736-40), ISSN 0923-7534

Molloy, FM., Floeter, MK., Syed, NA., Sandbrink, F., Culcea, E., Steinberg, SM., Dahut, W., Pluda, J., Kruger, EA., Reed, E., & Figg, WD. (2001). Thalidomide neuropathy in patients treated for metastatic prostate cancer. *Muscle Nerve,* Vol.24, No.8, (August 2001), pp. (1050-7), ISSN 0148-639X

Nabholtz, JM., Gelmon, K., Bontenbal, M.; Spielmann, M.; Catimel, G.; Conte, P.; Klaassen, U.; Namer, M.; Bonneterre, J.; Fumoleau, P., & Winograd, B. (1996). Multicenter randomized comparative study of two doses of paclitaxel in patients with metastatic breast cancer. *J Clin Oncol,* Vol.14, No.6, (June 1996), pp. (1858–67), ISSN 0732-183X

National Cancer Institute (2011). National Cancer Institute of the National Institutes of Health (NIH).Cancer topics, In: *Cancer Drug Information,* accessed 25 June 2011, Available from: *http://www.cancer.gov/cancertopics/druginfo/alphalist*

Ocean, AJ., & Vahdat, LT. (2004). Chemotherapy-induced peripheral neuropathy: pathogenesis and emerging therapies. *Support Care Cancer,* Vol.12, No.9, (September 2004), pp. (619-25), ISSN 0941-4355

Offidani, M., Corvatta, L., Marconi, M., Malerba, L., Mele, A., Olivieri, A., Brunori, M., Catarini, M., Candela, M., Capelli, D., Montanari, M., Rupoli, S., & Leoni, P. (2004). Common and rare side-effects of low-dose thalidomide in multiple myeloma: focus on the dose-minimizing peripheral neuropathy. *Eur J Haematol,* Vol.72, No.6, (June 2004), pp. (403-9), ISSN 0902-4441

Park, SB., Krishnan, AV., Lin, CS., Goldstein, D., Friedlander, M., & Kiernan, MC. (2008). Mechanisms underlying chemotherapy-induced neurotoxicity and the potential for neuroprotective strategies. *Curr Med Chem,* Vol.15, No.29, pp. (3081-94), ISSN 1568-0142

Pasetto, LM., D'Andrea, MR., Rossi, E., & Monfardini, S. (2006). Oxaliplatin-related neurotoxicity: how and why? *Crit Rev Oncol Hematol,* Vol.59, No.2, (August 2006), pp. (159-68), ISSN 1040-8428

Pei, XY., Dai ,Y., Grant, S.(2004). Synergistic induction of oxidative injury and apoptosis in human multiple myeloma cells by the proteasome inhibitor bortezomib and histone deacetylase inhibitors. *Clin Cancer Res,* Vol.10, No.11, (June 2004), pp. (3839-52), ISSN 1078-0432

Pietrangeli, A., Leandri, M., Terzoli, E., Jandolo, B., & Garufi, C. (2006). Persistence of high-dose oxaliplatin-induced neuropathy at long-term follow-up. *Eur Neurol,* Vol.56, No.1, pp. (13-6), ISSN 0014-3022

Ramanathan, RK., Rothenberg, ML., de Gramont, A., Tournigand, C., Goldberg, RM., Gupta, S., & André, T. (2010). Incidence and evolution of oxaliplatin-induced peripheral sensory neuropathy in diabetic patients with colorectal cancer: a pooled analysis of three phase III studies. *Ann Oncol,* Vol.21, No.4, (April 2010), pp. (754-8), ISSN 0923-7534

Rao, RD., Michalak, JC., Sloan, JA., Loprinzi, CL., Soori, GS., Nikcevich, DA., Warner, DO., Novotny, P., Kutteh, LA., & Wong, GY., North Central Cancer Treatment Group. (2007). Efficacy of gabapentin in the management of chemotherapy-induced peripheral neuropathy: a phase 3 randomized, double-blind, placebo-controlled crossover trial (N00C3). *Cancer,* Vol.110, No.9, (November 2007), pp. (2110-8), ISSN 0008-543X

Ravaglia, S., Corso, A., Piccolo, G., Lozza, A.; Alfonsi, E.; Mangiacavalli, S., Varettoni, M., Zappasodi, P., Moglia, A., Lazzarino, M., & Costa, A. (2008). Immune-mediated neuropathies in myeloma patients treated with bortezomib. *Clin Neurophysiol,* Vol.119, No.11, (November 2008), pp. (2507-12), ISSN 1388-2457

Ruzzo, A., Graziano, F., Loupakis, F., Rulli, E., Canestrari, E., Santini, D., Catalano, V., Ficarelli, R., Maltese, P., Bisonni, R., Masi, G., Schiavon, G., Giordani, P., Giustini, L., Falcone, A., Tonini, G., Silva, R., Mattioli, R., Floriani, I., & Magnani, M. (2007). Pharmacogenetic profiling in patients with advanced colorectal cancer treated with first-line FOLFOX-4 chemotherapy. *J Clin Oncol,* Vol.25, No.10, (April 2007), pp. (1247-54), ISSN 0732-183X

Sissung, TM., Mross, K., Steinberg, SM., Behringer, D., Figg, WD., Sparreboom, A., & Mielke, S. (2006). Association of ABCB1 genotypes with paclitaxel-mediated peripheral neuropathy and neutropenia. *Eur J Cancer,* Vol.42, No.17, (November 2006), pp. (2893-6), ISSN 0959-8049

Sissung, TM., Baum, CE., Deeken, J., Price, DK., Aragon-Ching, J., Steinberg, SM., Dahut, W., Sparreboom, A., & Figg, WD. (2008). ABCB1 genetic variation influences the toxicity and clinical outcome of patients with androgen-independent prostate cancer treated with docetaxel. *Clin Cancer Res,* Vol.14, No.14, (July 2008), pp. (4543-9) ISSN 1078-0432

Smith, RE., Brown, AM., Mamounas, EP., Anderson, SJ., Lembersky, BC., Atkins, JH., Shibata, HR., Baez, L., DeFusco, PA., Davila, E., Tipping, SJ., Bearden, JD., & Thirlwell, MP. (1999). Randomized trial of 3-hour versus 24-hour infusion of high-dose paclitaxel in patients with metastatic or locally advanced breast cancer: National Surgical Adjuvant Breast and Bowel Project Protocol B-26. *J Clin Oncol,* Vol.17, No.11, (November 1999), pp. (3403–11), ISSN 0732-183X

Souayah, N., & Khella, SL. (2010). A prospective double-blind, placebo-controlled study of thalidomide sensory symptoms in an elderly population with age-related macular degeneration. *J Clin Neurosci,* Vol.17, No.5, (May 2010), pp. (571-3), ISSN 0967-5868

Suyama, H., Kawamoto, M., Gaus, S., & Yuge, O. (2004). Effect of etodolac, a COX-2 inhibitor, on neuropathic pain in a rat model. *Brain Res,* Vol.1010, No.1-2, (June 2004), pp. (144-50), ISSN 0006-8993

Tosi, P., Zamagni, E., Cellini, C., Plasmati, R., Cangini, D., Tacchetti, P., Perrone, G., Pastorelli, F., Tura, S., Baccarani, M., & Cavo, M. (2005). Neurological toxicity of long-term (>1 yr) thalidomide therapy in patients with multiple myeloma. *Eur J Haematol,* Vol.74, No.3, (March 2005), pp. (212-6), ISSN 0902-4441

Tsavaris, N., Kopterides, P., Kosmas, C., Efthymiou, A., Skopelitis, H., Dimitrakopoulos, A., Pagouni, E., Pikazis, D., Zis, PV., & Koufos, C. (2008). Gabapentin monotherapy for the treatment of chemotherapy-induced neuropathic pain: a pilot study. *Pain Med,* Vol.9, No.8, (November 2008), pp. (1209-16), ISSN 1526-2375

Vanotti, A., Osio, M., Mailland, E., Nascimbene, C., Capiluppi, E., & Mariani, C. (2007). Overview on pathophysiology and newer approaches to treatment of peripheral neuropathies. *CNS Drugs,* Vol.21, Suppl 1, pp. (3-12), ISSN 1172-7047

Verstappen, CC., Koeppen, S., Heimans, JJ., Huijgens, PC., Scheulen, ME., Strumberg, D., Kiburg ,B., & Postma, TJ.(2005). Dose-related vincristine-induced peripheral neuropathy with unexpected off-therapy worsening. *Neurology,* Vol.64, No.6, (March 2005), pp. (1076-7), ISSN 0028-3878

Vo, T., Rice, AS., & Dworkin, RH. (2009). Non-steroidal anti-inflammatory drugs for neuropathic pain: how do we explain continued widespread use? *Pain,* Vol.143, No.3, (June 2009), pp. (169-71), ISSN 0304-3959

Vondracek, P., Oslejskova, H., Kepak, T., Mazanek, P., Sterba, J., Rysava, M., & Gal, P. (2009). Efficacy of pregabalin in neuropathic pain in paediatric oncological patients. *Eur J Paediatr Neurol,* Vol.13, No.4, (July 2009), pp. (332-6), ISSN 1090-3798

Walker, M., & Ni, O. (2007). Neuroprotection during chemotherapy: a systematic review. *Am J Clin Oncol* , Vol.30,No.1, (February 2007), pp. (82-92), ISSN 0277-3732

Watson, CP., Moulin, D., Watt-Watson, J., Gordon, A., & Eisenhoffer J. (2003). Controlled-release oxycodone relieves neuropathic pain: a randomized controlled trial in painful diabetic neuropathy. *Pain,* Vol.105, No.1-2, (September 2003), pp. (71-8), ISSN 0304-3959

Weintraub, M., Adde, MA., Venzon, DJ., Shad, AT., Horak, ID., Neely, JE., Seibel, NL., Gootenberg, J., Arndt, C., Nieder, ML., & Magrath, IT. (1996). Severe atypical neuropathy associated with administration of hematopoietic colony-stimulating factors and vincristine. *J Clin Oncol,* Vol.14, No.3, (March 1996), pp. (935-40), ISSN 0732-183X

Windebank, AJ., & Grisold, W. (2008). Chemotherapy-induced neuropathy. *J Peripher Nerv Syst,* Vol.13, No. 1, (March 2008), pp. (27-46), ISSN 1085-9489

Wolf, S., Barton, D., Kottschade L., Grothey A., & Loprinzi C. (2008). Chemotherapy-induced peripheral neuropathy: prevention and treatment strategies. *Eur J Cancer,* Vol.44, No.11, (July 2008), pp. (1507-15), ISSN 0961-5423

3

Targeting Molecular Chaperones in Diabetic Peripheral Neuropathy

Chengyuan Li and Rick T. Dobrowsky
*Department of Pharmacology & Toxicology,
University of Kansas, Lawrence, Kansas,
USA*

1. Introduction

1.1 Diabetic peripheral neuropathy

Diabetes Mellitus (DM) is estimated to affect 347 million patients globally as of 2008 (Danaei *et al.*, 2011) and this number is expected to double by 2030 (Wild *et al.*, 2004). DM results from the failure of our body to generate and/or respond to insulin, the principal hormone regulating uptake of glucose from the blood stream, leading to abnormally high blood glucose levels, termed hyperglycemia. Sensory neurons absorb glucose as a direct function of extracellular glucose concentration instead of insulin-mediated glucose uptake and are particularly susceptible to the cumulative metabolic insults imposed by chronic hyperglycemia (Tomlinson and Gardiner, 2008). This damage leads to secondary microvascular complications that contribute to the progression of diabetic neuropathy. Diabetic peripheral neuropathy (DPN) is the most prevalent complication of DM (Tahrani *et al.*, 2010), also comprises the most common form of peripheral neuropathy globally, surpassing leprosy in this aspect (Harati, 2010; Martyn and Hughes, 1997). Depending on the case definitions used, 30-70% of patients with either type 1 or type 2 DM are diagnosed with some form of peripheral neuropathy (National Institutes of Diabetes and Digestive and Kidney Diseases). A distal symmetric sensorimotor polyneuropathy is the most frequent manifestation of DPN. Patients with this form of DPN are predisposed to foot ulceration and increased risk of amputation; ulcerative complications from DPN account for approximately 87% of non-traumatic lower extremity amputations. In addition to this traumatic medical event, DPN is also a major contributing factor to the development of joint deformities, limb threatening ischemia as well as other various neurological dysfunctions (Harati, 2010). This greatly reduces the quality of life in people with DM through increased disability and is assuming more hospitalizations than all other diabetic complications combined (Mahmood *et al.*, 2009). As a consequence, approximately $15 billion are spent on DPN annually in the US, causing a major drain on healthcare expenditure (Rathmann and Ward, 2003). With the staggering individual, social and economic burden brought about by DPN-associated morbidity and mortality, development of effective treatments that prevent and/or reverse DPN are needed but currently unmet.

1.2 Clinical features

DPN encompasses a wide spectrum of clinical and subclinical syndromes differing in their pattern of neurological involvement, anatomic distribution, specific neuropathic alterations, risk covariates and course of development. As mentioned in the last section, distal symmetric sensorimotor polyneuropathy represents the most common type of involvement and affects 90% of patients with DPN (Harati, 2010). Damage to nerves initially begins with the longest axons, which accounts for the loss of sensation having a "stocking-glove" distribution. Degeneration continues to progress proximally in a dying-back, length-dependent pattern. (Boulton and Malik, 1998). Although post-mortem analysis indicates that all types and sizes of fibers are affected, sensory symptoms predominate over motor deficits at least in the early phase, likely due to the longer (and therefore more susceptible) axons needed to reach the epidermis. Patients diagnosed with this form of neuropathy often display symptoms such as paradoxical association of numbness with allodynia and dysesthesia associated with small fiber sensory dysfunction. As DPN advances, large sensory and motor fibers also become impaired which results in loss of vibratory sensation, proprioception, slowed nerve conduction velocities (NCV) and progressive fiber loss that culminates in irreversible neurodegeneration (Habib and Brannagan, 2010; Harati, 2010; Tahrani *et al.*, 2010).

1.3 Risk factors

Several landmark prospective studies enrolling a large cohort of type 1 diabetics, including the multicenter Diabetes Control and Complications Trial (DCCT) and Epidemiology of Diabetes Interventions and Complications (EDIC) observational study, have definitively established chronic hyperglycemia (mean glycosylated hemoglobin [HbA1c]> 6.5%) as a causative factor of DPN (Albers *et al.*, 2010; DCCT, 1988). This is strengthened by the fact that reduction in the incidence and progression of DPN can be achieved with rigorous glycemic control through intensified insulin therapy (DCCT, 1995; UK Prospective Diabetes Study Group, 1998). However, the fact that some patients still developed DPN even with good glucose control suggested the presence of other etiological factors. Indeed, duration of DM, age, obesity, hypertension, hyperlipidemia, cardiovascular disease, genetic predisposition and presence of other microvascular complications such as retinopathy and nephropathy also significantly increase an individual's susceptibility to DPN (Harati, 2010; Tesfaye and Selvarajah, 2009). Whether modifying some of these factors would help prevent or retard the development of DPN awaits further examination.

1.4 Pathogenesis

With years of ongoing efforts, a number of biochemical events have been identified as important mediators linking hyperglycemic stress to the development of DPN: increased oxidative stress, formation of advanced glycation end-products (AGEs), overflux of glucose through polyol and hexosamine pathways, abnormal activity of mitogen-activated protein kinases (MAPKs) and nuclear factor-κB (NK-κB), neuroinflammation as well as impaired neurotrophic support. Unfortunately, none of the compounds developed against these targets has shown unequivocal effectiveness in preventing, reversing, or even slowing the neuropathic process in humans (Mahmood *et al.*, 2009; Obrosova, 2009; Tahrani *et al.*, 2010). A principal reason to explain these failures is the complexity of the pathogenesis of DPN since this array of molecular targets and pathways do not contribute to its pathophysiological progression in a temporally and/or biochemically uniform fashion. To date, the only effective strategy and gold standard method for preventing and treating DPN remains aggressive glycemic control, supplemented by FDA-approved medications providing pain relief. However, many patients struggle to maintain normoglycemia and the eventual development of irreversible neurodegeneration has rendered our current management palliative at best. Clearly, the rational identification of new molecular paradigms that identify "druggable" targets is of high scientific impact to understanding the pathobiology of DPN and offers translational potential for improving its medical management. In this regard, emerging evidence has unraveled a fundamental but previously under-recognized alternative that modulating molecular chaperones, or heat shock proteins, affords a novel approach toward improving hyperglycemia as well as the function of myelinated and unmyelinated fibers in DPN. The remainder of this chapter will focus on a review of the functional, pathological and therapeutic implications of heat shock proteins in DM and DPN.

2. Scientific rationale for targeting molecular chaperones

2.1 Functions of heat shock proteins: "Molecular lifeguards"

Over 40 years ago, Ritossa observed that cells from the salivary gland of drosophila responded to an elevation in temperature with increased activation of certain sets of genes indicated by a "puffing" pattern of polytene chromosomes (Ritossa, 1962). A decade later, it was uncovered that the "puffs" were a result of a rapid and robust synthesis of a special group of proteins that are crucial for the protection and recovery from increased protein damage caused by heat stress, which would otherwise be lethal. These proteins were hence termed heat shock proteins (HSPs) and their induction was named the heat shock response (HSR). Abundant evidence has since accumulated suggesting that not only does this response exist in organisms ranging from prokaryotic bacteria to humans, but that it is also induced by a plethora of external and internal stimuli, including ischemic, hypoxic, chemical, inflammatory, oxidative and mechanical stress (Jaattela and Wissing, 1992). The universal nature of this phenomenon suggests that HSPs, or "stress proteins", play a critical role in cellular homeostasis. Indeed, blocking HSP induction mitigated the protective effect of mild heat-shock against subsequent death-inducing insults in cells (Park *et al.*, 2001). Most if not all HSPs function as "molecular chaperones", which provide a first line of defense against misfolded and/or aggregated proteins. By utilizing energy derived from ATP hydrolysis, molecular chaperones: 1) assist in the correct folding of nascent proteins during *de novo* synthesis or refolding of damaged proteins; 2) transport newly synthesized proteins to target organelles; 3) help maintain the correct tertiary structure of the protein, prevent and solubilize abnormal protein aggregates and 4) target severely damaged and irreparable proteins to proteasomal or lysosomal disposal. Apart from their "housekeeping" chaperoning function, increasing evidence suggests that HSPs are involved in other cellular processes such as inflammation and apoptosis. Transcription of HSPs during the HSR is regulated by heat shock factors (HSFs), of which HSF-1 is the prototype and master activator in vertebrates. Its importance to the HSR is underscored by the fact that genetic deletion of HSF-1 prevents HSP gene transactivation and development of thermotolerance as well as a loss of protection against inflammation (McMillan *et al.*, 1998; Pirkkala *et al.*, 2000; Xiao *et al.*, 1999; Zhang *et al.*, 2002). HSF-1 is largely repressed and kept as an inert monomer in the cytosol by the chaperone HSP90. This interaction is disrupted by certain types of cell stress and leads to the dissociation of HSF-1. Following homotrimerization, phosphorylation and translocation to the nucleus, HSF-1 activates transcription of HSPs by binding to highly conserved sequences known as heat shock elements (HSEs) within the promoter region of multiple heat-shock genes. However, the exact phoshorylation sites through which HSF-1 is activated is not settled (DeFranco *et al.*, 2004). Although different classifications can be ascribed based on function, cellular localization and expression pattern, HSPs are widely categorized according to their molecular sizes into five families, comprising HSP100, HSP90, HSP70, HSP60, HSP40 and small HSPs with a molecular mass less than 40 kilo-daltons (kDa) (Feder and Hofmann, 1999). Specific HSPs that are particularly implicated in the context of DM and DPN are briefly discussed below.

2.1.1 HSP90: Seeking effective pharmacological "heat-shock therapy"

HSP90 is one of the most prevalent cellular proteins as it accounts for 1-2% of total protein and is essential for the cell survival in most eukaryotes; the latter is clearly indicated by the embryonic lethality of HSP90 knockout mice (Yeyati and van Heyningen, 2008). HSP90 is ubiquitously expressed in the cytosol where it is responsible for post-translational maturation of a variety of nascent polypeptides as well as solubilization and refolding of misfolded and damaged proteins after stress. The most predominant isoforms are stress-inducible HSP90α and constitutive HSP90β that primarily localize in the cytoplasm. Other homologues include Grp94 in the endoplasmic reticulum and the mitochondria matrix protein HSP75/TRAP-1. All HSP90s are highly conserved evolutionarily in their structures and share an N-terminal ATPase domain, a connective linker region, a middle domain involved in binding substrates (client proteins). HSP90 also has a C-terminal domain that is responsible for interactions with various partner proteins and co-chaperones which provide a coordinate regulation over its diversified functions (Peterson and Blagg, 2009; Soti *et al.*, 2002). Because numerous HSP90 client proteins are involved in cell growth, differentiation, and survival secretion, inhibitors directed against the HSP90 N-terminal ATP binding domain induce simultaneous degradation of a wide variety of client proteins and are potent chemotherapeutic agents in cancer (Peterson and Blagg, 2009; Soti *et al.*, 2005). An important aspect of N-terminal HSP90 inhibitors in treating malignant phenotypes is that the drugs preferentially inhibit HSP90 and induce client protein degradation in malignant versus normal cells (Luo *et al.*, 2008). This selectivity may be due to the upregulation of HSP90 to accommodate the dependency of malignant cells on overexpressed oncogenic client proteins (Chiosis *et al.*, 2003) and/or an increased affinity of N-terminal inhibitors for HSP90-oncoprotein complexes in cancer cells (Kamal *et al.*, 2003). Although this selectivity aids the clinical efficacy of N-terminal HSP90 inhibitors, enthusiasm for their use has been hampered because induction of client protein degradation and cytotoxicity occurs at drug concentrations that also activate an antagonistic aspect of HSP90 biology, the promotion of the cytoprotective HSR.

Since N-terminal HSP90 inhibitors promote the HSR and decrease protein aggregation, they also have possible utility in treating neurodegenerative diseases associated with protein misfolding. In this regard, N-terminal HSP90 inhibitors decrease tau protein aggregation in Alzheimer's disease models (Dickey *et al.*, 2007; Luo *et al.*, 2007) and improve motor function in spinal and bulbar muscular atrophy (Waza *et al.*, 2005). Although a similar selectivity exists for the use of N-terminal inhibitors in treating neurodegenerative diseases (Dickey *et al.*, 2007), this selectivity does not circumvent the issue related to dissociating client protein degradation from induction of the HSR. Now, the inverse caveat exists; despite being neuroprotective, induction of client protein degradation may produce cytotoxicity. Thus, developing a highly effective HSP90 inhibitor for treating neurodegeneration requires establishing a sufficient therapeutic window that avoids increased client protein degradation that may antagonize a cytoprotective HSR. HSP90 also contains a C-terminus ATP binding domain that weakly binds the antibiotic novobiocin. Similar to N-terminal inhibitors, novobiocin can promote client protein degradation and induce a HSR. Through systematic modification of the coumarin ring pharmacophore of novobiocin, KU-32 was identified as a lead compound that exhibits at least a 500-fold divergence of client protein degradation from induction of HSP70 (Urban *et al.*, 2010). This divergence provides an excellent therapeutic window to promote neuroprotection in the absence of toxicity. Thus, non-selective uptake and off-target toxicity is not a confounding issue as discussed above. In support of this safety, administering 400 mg/kg of KU-32 to mice (20x > our typical dose) did not induce overt toxicity or histopathological changes on all organs examined. In our study with STZ-diabetic mice, treatment of mice with KU-32 effectively reversed the development of sensory hypoalgesia in an HSP70-dependent manner (Urban *et al.*, 2010). This study provides encouraging evidence that inhibition, or modulation of HSP90 offers a potent "heat-shock therapy" in treating DPN.

2.1.2 HSP70: Potent "cytoprotectant"

The 70-kDa HSPs are found in many of the major subcellular compartments: cytosolic heat shock cognate protein 70 (HSC70) with a molecular weight of 73kDa, the stress-inducible cytosolic HSP70 (HSP72 in humans), the endoplasmic-reticulum (ER)-localized glucose-regulated protein 78 (Grp78/BiP) and the mitochondrial glucose-regulated protein Grp75/mortalin. Although sharing 80% homology with HSP70, HSC70 is constitutively expressed and only moderately inducible whereas expression of HSP70, Grp78 and Grp75 can be induced by stressful stimuli to varying degrees, with HSP70 being the most robust. After cell stress, HSP70 appears in both the cytoplasm and nucleus and helps repair damaged proteins. Similarly, induction of Grp78/BiP and Grp75 are essential for maintenance of ER and mitochondrial proteostasis, respectively (Richter-Landsberg and Goldbaum, 2003). Chaperones rarely work alone, and usually associate with each other and/or other co-factors to carry out distinct functions. For example, binding of HSP40 co-chaperone to HSP70 often facilitates substrate folding and refolding (Michels *et al.*, 1997; Minami *et al.*, 1996) whereas association of HSP70 with HSP90 via HSP-organizing protein (HOP) typically targets proteins towards proteasomal degradation (Sajjad *et al.*, 2010). Due to the importance of HSP70 in the maintenance of cellular homeostasis and defense against various insults, its deficiency or dysfunction has been linked to numerous human diseases (Muchowski and Wacker, 2005). However, direct targeting of HSP70 as a pharmacological objective has been complicated by its high conservation and ubiquitous expression patterns. Nevertheless, there appear to be some compounds such as geranylgeranyl acetone (GGA) that directly modulate HSP70. GGA is currently the leading antiulcer drug in Japan (Ushijima *et al.*, 2005) and has been shown to be neuroprotective against cerebral ischemia, polyQ toxicity (Sajjad *et al.*, 2010) and recently in a diabetic monkey model to attenuate insulin resistance (Kavanagh *et al.*, 2011) via the induction of HSP70. As many of the other HSR inducers or co-inducers, the HSP induction mechanism of GGA is not elucidated but has been suggested via dissociation of HSF-1 from HSP70 by competitively interacting with HSP70 C-terminal peptide-binding domain, which is the HSF-1 binding sites during HSP70-HSF-1 negative feedback (Otaka *et al.*, 2007). If GGA indeed acts through this mechanism, a combination of GGA with HSP90 inhibitors might exert a robust "heat-shock paradigm".

2.2 HSP modulates insulin resistance

Skeletal muscle, heart, liver and adipocytes comprise about two-thirds of the cells in the body and depend on insulin for glucose uptake. Reduced or loss of response of these tissues to insulin, namely insulin resistance, is a key pathogenetic feature that leads to the development of frank type 2 DM and its complications, such as DPN. Since type 2 DM is accountable for more than 90% of all cases of DM worldwide (World Health Organization, 2011), inhibiting insulin resistance assumes an important role in managing DPN. Although the exact mechanisms leading to insulin resistance are yet to be elucidated, it has become apparent that excess free fatty acids, inflammatory cytokines, mitochondrial impairment and oxidative stress may activate multiple signaling pathways that negatively affect insulin signaling through inhibitory serine phosphorylation of insulin receptor substrate-1 (IRS-1). In obesity for instance, induction of protein kinase C (PKC)-ε/θ through increased synthesis of diacylglycerol (DAG) from fatty acids has been linked to impaired insulin activity in skeletal muscle and liver (Schmitz-Peiffer, 2002; Schmitz-Peiffer *et al.*, 1997), presumably through activation of serine-threonine kinases including inhibitor of nuclear factor κB kinase-β (IKK-β) (Itani *et al.*, 2002; Shoelson *et al.*, 2003) and/or c-jun N-terminal kinase (JNK) (Hirosumi *et al.*, 2002) (Fig.1.). Inflammatory cytokines, such as tumor necrosis factor-α (TNF-α) secreted from hypertrophied adipose tissue and/or macrophages, can also stimulate JNK and IKK-β in various insulin-sensitive tissues and promote insulin resistance (Wellen and Hotamisligil, 2005). Particularly, phosphorylation of serine 312 (S312) in humans or S307 in rats by JNK and IKK-β renders this crucial signaling intermediate a poor substrate for the insulin-stimulated receptor (McCarty, 2006).

2.2.1 HSP inhibits inflammation and stress kinases

As natural inhibitors of above damaging events and their catalyzing enzymes, HSPs may provide a broad defense against insulin resistance. The first supporting evidence came from a small clinical study performed by Hooper over ten years ago. In this study, heat therapy on patients with type 2 DM through hot tub immersion six days a week for three consecutive weeks dropped their fasting plasma glucose and mean glycosylated hemoglobin levels (Hooper, 1999). Although the HSP levels were not measured in this trial, it documented an average rise of 0.8°C in body temperature, which is sufficient for HSP induction (Okada *et al.*, 2004). Despite the lack of proper controls and its exploratory nature, the credibility of this early report has been substantiated by similar studies from animal models of DM. For example, whereas high-fat diet evoked significant hyperglycemia, hyperinsulinemia, insulin insensitivity, glucose intolerance as well as JNK and IKK-β activation in skeletal muscles in rodents, weekly heat therapy upregulated HSP70 which paralleled an apparent attenuation of these metabolic characteristics (Chung *et al.*, 2008; Gupte *et al.*, 2009b). Chung *et al* further demonstrated that targeted overexpression of HSP70 in mouse skeletal muscles mimicked the effects of heat therapy in preventing fat-induced JNK phosphorylation, insulin resistance and fat deposition, suggesting that HSP70 might mediate the beneficial effects afforded by heat therapy (Chung *et al.*, 2008). Indeed, pharmacological induction of HSP70 with the hydroxylamine derivative BGP-15, α-lipoic acid or GGA improved glucose tolerance in insulin-resistant mice (Chung *et al.*, 2008), rats (Gupte *et al.*, 2009a) and monkeys (Kavanagh *et al.*, 2011), respectively. Notably, administration of a HSP co-inducer BRX-220 to STZ-diabetic rats dose-dependently reduced insulin resistance and was associated with improved peripheral sensory and motor nerve deficits (Kurthy *et al.*, 2002).

In Gupte's study of rats fed with high-fat diet, addition of an HSP70 inhibitor diminished the heat-induced JNK depression, indicating that inhibition of JNK activation by heat-shock is largely HSP70-dependent (Gupte *et al.*, 2009b). In fact, a role for HSP70 as a JNK inhibitor has been well-established *in vitro* and appears to be of physiological significance. For example, heat-shock preconditioning suppressed JNK activity and apoptosis in fibroblasts upon ultra violet exposure. However, this effect was mitigated when cells were transfected with antisense HSP70 oligonucleotides (Park *et al.*, 2001). The precise mechanism by which HSP70 inhibits JNK is at dispute. HSP70 may directly bind to JNK and inhibit its activation by upstream activating kinases and preventing phosphorylation of its substrate, c-jun (Geiger and Gupte, 2011; Park *et al.*, 2001). On the other hand, others have failed to detect an HSP70-JNK physical interaction through immunoprecipitation (Chung *et al.*, 2008). This disparity is confounding and awaits further scrutiny. In addition to a direct modulation on JNK itself, other reports also suggest that HSP70 may regulate JNK activity via effects on upstream kinases (Daviau *et al.*, 2006) and/or phosphatases (Meriin *et al.*, 1999).

2.2.2 HSP enhances mitochondrial function

Although the exact role of mitochondrial dysfunction in the development of insulin resistance is controversial, mitochondrial dysfunction is frequently found in insulin-resistant human or animals (Bonnard *et al.*, 2008; Morino *et al.*, 2006; Petersen *et al.*, 2004). It is believed that with obesity and nutrient overload, there is excessive beta-oxidation of fatty acids that is unmatched with a concomitant elevation in downstream mitochondrial enzyme activities and ATP demand. This uncoupled mitochondrial flux produces a buildup of beta-oxidation intermediates which promote proton leak and increased reactive oxygen species (ROS) generation, which in turn stimulates the aforementioned stress kinases that contribute to insulin resistance (Koves *et al.*, 2008). One way in which insulin resistance is alleviated by heat therapy might be through enhancing mitochondrial energetic flux and oxidative capacity. This is supported by the observation that heat treatment maintained citrate synthase and cytochrome oxidase activity, which were decreased with fat feeding. Likewise, a single heat treatment prevented impaired mitochondrial oxygen consumption and fatty acid oxidation in L6 muscle cells treated with TNF-α and palmitate, respectively (Gupte *et al.*, 2009b). These results are consistent with previous studies demonstrating that heat shock protected mitochondrial function against oxidative and ischemic injury (Polla *et al.*, 1996; Sammut *et al.*, 2001). Independent of heat treatment, transgenic mice overexpressing HSP70 in skeletal muscles possess higher citrate synthase and β-hydroxyacyl-CoA-dehydrogenase activity and are refrained from insulin resistance (Chung *et al.*, 2008). HSP70 plays an important role in mitochondria proteostasis since it facilitates import of nuclear encoded proteins into mitochondria via interaction with the mitochondrial protein import receptor Tom70 (Young *et al.*, 2003). In addition, overexpression of HSP70 decreased ROS formation and maintained mitochondrial respiration in glucose-deprived astrocytes (Ouyang *et al.*, 2006). Clinically, poor HSP70 mRNA expression is found in diabetic humans and correlates with reduced mitochondrial enzyme activity (Bruce *et al.*, 2003), increased JNK activity (Chung *et al.*, 2008) and the degree of insulin resistance (Kurucz *et al.*, 2002). Evidence from animal models of DM also supports this finding at the protein level (Atalay *et al.*, 2004; Kavanagh *et al.*, 2011). Given the profound impact of HSP on stress kinases and mitochondrial integrity, it is conceivable that reduced HSP expression might have unfettered the deleterious inflammatory signaling and redox homeostasis which accelerate the development of insulin resistance.

Thus, increasing HSP could be a powerful tool in combating insulin resistance to help prevent diabetic complications such as DPN (see Fig.1.).

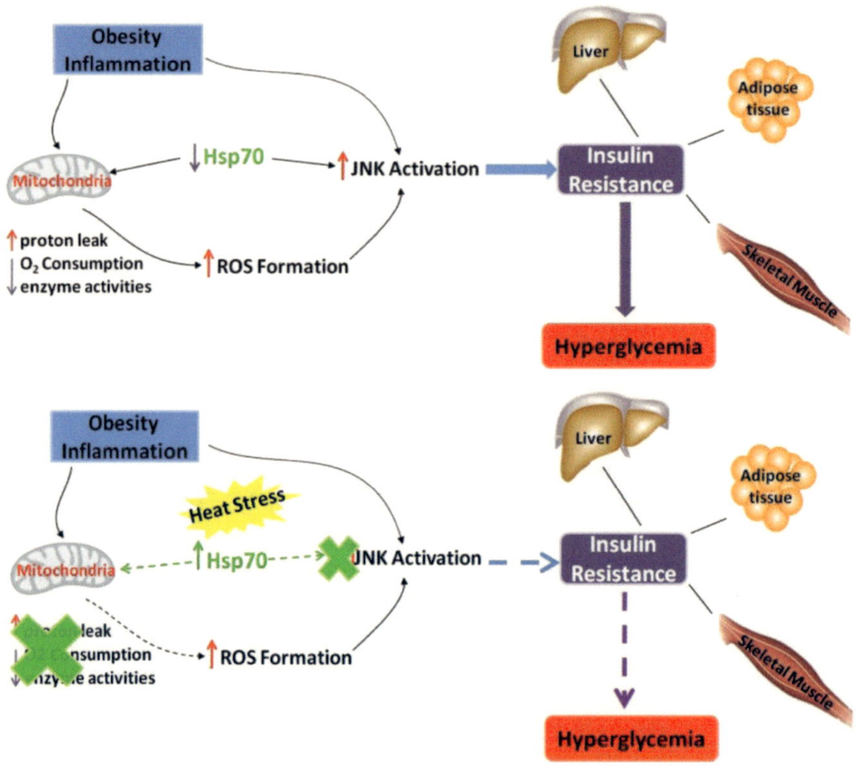

Fig. 1. Schematic of obesity and inflammation-induced insulin resistance and role for Hsp70 as an inhibitor of insulin resistance. Solid lines indicate stimulated pathways; dashed lines indicate inhibited pathways.

2.3 Impaired HSP Protection in DPN

Chronic hyperglycemia can trigger excess ischemic, hypoxic, oxidative and apoptotic stress. However, molecular chaperones, which normally respond by mounting a defense against such stresses, are often found paradoxically low in diabetic tissues. For example, in a couple of clinical studies enrolling type 2 diabetics and healthy controls, patients with DM had significantly lower mRNA levels of HSP70 and heme oxygenase-1 (HO-1, HSP32), a stress-inducible HSP that has antioxidant properties (Bruce *et al.*, 2003; Kurucz *et al.*, 2002). In a comparison of twins discordant for type 2 DM, muscle HSP70 levels are significantly lower in both diabetic twins and their non-diabetic but insulin-resistant monozygotic co-twins as compared to healthy controls. Particularly, the level of HSP70 mRNA inversely correlated with the severity of insulin-resistance and diabetic phenotype (Kurucz *et al.*, 2002). Chung *et al.* confirmed that there is a reduced expression of HSP70 protein in muscle from obese, insulin-resistant humans (Chung *et al.*, 2008). In type 1 diabetics diagnosed with polyneuropathy, a marked decreased in the HSP70 content in peripheral blood cells has also been reported (Strokov *et al.*, 2000). In contrast, this reduction was not observed in a recent study of non-insulin-dependent diabetic males who were free of diabetic complications (Brinkmann *et al.*, 2011). This discrepancy may indicate a positive correlation between lower HSP70 expression and the presence of diabetic complications. In line with this hypothesis, physical or pharmacological therapies that improved neuropathic symptoms in type 1 and type 2 diabetics have demonstrated significant restoration of HSP levels (Hooper, 1999; Strokov *et al.*, 2000).

The association of decreased HSP70 expression with DM is also supported by studies in a variety of animal models. In diabetic monkeys, hepatic and plasma HSP70 was reduced by hyperglycemia in a dose-dependent fashion. In addition, long-term hyperglycemia also dose-dependently impaired the activation of liver HSF-1 in response to heat-shock, with a concomitant compensatory increase in total HSF-1 protein (Kavanagh *et al.*, 2011). In mice fed a high-fat diet, the induction of HSP70 by heat therapy was attenuated compared to chow-fed mice (Chung *et al.*, 2008). Evaluation of HSP levels in rats rendered diabetic with the β-cell toxin streptozotocin (STZ) has generated equivocal results: HSP70 and HSF-1 protein content was reported to be both decreased (Atalay *et al.*, 2004) and unchanged (Najemnikova *et al.*, 2007; Swiecki *et al.*, 2003) in heart and liver. The effects of DM on muscle and kidney HSP expression may be more cell-type specific since diabetic rats showed increased renal HSP70 and HSP25 immunoreactivity in the outer medulla but not in glomeruli (Barutta *et al.*, 2008). Species and genotype, duration and severity of DM, tissue vulnerability and antibody specificity/sensitivity may serve as contributing variables that underpin these differing results. Alternatively, these seemingly contradictory observations might actually reflect the heterogeneous nature and pathological progression of DM. This is supported by findings in dorsal root ganglia of spontaneous diabetic BB/Wor rats (which develop β-cell dysfunction and neuropathy similar to that seen in human type 1 DM). Whereas an elevated expression of HSP70 and HSP25 was seen following 4-months of DM, HSP70 expression was significantly blunted after 10-months of DM and correlated with decreased neurotrophic components and degeneration of myelinated and unmyelinated fibers, indicative of advanced polyneuropathy (Kamiya *et al.*, 2006; Kamiya *et al.*, 2005). Therefore, despite the non-linear pattern of changing in HSP expression, the data suggest a possible inverse relationship between the level of HSP and neuropathological change in DM. Consistent with this notion, compounds known to co-induce HSP were able to improve diabetic peripheral neuropathy (Kurthy *et al.*, 2002) and wound healing (Vigh *et al.*, 1997). Although the development of diabetic complications is associated with a progressive decline in the expression of HSPs, mice with a genetic knock-out of the inducible isoforms of HSP70 (HSP70.1 and 70.3) did not develop any more severe neurophysiological deficits than were observed in wild-type diabetic mice (Urban *et al.*, 2010). Thus, HSP70 is not essential to the pathophysiologic development of DPN and the lack of a more severe neuropathy in the diabetic HSP70 knockout mice may suggest a compensatory involvement of other HSPs such as HSC70. Nevertheless, a genetic assessment in patients with DM identified an HSP70 gene polymorphism in association with an increased severity of diabetic foot ulceration, need for amputation and greater duration of hospitalization (Mir *et al.*, 2009). Similar to that observed in spontaneous diabetic BB/Wor rats, short-term DM (30 days) enhanced HSP induction in response to heat treatment in STZ-injected rats versus control (Najemnikova *et al.*, 2007). However, prolonged (8 weeks) hyperglycemia significantly blunted the HSR stimulated by endurance exercise training or heat stress in the same model (Atalay *et al.*, 2004; Swiecki *et al.*, 2003). On the other hand, although a 15-min heat-shock upregulated HSP70 in diabetic rat heart, it failed to protect against myocardial ischemia/reperfusion injury (Joyeux *et al.*, 1999). Therefore, DM may have impaired the cytoprotective function of chaperones and some of the enhanced expression of HSP might reflect an overwhelmed cellular stress defense or overall failure of chaperones to function properly. Although a systemic and in-depth characterization of expression and functional change of nerve HSPs throughout the course of DPN is needed, it is tempting to speculate that chronic metabolic stress in DM produces a disturbed endogenous defense system and results in widespread tissue vulnerability to various insults which contribute to diabetic complications such as DPN. Despite the ambiguity cited above, these results collectively support that modulating chaperone function can have potential benefit on the progression of DM and its complications.

2.4 Direct role for HSP in neuroprotection

A direct cytoprotective effect of HSPs in nerves has been extensively characterized in an array of neurodegenerative disease models. For instance, transgenic overexpression of HSP70, HSP40 or HSP27, either separately or in combination, protected neurons from mutant or misfolded protein-induced toxicity in cell culture and animal models of familial amyotrophic lateral sclerosis (Bruening *et al.*, 1999; Takeuchi *et al.*, 2002), Alzheimer's (Magrane *et al.*, 2004; Shimura *et al.*, 2004a), Parkinson's (Klucken *et al.*, 2004) and polyglutamine (polyQ) expansion diseases (Jana *et al.*, 2000; Wyttenbach *et al.*, 2002). A large part of this protection was attributed to the ability of HSPs to decrease toxic protein aggregates through refolding or targeted degradation (Cuervo *et al.*, 2004; Klucken *et al.*, 2004; Shimura *et al.*, 2004b). Apart from chaperone function, both heat-shock preconditioning and overexpression of HSP70 and HSP27 improved neuronal survival in mice following focal or global cerebral ischemia (Kelly and Yenari, 2002); this protection was linked to HSPs interfering with inflammatory and apoptotic signaling pathways.

In contrast to the extensive evidence characterizing the neuroprotective effects of HSPs in protein conformational and neurodegenerative disorders, scant data has been published with regard to their possible benefit in diabetic nerve. To date, most relevant evidence is largely correlative in nature and comes from indirect evaluation of pharmacological HSP co-inducers. In STZ-induced diabetic Wistar rats, two known HSP co-inducing compounds, bimoclomol (Biro *et al.*, 1997) and BRX-220 (Kurthy *et al.*, 2002), independently reversed the slowing of motor and sensory conduction deficits as well as the ischemic conduction failure in sciatic nerve. Substantially advancing these findings, studies in our laboratory also demonstrated a potent reversal of pre-existing mechanical and thermal hypoalgesia in addition to an improved motor and sensory NCV in STZ-mice administered a small molecule HSP90 inhibitor, KU-32 (Urban *et al.*, 2010). This protection occurred without an obvious improvement in serum glucose or insulin levels, indicating that it is likely to be a direct effect in nerves, Schwann cells (SCs) or endothelium. Importantly, HSP70 appeared to be a critical component in the mechanism of protection by KU-32 as this compound showed no sign of ameliorating any of the clinical indices of DPN that developed in diabetic HSP70 knockout mice (Urban *et al.*, 2010). These studies, however, do not provide mechanistic insight as to whether and how HSP70 elicits a protective effect in diabetic peripheral nerves. Part of the reason comes from the fact that unlike most other neurodegenerative disorders that have been the focus of chaperone therapy, the etiology of DPN is not associated with the accumulation of a specific misfolded or aggregated protein. However, the efficacy of KU-32 in reversing several clinically relevant physiologic indices of nerve dysfunction strongly supports that damaged proteins contribute to DPN. Although DPN is primarily a metabolic disease that encompasses a panoply of physiological and biochemical disturbances, hyperglycemic stress can increase oxidative modification of amino acids (Akude *et al.*, 2009; Obrosova, 2009) that can impair protein folding, decrease refolding or induce protein aggregation (Muchowski and Wacker, 2005). Oxidative stress can also contribute to mitochondrial dysfunction (Chowdhury et al., 2011) and aggregation within sensory axons in DPN (Zherebitskaya *et al.*, 2009). In this regard, increasing chaperones in nerves may provide an excellent endogenous protein "quality control" defense by enhancing protein folding and/or refolding. Additionally, evidence is accumulating that HSPs are capable of intersecting with multiple other molecular targets that contribute to DPN.

2.4.1 JNK inhibition

JNK activation has been suggested to mediate neurotrophic factor deprivation-induced apoptosis in cultured sympathetic, motor or cerebral granule neurons (Eilers *et al.*, 1998; Maroney *et al.*, 1998; Watson *et al.*, 1998). As mentioned earlier, the inhibition of JNK-mediated inflammation and apoptosis by HSP70 is well-established in non-neuronal cells. This anti-apoptotic effect of HSP70 was further extended in sympathetic neurons where virally-directed (Bienemann *et al.*, 2008) or compound-induced expression (Salehi *et al.*, 2006) of HSP70 suppressed JNK activity and subsequent apoptosis. Although the contribution of neuronal apoptosis to DPN is controversial (Cheng and Zochodne, 2003), high concentrations of glucose induced apoptotic change in superior cervical gangalion neurons (Russell and Feldman, 1999). JNK inhibition might therefore partially contribute to nerve protection by HSP70 (see Fig.2.). In agreement, pretreatment of rat embryonic sensory neurons with KU-32 prevented glucose-induced cell death (Urban *et al.*, 2010). In amputated limbs from type 1 diabetic patients, sural nerve biopsies revealed a 2.5-fold increase in JNK activity (Purves *et al.*, 2001). Both hyperglycemically stressed adult sensory neurons (Purves *et al.*, 2001) and diabetic rat DRGs and sural nerve (Fernyhough *et al.*, 1999) underwent prolonged JNK activation that correlated with increased hyperphosphorylation of neurofilaments, the latter has been linked to axonal dystrophy seen in DPN (Fernyhough *et al.*, 1999). In addition, there is compelling evidence that the JNK pathway contributes to the pain sensitization of mechanical allodynia (Gao and Ji, 2008; Zhuang *et al.*, 2006), inflammatory hyperalgesia (Doya *et al.*, 2005) and diabetic neuropathic pain (Daulhac *et al.*, 2006). These observations support that JNK inhibition by HSP70 might help prevent development of distal axonopathy or neuropathic pain in DM.

2.4.2 Mitochondria protection

Investigation on mitochondrial dysfunction in diabetic nerves is a rapidly developing field. Sensory neurons from diabetic rats demonstrate significant decreases in mitochondrial respiration rate and complex I and IV enzyme activity, which is associated with impaired oxidative phosphorylation and diminished ROS formation (Akude *et al.*, 2011; Fernyhough *et al.*, 2010). Since HSP70 was closely linked to the maintenance and enhancement of mitochondrial function in diabetic muscle (Chung *et al.*, 2008; Gupte *et al.*, 2009b), it is reasonable to test the hypothesis that HSP70 might help preserve the competency of mitochondrial bioenergetics in neurons under glucose-driven metabolic stress. In support of this, over-expression of HSP70 increased the activity of complexes III and IV of the respiratory chain from hypoxia/reoxygenation injury in heart (Williamson *et al.*, 2008).

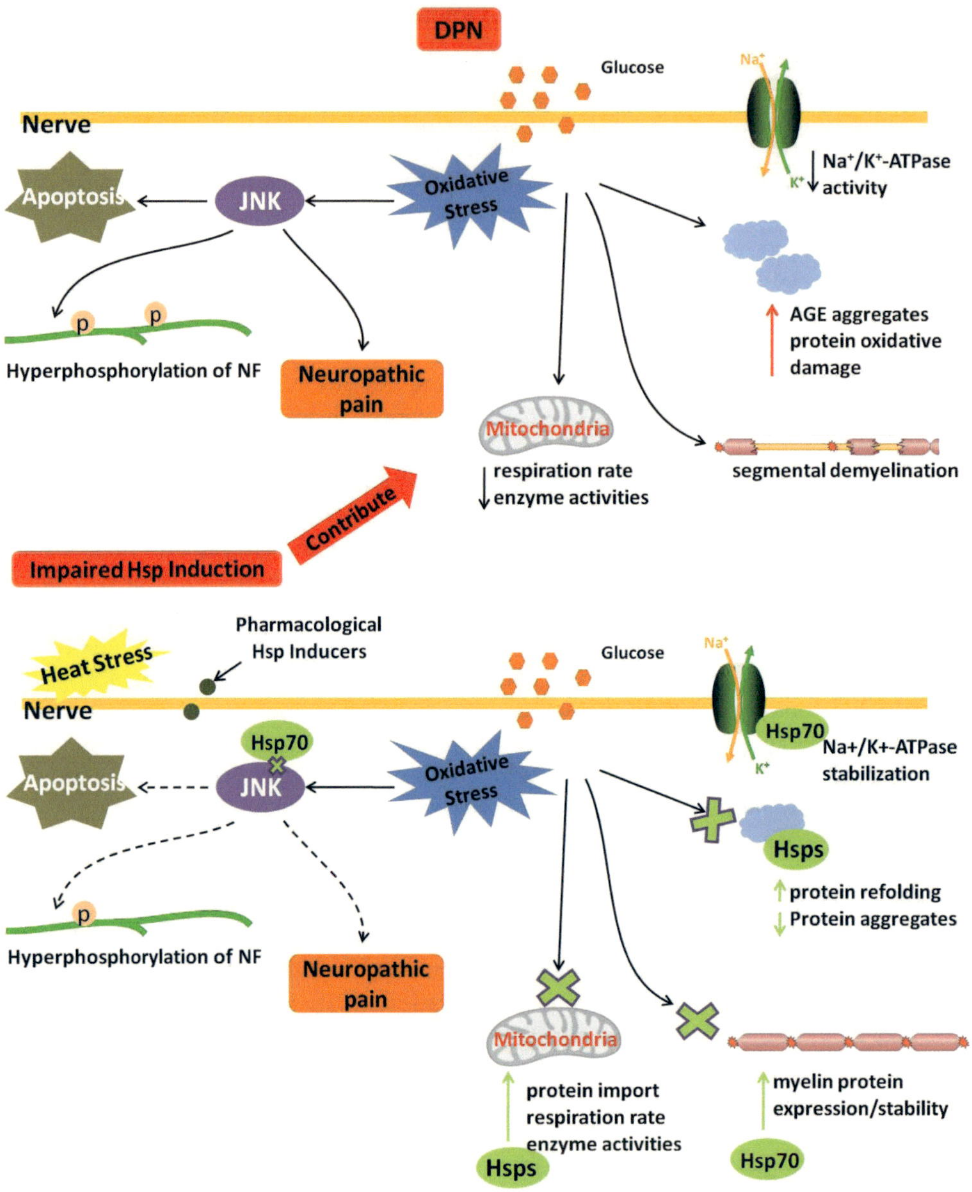

Fig. 2. Potential mechanisms underlying Hsps-mediated neuroprotection in diabetic nerve. Solid lines indicate stimulated pathways; dashed lines indicate inhibited pathways.

A study in *ex vivo* rat heart also found HSP90 was necessary for targeted mitochondrial import of PKCε and was critical for cardioprotection from ischemia/reperfusion injury (Budas *et al.*, 2010). It is also worth-mentioning that the expression of HSP60 and Grp75, two mitochondria-localized chaperones involved in organelle proteostasis, were decreased in myocardial mitochondria from STZ-rats (Turko and Murad, 2003). Decreased expression of Grp75 correlated with a decrease in the rate of protein import in interfibrillar mitochondria isolated from diabetic heart (Baseler et al., 2011). Since Grp75 is a key component of the molecular motor complex involved in mitochondrial protein import, these data suggest that increasing HSP70 paralogs may have beneficial effects on mitochondrial dysfunction in DPN. Along this line, we have observed that KU-32 can translationally induce Grp75 in hyperglycemically stressed sensory neurons and are examining if this may contribute to improving mitochondrial function (unpublished observation). Recent work has also shown that genetic over-expression of Grp75 can increase Mn superoxide dismutase (MnSOD) expression, reduce markers of oxidative stress and decrease cell death induced by ischemia/reperfusion (Williamson *et al.*, 2008; Xu *et al.*, 2009). Since increased expression of MnSOD correlated with improved mitochondrial respiratory function in sensory neurons of diabetic mice treated with insulin (Akude et al 2011, Zherebitskaya etal., 2009), these data provide a potential mechanism by which increasing Grp75 may decrease oxidative stress and improve mitochondrial function in diabetic neurons. Interestingly, our unpublished preliminary data indicates that KU-32 also increased the translation of MnSOD and its expression in mitochondria of hyperglycemically stressed sensory neurons (unpublished data). Similarly, increasing expression of HSP60 with heat stress in myocardium was associated with enhanced mitochondrial complex activity which was believed to partially confer the protection against subsequent ischemia/reperfusion injury (Sammut *et al.*, 2001). Thus, increasing the expression of mitochondrial chaperones might offer a defense against mitochondrial dysfunction in diabetic neurons (Fig.2.).

2.4.3 Myelin protection

Segmental demyelination is a well characterized outcome of severe DPN in humans (Mizisin and Powell, 2003). However, it is difficult to assess the efficacy of increasing HSP70 in ameliorating diabetes-induced myelin degeneration since most diabetic rodent models do not recapitulate the observed myelinopathy in humans. Nonetheless, the ability of KU-32 to improve mechanical sensitivity in diabetic mice suggests that modulating chaperones can improve the function of myelinated fiber subtypes. Along this line, HSP70 is expressed in SCs of sciatic nerve but did not have a strong expression in axons (Fig.3.).

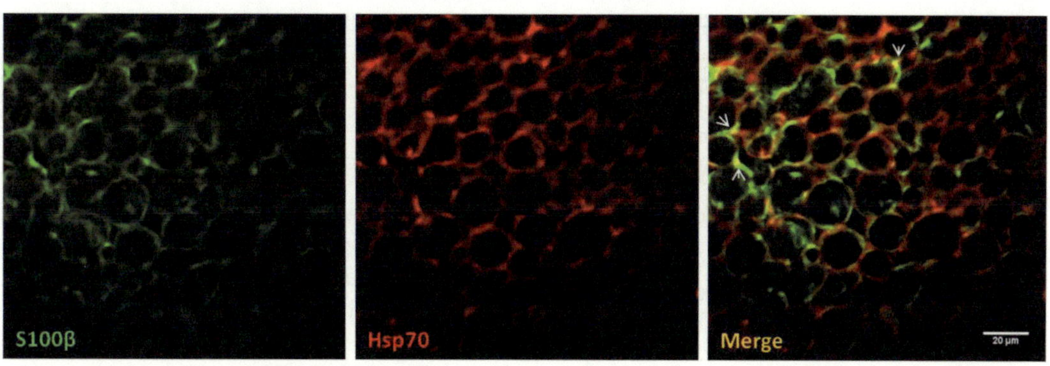

Fig. 3. Co-localization of HSP70 and SC marker in sciatic nerve. Sciatic nerves were removed from ~1 month-old C57Bl mice, fixed using 4% paraformaldehyde and cryoprotected using 30% sucrose before being embedded with tissue tek for freeze-sectioning (cross-section [10-micron]). Sections were then stained for HSP70 (red) and SC marker S100β (green). Arrowheads provide examples of co-localization of protein expression.

To more clearly localize the induction of HSP70 in peripheral nerve in response to KU-32 treatment, we are using transgenic mice that express green fluorescent protein under the control of the HSP70 promoter. However, our in vitro results using myelinated Schwann cell (SC)-sensory neuron co-cultures demonstrate that KU-32 pre-treatment effectively inhibits neuregulin-induced demyelination (Urban *et al.*, 2010). Similar to the result obtained in diabetic mice, HSP70 was required for this neuroprotection since KU-32 was unable to prevent neuregulin-induced demyelination in co-cultures prepared form HSP70 knockout mice. Although the mechanism by which HSP70 may prevent demyelination is unclear, induction of HSP70 in SCs by a small molecule HSP90 inhibitor significantly improved the myelination of DRG explants from a mouse model of hereditary demyelinating neuropathy, possibly via preventing the pathological misfolding and aggregation of myelin protein PMP22 (Rangaraju *et al.*, 2008).

2.4.4 Na^+/K^+-ATPase stabilization

Impaired Na^+/K^+-ATPase activity has been a frequent finding in nerves of diabetic humans and animals and strongly correlates with defects in NCV (Coste *et al.*, 1999; Greene *et al.*, 1987; Raccah *et al.*, 1994; Scarpini *et al.*, 1993). HSP70 directly interacts with the Na^+/K^+-ATPase and stabilizes its cytoskeletal anchorage in renal outer medulla (Ruete *et al.*, 2008) and epithelial cells (Riordan *et al.*, 2005) after ATP depletion. Whether this interaction may represent a fundamental mechanism underlying cellular protection is unknown, but warrants investigating if stabilization of Na^+/K^+-ATPase by HSP70 contributes to restoring NCV in diabetic nerves.

2.4.5 Protein chaperoning

Lastly, although protein misfolding or aggregation is not a primary pathological factor in DPN, excessive ROS production and protein glycation would unavoidably destabilize and damage cellular proteins and lead to their functional disruption and aggregation (Fig.2.). Indeed, deposition of advanced glycation end-products have been detected at the submicroscopic level as irregular aggregates in the cytoplasm of endothelial cells, pericytes, axoplasm and SCs of both myelinated and unmyelinated fibers in sural nerve biopsies of diabetic patients (Sugimoto *et al.*, 1997). Glycation of myelin also occurs and has been linked to abnormal NCV (Vlassara *et al.*, 1981). Hence, the chaperoning function of HSPs in promoting the health of diabetic nerve should not be overlooked.

3. Concluding remarks

With the climbing global prevalence of DPN and relatively scarcity of effective therapeutic strategies, novel approaches are needed to improve its medical management. The promising effects demonstrated by HSP70 in improving insulin resistance and DPN offers the exciting potential that induction of HSPs may be effective in improving both glycemic control and indirectly delaying the development of complications such as DPN in type 2 diabetics. However, the ability of HSP70 induction to ameliorate clinically relevant indices of DPN in the absence of improving metabolic control in models of type 1 DM also suggests that chaperones can directly affect neurons and SCs and retard disease progression. Given the decades long natural history of DPN, it is possible that, coupled with good glycemic control, combining inhibitors that target specific pathogenetic pathways with small molecule inducers of the inherently cytoprotective biology associated with molecular chaperones may provide a powerful approach to decrease neuronal glucotoxicity and increase tolerance to recurring hyperglycemic stress.

4. Acknowledgements

This work was supported by grants from the Juvenile Diabetes Research Foundation and The National Institutes of Health [NS054847].

5. References

Akude, E., Zherebitskaya, E., Chowdhury, S. K., Smith, D. R., Dobrowsky, R. T. &Fernyhough, P. (2011). Diminished superoxide generation is associated with respiratory chain dysfunction and changes in the mitochondrial proteome of sensory neurons from diabetic rats. *Diabetes* 60(1): 288-297.

Akude, E., Zherebitskaya, E., Roy Chowdhury, S. K., Girling, K. &Fernyhough, P. (2009). 4-Hydroxy-2-Nonenal Induces Mitochondrial Dysfunction and Aberrant Axonal Outgrowth in Adult Sensory Neurons that Mimics Features of Diabetic Neuropathy. *Neurotox Res* 1: 28-38.

Albers, J. W., Herman, W. H., Pop-Busui, R., Feldman, E. L., Martin, C. L., Cleary, P. A., Waberski, B. H. &Lachin, J. M. (2010). Effect of prior intensive insulin treatment during the Diabetes Control and Complications Trial (DCCT) on peripheral neuropathy in type 1 diabetes during the Epidemiology of Diabetes Interventions and Complications (EDIC) Study. *Diabetes Care* 33(5): 1090-1096.

Atalay, M., Oksala, N. K., Laaksonen, D. E., Khanna, S., Nakao, C., Lappalainen, J., Roy, S., Hanninen, O. &Sen, C. K. (2004). Exercise training modulates heat shock protein response in diabetic rats. *Journal of applied physiology* 97(2): 605-611.

Barutta, F., Pinach, S., Giunti, S., Vittone, F., Forbes, J. M., Chiarle, R., Arnstein, M., Perin, P. C., Camussi, G., Cooper, M. E. &Gruden, G. (2008). Heat shock protein expression in diabetic nephropathy. *American journal of physiology. Renal physiology* 295(6): F1817-1824.

Bienemann, A. S., Lee, Y. B., Howarth, J. &Uney, J. B. (2008). Hsp70 suppresses apoptosis in sympathetic neurones by preventing the activation of c-Jun. *Journal of neurochemistry* 104(1): 271-278.

Biro, K., Jednakovits, A., Kukorelli, T., Hegedus, E. &Koranyi, L. (1997). Bimoclomol (BRLP-42) ameliorates peripheral neuropathy in streptozotocin-induced diabetic rats. *Brain research bulletin* 44(3): 259-263.

Bonnard, C., Durand, A., Peyrol, S., Chanseaume, E., Chauvin, M. A., Morio, B., Vidal, H. &Rieusset, J. (2008). Mitochondrial dysfunction results from oxidative stress in the skeletal muscle of diet-induced insulin-resistant mice. *The Journal of clinical investigation* 118(2): 789-800.

Boulton, A. J. &Malik, R. A. (1998). Diabetic neuropathy. *The Medical clinics of North America* 82(4): 909-929.

Brinkmann, C., Chung, N., Schmidt, U., Kreutz, T., Lenzen, E., Schiffer, T., Geisler, S., Graf, C., Montiel-Garcia, G., Renner, R., Bloch, W. &Brixius, K. (2011). Training alters the skeletal muscle antioxidative capacity in non-insulin-dependent type 2 diabetic men. *Scandinavian journal of medicine & science in sports.*

Bruce, C. R., Carey, A. L., Hawley, J. A. &Febbraio, M. A. (2003). Intramuscular heat shock protein 72 and heme oxygenase-1 mRNA are reduced in patients with type 2 diabetes: evidence that insulin resistance is associated with a disturbed antioxidant defense mechanism. *Diabetes* 52(9): 2338-2345.

Bruening, W., Roy, J., Giasson, B., Figlewicz, D. A., Mushynski, W. E. &Durham, H. D. (1999). Up-regulation of protein chaperones preserves viability of cells expressing toxic Cu/Zn-superoxide dismutase mutants associated with amyotrophic lateral sclerosis. *Journal of neurochemistry* 72(2): 693-699.

Budas, G. R., Churchill, E. N., Disatnik, M. H., Sun, L. &Mochly-Rosen, D. (2010). Mitochondrial import of PKCepsilon is mediated by HSP90: a role in cardioprotection from ischaemia and reperfusion injury. *Cardiovascular research* 88(1): 83-92.

Cheng, C. &Zochodne, D. W. (2003). Sensory neurons with activated caspase-3 survive long-term experimental diabetes. *Diabetes* 52(9): 2363-2371.

Chiosis, G., Huezo, H., Rosen, N., Mimnaugh, E., Whitesell, L. &Neckers, L. (2003). 17AAG: low target binding affinity and potent cell activity--finding an explanation. *Molecular cancer therapy* 2(2): 123-129.

Chowdury, S.K.R., Dobrowsky, R.T. & Fernyhough, P (2011) Nutrient excess and altered mitochondrial proteome and functin contribute to neurodegeneration in diabetes. *Mitochondrion*, doi:10.1016/j.mito.2011.06.007

Chung, J., Nguyen, A. K., Henstridge, D. C., Holmes, A. G., Chan, M. H., Mesa, J. L., Lancaster, G. I., Southgate, R. J., Bruce, C. R., Duffy, S. J., Horvath, I., Mestril, R., Watt, M. J., Hooper, P. L., Kingwell, B. A., Vigh, L., Hevener, A. &Febbraio, M. A. (2008). HSP72 protects against obesity-induced insulin resistance. *Proceedings of the National Academy of Sciences* 105(5): 1739-1744.

Coste, T., Pierlovisi, M., Leonardi, J., Dufayet, D., Gerbi, A., Lafont, H., Vague, P. &Raccah, D. (1999). Beneficial effects of gamma linolenic acid supplementation on nerve conduction velocity, Na+, K+ ATPase activity, and membrane fatty acid composition in sciatic nerve of diabetic rats. *The Journal of nutritional biochemistry* 10(7): 411-420.

Cuervo, A. M., Stefanis, L., Fredenburg, R., Lansbury, P. T. &Sulzer, D. (2004). Impaired degradation of mutant alpha-synuclein by chaperone-mediated autophagy. *Science* 305(5688): 1292-1295.

Danaei, G., Finucane, M. M., Lu, Y., Singh, G. M., Cowan, M. J., Paciorek, C. J., Lin, J. K., Farzadfar, F., Khang, Y. H., Stevens, G. A., Rao, M., Ali, M. K., Riley, L. M., Robinson, C. A. &Ezzati, M. (2011). National, regional, and global trends in fasting plasma glucose and diabetes prevalence since 1980: systematic analysis of health examination surveys and epidemiological studies with 370 country-years and 2.7 million participants. *Lancet.*

Daulhac, L., Mallet, C., Courteix, C., Etienne, M., Duroux, E., Privat, A. M., Eschalier, A. &Fialip, J. (2006). Diabetes-induced mechanical hyperalgesia involves spinal mitogen-activated protein kinase activation in neurons and microglia via N-methyl-D-aspartate-dependent mechanisms. *Molecular pharmacology* 70(4): 1246-1254.

Daviau, A., Proulx, R., Robitaille, K., Di Fruscio, M., Tanguay, R. M., Landry, J., Patterson, C., Durocher, Y. &Blouin, R. (2006). Down-regulation of the mixed-lineage dual leucine zipper-bearing kinase by heat shock protein 70 and its co-chaperone CHIP. *The Journal of biological chemistry* 281(42): 31467-31477.

DCCT (1988). Factors in development of diabetic neuropathy. Baseline analysis of neuropathy in feasibility phase of Diabetes Control and Complications Trial (DCCT). The DCCT Research Group. *Diabetes* 37(4): 476-481.

DCCT (1995). The effect of intensive diabetes therapy on the development and progression of neuropathy. The Diabetes Control and Complications Trial Research Group. *Annals of internal medicine* 122(8): 561-568.

DeFranco, D. B., Ho, L., Falke, E. &Callaway, C. W. (2004). Small molecule activators of the heat shock response and neuroprotection from stroke. *Current atherosclerosis reports* 6(4): 295-300.

Dickey, C. A., Kamal, A., Lundgren, K., Klosak, N., Bailey, R. M., Dunmore, J., Ash, P., Shoraka, S., Zlatkovic, J., Eckman, C. B., Patterson, C., Dickson, D. W., Nahman, N. S., Jr., Hutton, M., Burrows, F. &Petrucelli, L. (2007). The high-affinity HSP90-CHIP complex recognizes and selectively degrades phosphorylated tau client proteins. *Journal of clincial investigation* 117(3): 648-658.

Doya, H., Ohtori, S., Fujitani, M., Saito, T., Hata, K., Ino, H., Takahashi, K., Moriya, H. &Yamashita, T. (2005). c-Jun N-terminal kinase activation in dorsal root ganglion contributes to pain hypersensitivity. *Biochemical and biophysical research communications* 335(1): 132-138.

Eilers, A., Whitfield, J., Babij, C., Rubin, L. L. &Ham, J. (1998). Role of the Jun kinase pathway in the regulation of c-Jun expression and apoptosis in sympathetic neurons. *The Journal of neuroscience* 18(5): 1713-1724.

Feder, M. E. &Hofmann, G. E. (1999). Heat-shock proteins, molecular chaperones, and the stress response: evolutionary and ecological physiology. *Annual review of physiology* 61: 243-282.

Fernyhough, P., Gallagher, A., Averill, S. A., Priestley, J. V., Hounsom, L., Patel, J. &Tomlinson, D. R. (1999). Aberrant neurofilament phosphorylation in sensory neurons of rats with diabetic neuropathy. *Diabetes* 48(4): 881-889.

Fernyhough, P., Roy Chowdhury, S. K. &Schmidt, R. E. (2010). Mitochondrial stress and the pathogenesis of diabetic neuropathy. *Expert review of endocrinology & metabolism* 5(1): 39-49.

Gao, Y. J. &Ji, R. R. (2008). Activation of JNK pathway in persistent pain. *Neuroscience letters* 437(3): 180-183.

Geiger, P. C. &Gupte, A. A. (2011). Heat shock proteins are important mediators of skeletal muscle insulin sensitivity. *Exercise and sport sciences reviews* 39(1): 34-42.

Greene, D. A., Lattimer, S. A. &Sima, A. A. (1987). Sorbitol, phosphoinositides, and sodium-potassium-ATPase in the pathogenesis of diabetic complications. *The New England journal of medicine* 316(10): 599-606.

Gupte, A. A., Bomhoff, G. L., Morris, J. K., Gorres, B. K. &Geiger, P. C. (2009a). Lipoic acid increases heat shock protein expression and inhibits stress kinase activation to improve insulin signaling in skeletal muscle from high-fat-fed rats. *Journal of applied physiology* 106(4): 1425-1434.

Gupte, A. A., Bomhoff, G. L., Swerdlow, R. H. &Geiger, P. C. (2009b). Heat treatment improves glucose tolerance and prevents skeletal muscle insulin resistance in rats fed a high-fat diet. *Diabetes* 58(3): 567-578.

Habib, A. A. &Brannagan, T. H., 3rd (2010). Therapeutic strategies for diabetic neuropathy. *Current neurology and neuroscience reports* 10(2): 92-100.

Harati, Y. (2010). Diabetic peripheral neuropathies. *Methodist DeBakey cardiovascular journal* 6(2): 15-19.

Hirosumi, J., Tuncman, G., Chang, L., Gorgun, C. Z., Uysal, K. T., Maeda, K., Karin, M. &Hotamisligil, G. S. (2002). A central role for JNK in obesity and insulin resistance. *Nature* 420(6913): 333-336.

Hooper, P. L. (1999). Hot-tub therapy for type 2 diabetes mellitus. *The New England journal of medicine* 341(12): 924-925.

Itani, S. I., Ruderman, N. B., Schmieder, F. &Boden, G. (2002). Lipid-induced insulin resistance in human muscle is associated with changes in diacylglycerol, protein kinase C, and IkappaB-alpha. *Diabetes* 51(7): 2005-2011.

Jaattela, M. &Wissing, D. (1992). Emerging role of heat shock proteins in biology and medicine. *Annals of medicine* 24(4): 249-258.

Jana, N. R., Tanaka, M., Wang, G. &Nukina, N. (2000). Polyglutamine length-dependent interaction of Hsp40 and Hsp70 family chaperones with truncated N-terminal huntingtin: their role in suppression of aggregation and cellular toxicity. *Human molecular genetics* 9(13): 2009-2018.

Joyeux, M., Faure, P., Godin-Ribuot, D., Halimi, S., Patel, A., Yellon, D. M., Demenge, P. &Ribuot, C. (1999). Heat stress fails to protect myocardium of streptozotocin-induced diabetic rats against infarction. *Cardiovascular research* 43(4): 939-946.

Kamal, A., Thao, L., Sensintaffar, J., Zhang, L., Boehm, M. F., Fritz, L. C. &Burrows, F. J. (2003). A high-affinity conformation of Hsp90 confers tumour selectivity on Hsp90 inhibitors. *Nature* 425(6956): 407-410.

Kamiya, H., Zhangm, W. &Sima, A. A. (2005). Apoptotic stress is counterbalanced by survival elements preventing programmed cell death of dorsal root ganglions in subacute type 1 diabetic BB/Wor rats. *Diabetes* 54(11): 3288-3295.

Kamiya, H., Zhang, W. &Sima, A. A. (2006). Degeneration of the Golgi and neuronal loss in dorsal root ganglia in diabetic BioBreeding/Worcester rats. *Diabetologia* 49(11): 2763-2774.

Kavanagh, K., Flynn, D. M., Jenkins, K. A., Zhang, L. &Wagner, J. D. (2011). Restoring HSP70 deficiencies improves glucose tolerance in diabetic monkeys. *American journal of physiology. Endocrinology and metabolism* 300(5): E894-901.

Kelly, S. &Yenari, M. A. (2002). Neuroprotection: heat shock proteins. *Current medical research and opinion* 18 Suppl 2: s55-60.

Klucken, J., Shin, Y., Masliah, E., Hyman, B. T. &McLean, P. J. (2004). Hsp70 Reduces alpha-Synuclein Aggregation and Toxicity. *The Journal of biological chemistry* 279(24): 25497-25502.

Koves, T. R., Ussher, J. R., Noland, R. C., Slentz, D., Mosedale, M., Ilkayeva, O., Bain, J., Stevens, R., Dyck, J. R., Newgard, C. B., Lopaschuk, G. D. &Muoio, D. M. (2008). Mitochondrial overload and incomplete fatty acid oxidation contribute to skeletal muscle insulin resistance. *Cell metabolism* 7(1): 45-56.

Kurthy, M., Mogyorosi, T., Nagy, K., Kukorelli, T., Jednakovits, A., Talosi, L. &Biro, K. (2002). Effect of BRX-220 against peripheral neuropathy and insulin resistance in diabetic rat models. *Annals of the New York Academy of Sciences* 967: 482-489.

Kurucz, I., Morva, A., Vaag, A., Eriksson, K. F., Huang, X., Groop, L. &Koranyi, L. (2002). Decreased expression of heat shock protein 72 in skeletal muscle of patients with type 2 diabetes correlates with insulin resistance. *Diabetes* 51(4): 1102-1109.

Luo, W., Dou, F., Rodina, A., Chip, S., Kim, J., Zhao, Q., Moulick, K., Aguirre, J., Wu, N., Greengard, P. &Chiosis, G. (2007). Roles of heat-shock protein 90 in maintaining and facilitating the neurodegenerative phenotype in tauopathies. *Proceeding of the national academy of science* 104(22): 9511-9516.

Luo, W., Rodina, A. &Chiosis, G. (2008). Heat shock protein 90: translation from cancer to Alzheimer's disease treatment? *BMC Neuroscience* 9 Suppl 2: S7.

Magrane, J., Smith, R. C., Walsh, K. &Querfurth, H. W. (2004). Heat shock protein 70 participates in the neuroprotective response to intracellularly expressed beta-amyloid in neurons. *The Journal of neuroscience* 24(7): 1700-1706.

Mahmood, D., Singh, B. K. &Akhtar, M. (2009). Diabetic neuropathy: therapies on the horizon. *The Journal of pharmacy and pharmacology* 61(9): 1137-1145.

Maroney, A. C., Glicksman, M. A., Basma, A. N., Walton, K. M., Knight, E., Jr., Murphy, C. A., Bartlett, B. A., Finn, J. P., Angeles, T., Matsuda, Y., Neff, N. T. &Dionne, C. A. (1998). Motoneuron apoptosis is blocked by CEP-1347 (KT 7515), a novel inhibitor of the JNK signaling pathway. *The Journal of neuroscience* 18(1): 104-111.

Martyn, C. N. &Hughes, R. A. (1997). Epidemiology of peripheral neuropathy. *Journal of neurology, neurosurgery, and psychiatry* 62(4): 310-318.

McCarty, M. F. (2006). Induction of heat shock proteins may combat insulin resistance. *Medical Hypotheses* 66(3): 527-534.

McMillan, D. R., Xiao, X., Shao, L., Graves, K. &Benjamin, I. J. (1998). Targeted disruption of heat shock transcription factor 1 abolishes thermotolerance and protection against heat-inducible apoptosis. *The Journal of biological chemistry* 273(13): 7523-7528.

Meriin, A. B., Yaglom, J. A., Gabai, V. L., Zon, L., Ganiatsas, S., Mosser, D. D. &Sherman, M. Y. (1999). Protein-damaging stresses activate c-Jun N-terminal kinase via inhibition of its dephosphorylation: a novel pathway controlled by HSP72. *Molecular and cellular biology* 19(4): 2547-2555.

Michels, A. A., Kanon, B., Konings, A. W., Ohtsuka, K., Bensaude, O. &Kampinga, H. H. (1997). Hsp70 and Hsp40 chaperone activities in the cytoplasm and the nucleus of mammalian cells. *The Journal of biological chemistry* 272(52): 33283-33289.

Minami, Y., Hohfeld, J., Ohtsuka, K. &Hartl, F. U. (1996). Regulation of the heat-shock protein 70 reaction cycle by the mammalian DnaJ homolog, Hsp40. *The Journal of biological chemistry* 271(32): 19617-19624.

Mir, K. A., Pugazhendhi, S., Paul, M. J., Nair, A. &Ramakrishna, B. S. (2009). Heat-shock protein 70 gene polymorphism is associated with the severity of diabetic foot ulcer and the outcome of surgical treatment. *The British journal of surgery* 96(10): 1205-1209.

Mizisin, A. P. &Powell, H. C. (2003).Pathogenesis and Pathology of Diabetic Neuropathy-Histopathology. In *Textbook of Diabetic Neuropathy*, 83-87 (Ed F. A. G. N. E. C. P. A. L. D. Ziegler). Stuttgart: Georg Thieme Verlag.

Morino, K., Petersen, K. F. &Shulman, G. I. (2006). Molecular mechanisms of insulin resistance in humans and their potential links with mitochondrial dysfunction. *Diabetes* 55 Suppl 2: S9-S15.

Muchowski, P. J. &Wacker, J. L. (2005). Modulation of neurodegeneration by molecular chaperones. *Nature reviews. Neuroscience* 6(1): 11-22.

Najemnikova, E., Rodgers, C. D. &Locke, M. (2007). Altered heat stress response following streptozotocin-induced diabetes. *Cell stress & chaperones* 12(4): 342-352.

NIDDK (2009). What are diabetic neuropathies? In *Diabetic Neuropathies: The Nerve Damage of Diabetes*: National Institutes of Diabetes and Digestive and Kidney Diseases.

Obrosova, I. G. (2009). Diabetes and the peripheral nerve. *Biochimica biophysica acta* 10: 931-940.

Okada, M., Hasebe, N., Aizawa, Y., Izawa, K., Kawabe, J. &Kikuchi, K. (2004). Thermal treatment attenuates neointimal thickening with enhanced expression of heat-shock protein 72 and suppression of oxidative stress. *Circulation* 109(14): 1763-1768.

Otaka, M., Yamamoto, S., Ogasawara, K., Takaoka, Y., Noguchi, S., Miyazaki, T., Nakai, A., Odashima, M., Matsuhashi, T., Watanabe, S. &Itoh, H. (2007). The induction mechanism of the molecular chaperone HSP70 in the gastric mucosa by Geranylgeranylacetone (HSP-inducer). *Biochemical and biophysical research communications* 353(2): 399-404.

Ouyang, Y. B., Xu, L. J., Sun, Y. J. &Giffard, R. G. (2006). Overexpression of inducible heat shock protein 70 and its mutants in astrocytes is associated with maintenance of mitochondrial physiology during glucose deprivation stress. *Cell stress & chaperones* 11(2): 180-186.

Park, H. S., Lee, J. S., Huh, S. H., Seo, J. S. &Choi, E. J. (2001). Hsp72 functions as a natural inhibitory protein of c-Jun N-terminal kinase. *The EMBO journal* 20(3): 446-456.

Petersen, K. F., Dufour, S., Befroy, D., Garcia, R. &Shulman, G. I. (2004). Impaired mitochondrial activity in the insulin-resistant offspring of patients with type 2 diabetes. *The New England journal of medicine* 350(7): 664-671.

Peterson, L. B. &Blagg, B. S. (2009). To fold or not to fold: modulation and consequences of Hsp90 inhibition. *Future medicinal chemistry* 1(2): 267-283.

Pirkkala, L., Alastalo, T. P., Zuo, X., Benjamin, I. J. &Sistonen, L. (2000). Disruption of heat shock factor 1 reveals an essential role in the ubiquitin proteolytic pathway. *Molecular and cellular biology* 20(8): 2670-2675.

Polla, B. S., Kantengwa, S., Francois, D., Salvioli, S., Franceschi, C., Marsac, C. &Cossarizza, A. (1996). Mitochondria are selective targets for the protective effects of heat shock against oxidative injury. *Proceedings of the national academy of sciences* 93(13): 6458-6463.

Purves, T., Middlemas, A., Agthong, S., Jude, E. B., Boulton, A. J., Fernyhough, P. &Tomlinson, D. R. (2001). A role for mitogen-activated protein kinases in the etiology of diabetic neuropathy. *The FASEB journal* 15(13): 2508-2514.

Raccah, D., Lamotte-Jannot, M. F., Issautier, T. &Vague, P. (1994). Effect of experimental diabetes on Na/K-ATPase activity in red blood cells, peripheral nerve and kidney. *Diabete & metabolisme* 20(3): 271-274.

Rangaraju, S., Madorsky, I., Pileggi, J. G., Kamal, A. &Notterpek, L. (2008). Pharmacological induction of the heat shock response improves myelination in a neuropathic model. *Neurobiology of disease* 32(1): 105-115.

Rathmann, W. &Ward, J. (2003).Socioeconomic Aspects. In *Textbook of Diabetic Neuropathy*, 361-372 (Ed F. A. G. N. E. C. P. A. L. D. Ziegler). Stuttgart: Georg Thieme Verlag.

Richter-Landsberg, C. &Goldbaum, O. (2003). Stress proteins in neural cells: functional roles in health and disease. *Cellular and molecular life sciences : CMLS* 60(2): 337-349.

Riordan, M., Sreedharan, R., Wang, S., Thulin, G., Mann, A., Stankewich, M., Van Why, S., Kashgarian, M. &Siegel, N. J. (2005). HSP70 binding modulates detachment of Na-K-ATPase following energy deprivation in renal epithelial cells. *American journal of physiology. Renal physiology* 288(6): F1236-1242.

Ritossa, F. (1962). A new puffing pattern induced by temperature shock and DNP in drosophila. *Cellular and Molecular Life Sciences* 18(12): 571-573.

Ruete, M. C., Carrizo, L. C. &Valles, P. G. (2008). Na+/K+ -ATPase stabilization by Hsp70 in the outer stripe of the outer medulla in rats during recovery from a low-protein diet. *Cell stress & chaperones* 13(2): 157-167.

Russell, J. W. &Feldman, E. L. (1999). Insulin-like growth factor-I prevents apoptosis in sympathetic neurons exposed to high glucose. *Hormone and metabolism research* 31(2-3): 90-96.

Sajjad, M. U., Samson, B. &Wyttenbach, A. (2010). Heat shock proteins: therapeutic drug targets for chronic neurodegeneration? *Current pharmaceutical biotechnology* 11(2): 198-215.

Salehi, A. H., Morris, S. J., Ho, W. C., Dickson, K. M., Doucet, G., Milutinovic, S., Durkin, J., Gillard, J. W. &Barker, P. A. (2006). AEG3482 is an antiapoptotic compound that inhibits Jun kinase activity and cell death through induced expression of heat shock protein 70. *Chemistry & biology* 13(2): 213-223.

Sammut, I. A., Jayakumar, J., Latif, N., Rothery, S., Severs, N. J., Smolenski, R. T., Bates, T. E. &Yacoub, M. H. (2001). Heat stress contributes to the enhancement of cardiac mitochondrial complex activity. *The American journal of pathology* 158(5): 1821-1831.

Scarpini, E., Bianchi, R., Moggio, M., Sciacco, M., Fiori, M. G. &Scarlato, G. (1993). Decrease of nerve Na+,K(+)-ATPase activity in the pathogenesis of human diabetic neuropathy. *Journal of the neurological sciences* 120(2): 159-167.

Schmitz-Peiffer, C. (2002). Protein kinase C and lipid-induced insulin resistance in skeletal muscle. *Annals of the New York Academy of Sciences* 967: 146-157.

Schmitz-Peiffer, C., Browne, C. L., Oakes, N. D., Watkinson, A., Chisholm, D. J., Kraegen, E. W. &Biden, T. J. (1997). Alterations in the expression and cellular localization of protein kinase C isozymes epsilon and theta are associated with insulin resistance in skeletal muscle of the high-fat-fed rat. *Diabetes* 46(2): 169-178.

Shimura, H., Miura-Shimura, Y. &Kosik, K. S. (2004a). Binding of tau to heat shock protein 27 leads to decreased concentration of hyperphosphorylated tau and enhanced cell survival. *The Journal of biological chemistry* 279(17): 17957-17962.

Shimura, H., Schwartz, D., Gygi, S. P. &Kosik, K. S. (2004b). CHIP-Hsc70 complex ubiquitinates phosphorylated tau and enhances cell survival. *The Journal of biological chemistry* 279(6): 4869-4876.

Shoelson, S. E., Lee, J. &Yuan, M. (2003). Inflammation and the IKK beta/I kappa B/NF-kappa B axis in obesity- and diet-induced insulin resistance. *International journal of obesity and related metabolic disorders* 27 Suppl 3: S49-52.

Soti, C., Racz, A. &Csermely, P. (2002). A Nucleotide-dependent molecular switch controls ATP binding at the C-terminal domain of Hsp90. N-terminal nucleotide binding unmasks a C-terminal binding pocket. *The Journal of biological chemistry* 277(9): 7066-7075.

Soti, C., Nagy, E., Giricz, Z., Vigh, L., Csermely, P. &Ferdinandy, P. (2005). Heat shock proteins as emerging therapeutic targets. *British journal of pharmacology* 146(6): 769-780.

Strokov, I. A., Manukhina, E. B., Bakhtina, L. Y., Malyshev, I. Y., Zoloev, G. K., Kazikhanova, S. I. &Ametov, A. S. (2000). The function of endogenous protective systems in patients with insulin-dependent diabetes mellitus and polyneuropathy: effect of antioxidant therapy. *Bulletin of experimental biology and medicine* 130(10): 986-990.

Sugimoto, K., Nishizawa, Y., Horiuchi, S. &Yagihashi, S. (1997). Localization in human diabetic peripheral nerve of N(epsilon)-carboxymethyllysine-protein adducts, an advanced glycation endproduct. *Diabetologia* 40(12): 1380-1387.

Swiecki, C., Stojadinovic, A., Anderson, J., Zhao, A., Dawson, H. &Shea-Donohue, T. (2003). Effect of hyperglycemia and nitric oxide synthase inhibition on heat tolerance and induction of heat shock protein 72 kDa in vivo. *The American surgeon* 69(7): 587-592.

Tahrani, A. A., Askwith, T. &Stevens, M. J. (2010). Emerging drugs for diabetic neuropathy. *Expert opinion on emerging drugs* 15(4): 661-683.

Takeuchi, H., Kobayashi, Y., Yoshihara, T., Niwa, J., Doyu, M., Ohtsuka, K. &Sobue, G. (2002). Hsp70 and Hsp40 improve neurite outgrowth and suppress intracytoplasmic aggregate formation in cultured neuronal cells expressing mutant SOD1. *Brain research* 949(1-2): 11-22.

Tesfaye, S. &Selvarajah, D. (2009). The Eurodiab study: what has this taught us about diabetic peripheral neuropathy? *Current diabetes reports* 9(6): 432-434.

Tomlinson, D. R. &Gardiner, N. J. (2008). Glucose neurotoxicity. *Nature reviews. Neuroscience* 9(1): 36-45.

Turko, I. V. &Murad, F. (2003). Quantitative protein profiling in heart mitochondria from diabetic rats. *The Journal of biological chemistry* 278(37): 35844-35849.

UKPDS (1998). Intensive blood-glucose control with sulphonylureas or insulin compared with conventional treatment and risk of complications in patients with type 2 diabetes (UKPDS 33). UK Prospective Diabetes Study (UKPDS) Group. *Lancet* 352(9131): 837-853.

Urban, M. J., Li, C., Yu, C., Lu, Y., Krise, J. M., McIntosh, M. P., Rajewski, R. A., Blagg, B. S. &Dobrowsky, R. T. (2010). Inhibiting heat-shock protein 90 reverses sensory hypoalgesia in diabetic mice. *ASN neuro* 2(4) 189-199.

Ushijima, H., Tanaka, K., Takeda, M., Katsu, T., Mima, S. &Mizushima, T. (2005). Geranylgeranylacetone protects membranes against nonsteroidal anti-inflammatory drugs. *Molecular pharmacology* 68(4): 1156-1161.

Vigh, L., Literati, P. N., Horvath, I., Torok, Z., Balogh, G., Glatz, A., Kovacs, E., Boros, I., Ferdinandy, P., Farkas, B., Jaszlits, L., Jednakovits, A., Koranyi, L. &Maresca, B. (1997). Bimoclomol: a nontoxic, hydroxylamine derivative with stress protein-inducing activity and cytoprotective effects. *Nature medicine* 3(10): 1150-1154.

Vlassara, H., Brownlee, M. &Cerami, A. (1981). Nonenzymatic glycosylation of peripheral nerve protein in diabetes mellitus. *Proceedings of the National Academy of Sciences* 78(8): 5190-5192.

Watson, A., Eilers, A., Lallemand, D., Kyriakis, J., Rubin, L. L. &Ham, J. (1998). Phosphorylation of c-Jun is necessary for apoptosis induced by survival signal withdrawal in cerebellar granule neurons. *The Journal of neuroscience* 18(2): 751-762.

Waza, M., Adachi, H., Katsuno, M., Minamiyama, M., Sang, C., Tanaka, F., Inukai, A., Doyu, M. &Sobue, G. (2005). 17-AAG, an Hsp90 inhibitor, ameliorates polyglutamine-mediated motor neuron degeneration. *Nature medicine* 11(10): 1088-1095.

Wellen, K. E. &Hotamisligil, G. S. (2005). Inflammation, stress, and diabetes. *The Journal of clinical investigation* 115(5): 1111-1119.

WHO (2011).Diabetes. World Health Organization Media centre.

Wild, S., Roglic, G., Green, A., Sicree, R. &King, H. (2004). Global prevalence of diabetes: estimates for the year 2000 and projections for 2030. *Diabetes Care* 27(5): 1047-1053.

Williamson, C. L., Dabkowski, E. R., Dillmann, W. H. &Hollander, J. M. (2008). Mitochondria protection from hypoxia/reoxygenation injury with mitochondria heat shock protein 70 overexpression. *American journal of physiology. Heart and circulatory physiology* 294(1): H249-256.

Wyttenbach, A., Sauvageot, O., Carmichael, J., Diaz-Latoud, C., Arrigo, A. P. &Rubinsztein, D. C. (2002). Heat shock protein 27 prevents cellular polyglutamine toxicity and suppresses the increase of reactive oxygen species caused by huntingtin. *Human molecular genetics* 11(9): 1137-1151.

Xiao, X., Zuo, X., Davis, A. A., McMillan, D. R., Curry, B. B., Richardson, J. A. &Benjamin, I. J. (1999). HSF1 is required for extra-embryonic development, postnatal growth and protection during inflammatory responses in mice. *The EMBO journal* 18(21): 5943-5952.

Xu, L., Voloboueva, L. A., Ouyang, Y., Emery, J. F., Giffard, R. G. (2009). Overexpression of mitochondrial Hsp70/Hsp75 in rat brain protects mitochondria, reduces oxidative stress, and protects from focal ischemia. *Journal of cerebral blood flow and metabolism* 29(2):365-374.

Yang H, Zhou X, Liu X, Yang L, Chen Q, Zhao D, Zuo J, Liu W (2011). Mitochondrial dysfunction induced by knockdown of mortalin is rescued by Parkin. *Biochemical biophysical research communications.* 410(1):114-20.

Yeyati, P. L. &van Heyningen, V. (2008). Incapacitating the evolutionary capacitor: Hsp90 modulation of disease. *Current opinion in genetics & development* 18(3): 264-272.

Young, J. C., Hoogenraad, N. J. &Hartl, F. U. (2003). Molecular chaperones Hsp90 and Hsp70 deliver preproteins to the mitochondrial import receptor Tom70. *Cell* 112(1): 41-50.

Zhang, Y., Huang, L., Zhang, J., Moskophidis, D. &Mivechi, N. F. (2002). Targeted disruption of hsf1 leads to lack of thermotolerance and defines tissue-specific regulation for stress-inducible Hsp molecular chaperones. *Journal of cellular biochemistry* 86(2): 376-393.

Zherebitskaya, E., Akude, E., Smith, D. R. &Fernyhough, P. (2009). Development of selective axonopathy in adult sensory neurons isolated from diabetic rats: role of glucose-induced oxidative stress. *Diabetes* 58(6): 1356-1364.

Zhuang, Z. Y., Wen, Y. R., Zhang, D. R., Borsello, T., Bonny, C., Strichartz, G. R., Decosterd, I. &Ji, R. R. (2006). A peptide c-Jun N-terminal kinase (JNK) inhibitor blocks mechanical allodynia after spinal nerve ligation: respective roles of JNK activation in primary sensory neurons and spinal astrocytes for neuropathic pain development and maintenance. *The Journal of neuroscience* 26(13): 3551-3560.

Part 2

Methods of Investigation of Peripheral Neuropathies

4

Role of Skeletal Muscle MRI in Peripheral Nerve Disorders

Nozomu Matsuda, Shunsuke Kobayashi and Yoshikazu Ugawa
Fukushima Medical University, Department of Neurology
Japan

1. Introduction

In diagnosing peripheral nerve disorders, the involved nerves can usually be determined based on clinical history and neurological findings with the aid of electrophysiological examinations. Despite the principle, we often encounter diagnostic challenges. In this chapter, we describe the clinical utility of magnetic resonance imaging (MRI) for the evaluation of peripheral nerve disorders. MRI can visualize pathological changes in skeletal muscles secondary to lesions of the peripheral nerve, plexus or nerve root. The lesion sites may be inferred based on the distribution of the involved muscles.

After the first report in 1987 (Shabas et al., 1987), MRI has increasingly been used to evaluate denervated muscles (West et al., 1994; Fleckenstein et al., 1993; Uetani et al., 1993). In particular, studies of entrapment or compressive neuropathy have greatly contributed to the understanding of clinical-radiological correlations in peripheral nerve damage. Animal experiments have also been conducted, in which muscle MRI was examined after peripheral nerve transection.

MRI has several distinct advantages over needle electromyography (EMG), including non-invasiveness, accessibility to deep muscles and interexaminer reliability (Koltzenburg and Bendszus, 2004; Bendszus et al., 2003; McDonald et al., 2000). MRI is particularly useful as needle EMG is difficult to perform on children or patients on anticoagulation. Excellent spatial resolution allows MRI to detect atrophy of the small muscles, moreover, different MRI pulse sequences show sensitivity to different stages of denervation, thus, MRI can provide valuable information about the duration of muscle denervation (Kamath et al., 2008). MRI has a potential to visualize mass lesions causing nerve damage, such as tumours, which is useful for the clinical judgment of surgical resectability (Grant et al., 2002).

An abnormal MR signal in muscles is not specific to denervation and may also be seen in any condition that causes muscle edema, including severe muscle strains, blunt trauma and acute myositis. Thus, MRI findings need to be interpreted in combination with other clinical information. Previous muscle MRI studies of peripheral nerve disorders have mostly focused on entrapment or compression neuropathy (Andreisek et al., 2006; Petchprapa et al., 2010; Donovan et al., 2010). However, given its capability in visualizing pathological changes and mapping the distributions of the involved muscles, the use of MRI can be extended to a variety of peripheral nerve disorders. We will give a theoretical background of muscle MRI and describe its clinical applications in peripheral nerve disorders with some representative cases. We will also mention non-muscular features of MRI, e.g. nerve signal and mass lesions causing nerve damage, which contribute to the diagnosis of peripheral nerve disorders.

2. Radiological basis of muscle MRI

Normal muscles have intermediate to long T1 and short T2 relaxation times of MRI relative to the surrounding soft tissue. The spin-echo decay curve of skeletal muscle has been modelled to fit into a multi-exponent curve, in which the longer component is extracellular water and the shorter component is intracellular water (Hazlewood et al., 1974). The other determinants of MR relaxation times in muscle include tissue fat, total water content and blood volume. In theory, increased extracellular fluid in denervated muscles causes prolongation of both T1 and T2 relaxation times, because the relaxation time of water in the extracellular space of muscle is about four times that of the myoplasm (Polak et al., 1988). Most clinical studies show a normal T1 signal in the denervated muscles in the acute phase, thus sensitivity of the T1-weighted sequence appears to be low for detection of early stage denervation. By contrast, T2-weighted images reliably detect muscle denervation in the acute phase. A longitudinal imaging study in rats showed T2 signal changes as early as 48 hours after complete transection of the sciatic nerve and the signal intensity continued to increase until two months after denervation (Bendszus et al., 2002; Table 1).

Another factor that may contribute to MRI signal changes in denervated muscles is the altered blood flow caused by an interruption of the sympathetic vasoconstriction. Blood flow increases immediately after denervation, with a subsequent decline in the following week. An experimental nerve compression study found a strong correlation between T2 signal intensity and blood volume *in vivo* (Hayashi et al., 1997; Wessig et al., 2004). However, the time course of the blood flow changes was not in parallel to that of the MR signal changes. Thus, it remains unclear as to how much the blood flow changes explain MR signals in denervated muscles.

Several MR sequences are known to be particularly sensitive to early changes in denervated muscles. Inversion-recovery imaging, including turbo inversion recovery magnitude (TIRM) and short tau inversion recovery (STIR), suppresses the fat signal based on differences in the T1 relaxation time of the tissues and enhances differences between the water content of the tissues. In an experimental nerve transection study with rats, the TIRM signal started to increase as early as 24 hours after denervation (Bendszus et al., 2002). In clinical studies, an abnormal STIR signal in the denervated muscles has been demonstrated within four days after the onset of clinical symptoms (West et al., 1994). Generally, the threshold for producing an increased STIR signal is weakness graded at '3' (antigravity) or less out of '5' on the Medical Research Council's (MRC) scale.

Use of a contrast medium, such as gadolinium (Gd) diethyltriaminepentaacetic acid, may increase sensitivity for detecting muscle denervation. Gd uptake appears to start within days after symptom onset and the extent of the enhancement correlates with electrophysiological signs of denervation. A rat experiment showed the Gd enhancement as early as 24 hours after nerve lesion and the effect increased over time until it reached a plateau on day 21 (Bendszus and Koltzenburg, 2001). Gd enhancement could be caused by a dilatation of the vascular bed, an enlargement of the extracellular space or both. Therefore, fluid accumulation appears to contribute to both Gd uptake and T2 prolongation.

Traditionally, nerve injury is classified into three grades. In neurapraxic nerve injuries, axons are spared but myelin sheath is damaged causing conduction delay or block. The damage is usually transient and self-limiting with complete recovery. Axonotmesis is the intermediate grade of nerve injury, in which axons distal to the site of injury are disrupted with preserved connective tissue framework of the nerve. Neurotmesis is the most severe form of nerve injury, characterized by loss of axonal continuity along with disruption of the surrounding myelin sheath and connective tissue. The aforementioned signal changes in T2, TIRM and STIR sequences are observed in severe axonotmetic and neurotmetric injuries, in which the axons are disrupted and Wallerian degeneration follows. In axonotmetic nerve injuries, the abnormal signal of muscle MRI will return to normal as axons regenerate (Kikuchi et al., 2003). In neurotmetic injuries, the increased MR signal in the involved muscles will eventually decrease with atrophy and fatty infiltration, which is best visualized with the T1-weighted sequence. MRI may be able to differentiate axonotmetic from neurotmetic nerve injury, because the increased T2 signal persists longer in neurotmesis than in axonotmesis. In predominantly neurapraxic injuries with minimal axonal loss, the involved muscles exhibit normal signal characteristics on T2 and STIR pulse sequences.

	T1-weighted	T2-weighted	STIR	Gadolinium
Acute (< 1 month)	Unchanged	Increased	Increased	Enhancement
Subacute (1-6 months)	Unchanged	Increased	Increased or Normalized	No enhancement
Chronic (> 6 months)	Increased (fatty degeneration) or Unchanged (fair reinnervation)	Increased or Normalized	Normalized	No enhancement

Table 1. MRI findings of denervated muscles at different stages.

3. Correlations between muscle MRI and electrophysiological findings

The EMG findings in peripheral nerve disorders reflect the functional processes of denervation and reinnervation. Active denervation causes spontaneous discharge of single muscle fibres, which is observed as fibrillation potentials and positive sharp waves. Spontaneous motor unit potentials caused by irritability of motor neurons are observed as fasciculation. In the case of traumatic nerve injuries, EMG evidence of denervation usually develops in two to three weeks. On the other hand, early change of MRI signal in denervated muscles is observed as early as four days after the onset of clinical symptoms (West et al., 1994). Thus, MRI signal change appears to develop no later than EMG change. Good time sensitivity of MRI may reflect early development of the myoplasm-to-extracellular fluid shift in denervated muscles as compared with delayed electrophysiological manifestation of spontaneous EMG activity.

Beside the time sensitivity, detection sensitivity is also important when considering radiological-physiological correlations. McDonald and colleagues directly compared the findings of MRI and needle EMG in 90 patients with peripheral nerve injury or radiculopathy of one to four months duration (McDonald et al., 2000). The results of the two

methods matched anatomically in 49 subjects, i.e. the specific muscles showing abnormal spontaneous EMG activity correlated directly with the increased STIR signal on MRI. Moreover, the STIR intensity tended to increase with the higher degree of spontaneous activity as measured with EMG. It should be noted that, in 16 (18%) subjects, abnormal spontaneous EMG activity was present in the muscles that did not show increased STIR. The results indicate that the STIR has lower sensitivity than needle EMG. Bendszus and colleagues conducted a similar study with Gd-enhanced MRI in patients with a foot drop caused by L5 radiculopathy, common peroneal nerve palsy and sciatic nerve palsy. They found that Gd enhancement was more prominent in the muscles with EMG signs of denervation compared to those without denervation signs (Bendszus and Koltzenburg, 2001; Bendszus et al., 2003). To summarise, the STIR and Gd-enhanced MRI have good sensitivity for detecting denervated muscles, if not better than needle EMG.
After acute denervation, reinnervation occurs by collateral sprouting, which manifests on EMG as polyphasic motor unit action potentials (MUPs) with a prolonged duration. During the chronic stage, reinnervated muscle fibres are integrated into large MUPs. In a study that examined EMG and MRI in patients with axonal motor sensory polyneuropathy, the MUP size showed a positive correlation with T1 signal intensity. Thus, the increase of T1 signal may well reflect the fatty replacement of those muscle fibres that are not reinnervated and thus not integrated into working motor units (Jonas et al., 2000).

4. Basics of peripheral nerve imaging

The standard evaluation of a peripheral nerve is based on morphological image analysis on T1-weighted sequences and on signal change analysis on fat-suppressed sequences. T2-weighted images have exquisite resolution, but pathologic findings are generally not as conspicuous as on STIR imaging. Normal peripheral nerves appear isointense compared to muscle, surrounded by a small rim of fat tissue. An entrapped nerve generally shows increased signal on T2-weighted and STIR images over the abnormal segment (Hof et al., 2008; Stoll et al., 2009; Thawait et al., 2011; Table 2). Distal extension of the high intensity signal in an injured nerve may indicate axonal damage due to Wallerian degeneration.

	Normal peripheral nerve	Abnormal peripheral nerve
Size	Smaller than accompanying artery	Larger than accompanying artery Focal or diffuse enlargement
Fascicular pattern	Seen in especially large nerves	Loss of normal fascicular pattern
T1-weighted	Isointensity to muscle	Isointensity to muscle
T2-weighted	Iso to minimal high intensity	Moderate to marked high intensity
Gadolinium	No enhancement	Enhancement (when blood-nerve barrier is disturbed)

Table 2. MRI findings of a normal and abnormal peripheral nerve (modified from Thawait et al., 2011 with permission).

The signal changes of injured nerves on T2-weighted and STIR images may reflect changes in water content due to altered axoplasmic flow, endoneurial or perineurial edema as a result of changes in the blood-nerve barrier or axonal myelin degeneration (Filler et al., 1996).

5. Clinical application of MRI in peripheral nerve disorders

MRI has been used to detect mass lesions and inflammation causing entrapment or compression neuropathy. MRI can also evaluate muscle denervation secondary to nerve damage. Thus it is applied to a wide range of peripheral nerve disorders, including polyneuropathy, radiculopathy and plexopathy. MRI may show a specific pattern of denervated muscles depending on the level of peripheral nerve damage. Here we describe the MRI findings of common peripheral nerve disorders and discuss the clinical utility of MRI.

5.1 Mononeuropathy

The common causes of mononeuropathy include entrapment, compression and stretch of the nerves. Nerve entrapment often occurs at the sites where the nerve courses through fibro-osseous or fibromuscular tunnels or penetrates a muscle. Nerve compression may be due to an adjacent mass, such as ganglion, synovial cyst, lipoma and tumour. Inflammation from tenosynovitis and bursitis may also cause mononeuropathy. It is clinically important to determine the lesion sites and evaluate the severity and prognosis. MRI is useful for the diagnosis of mononeuropathy because: i) a mass lesion causing nerve compression may be directly depicted, ii) a localized abnormal T2 signal may be seen within the injured segment of the nerves, and iii) involved muscles may show an abnormal MR signal, indicating the severity and duration of denervation. This section focuses on common types of mononeuropathy with special emphasis on MRI findings (Sallomi et al., 1998; Lisle and Johnstone, 2007; Kim et al., 2011).

5.1.1 Median nerve

Carpal tunnel syndrome (CTS) is the most common entrapment neuropathy. CTS presents with intermittent pain and numbness of the thumb, index, middle and radial half of the ring finger. Long-standing CTS leads to weakness and atrophy of the abductor pollicis brevis, opponens pollicis, flexor pollicis brevis and the first and second lumbrical muscles. Occasionally, sensory symptoms of the CTS may present beyond the median nerve territory, sometimes mimicking radicular pain in cervical radiculopathy. Differential diagnosis of CTS includes C6-7 radiculopathy, polyneuropathy and proximal entrapment of the median nerve. Electrodiagnostic tests are 85-90% accurate in patients with CTS, with a false-negative rate of 10-15%. Therefore, in cases of clinically symptomatic CTS with normal electrophysiological findings, MRI has a complementary role in diagnosis. The denervated thenar muscle may show an increased STIR signal (West et al., 1994; Jarvik et al., 2002). It has been reported that the median nerve itself shows an abnormal MRI signal in CTS. The common findings are isolated prestenotic and intracarpal swelling and an increased T2 signal retrograde to the distal radius (Mesgarzadeh et al., 1989). Anatomical constriction of the median nerve may also be revealed by MRI. Pronounced palmar bowing of the flexor retinaculum (transverse carpal ligament) observed in the MRI of CTS patients show a significant correlation with subjective reports of pain severity (Tsujii et al., 2009). Horch and colleagues conducted a dynamic MRI study of 20 wrists of CTS patients (Horch et al., 1997). They measured the cross-sectional area of the carpal tunnel with different angles of wrist flexion and extension. They demonstrated that the carpal tunnel was smaller during wrist flexion, but the size was not significantly smaller in CTS patients as compared with normal volunteers. They also conducted a longitudinal study of CTS after surgical decompression. They found that the distal flattening of the median nerve, as visualized by MRI, normalized in 94% of the patients and the abnormal T2 signal decreased in 67% of the patients within six months postoperatively. Jarvik and colleagues prospectively studied a large cohort of 120 subjects with clinically suspected CTS (Jarvik et al., 2002). They checked five MRI parameters, namely median nerve signal, degree of nerve compression, bowing of the flexor retinaculum, thickening of the flexor tendon interspace and thenar muscle signal. An increased median nerve signal in the STIR sequence had a high sensitivity (88%), but specificity was low (39%). By contrast, an increased thenar muscle signal had a low sensitivity (10%), but specificity was high (90%). A combination of all parameters yielded high sensitivity (92%), but specificity was low (39%). To recap, electrophysiological tests are still the gold standard, but MRI plays a complementary role in the diagnosis of CTS.

The anterior interosseous nerve is the largest branch of the median nerve, innervating the flexor pollicis longus (FPL), pronator quadratus and the radial half of the flexor digitorum profundus (FDP) muscles. Anterior interosseous nerve syndrome, also known as Kiloh-Nevin syndrome, is usually caused by entrapment or compression of the median nerve in the proximal forearm. The patients show pinching deformity due to weakness of the FPL or FDP muscle. Because the anterior interosseous nerve is purely a motor nerve, its damage will not cause sensory loss, though dull pain may be present in the volar aspect of the forearm. During the acute to subacute stages, axial T2 or STIR images may depict a high intensity signal in the FPL, FDP and pronator quadratus muscles (Grainger et al., 1998; Spratt et al., 2002). However, the MRI findings have to be interpreted carefully, because a recent study showed that high intensity in the pronator quadratus muscle is sometimes observed in subjects without evidence of anterior interosseous nerve syndrome (Gyftopoulos et al., 2010). Over diagnosis of the anterior interosseous nerve syndrome should be avoided by knowing the prevalence of increased MR signals in the pronator quadratus muscle.

5.1.2 Ulnar nerve

The cubital tunnel, located posterior to the medial epicondyle of the humerus, is the most common site of ulnar nerve palsy. The possible causes of cubital tunnel syndrome include external compression (e.g. sleep palsy, perioperative damage), prolonged and excessive elbow flexion, trauma (e.g. from using jackhammers, humeral fracture with loose bodies or callus formation), a nerve-compressing lesion (e.g. ganglionic cysts, lipoma) and infection (Kato et al., 2002). Clinically, cubital tunnel syndrome presents with weakness and atrophy of hand intrinsic muscles, and sensory loss at the ring and little fingers. The MRI shows high intensity signals with a T2-weighted or STIR pulse sequence in the flexor carpi ulnaris and the ulnar half of the FDP muscles. Dynamic compression and inflammation will be seen on MRI as thickening and high intensity of the ulnar nerve on sagittal T2-weighted images (Rosenberg et al., 1993). Compression by a soft tissue mass may also be well depicted with

MRI. Dislocation and subluxation of the ulnar nerve would be detected on axial images during elbow flexion.
Guyon canal syndrome results from entrapment of the ulnar nerve as it passes through the wrist. Possible causes of ulnar nerve lesions at the Guyon canal include cystic lesions and chronic repetitive trauma (e.g. handlebar palsy in cyclists). Patients of Guyon canal syndrome experience wrist pain, sensory deficit in the ulnar nerve territory and weakness of ulnar intrinsic hand muscles. The hypothenar muscle may be spared in a distal lesion of the deep motor branch. A MRI may help exclude the presence of a mass lesion (Pearce et al., 2009) and an axial MRI at the level of the metacarpal bones is useful for detecting denervation of the intrinsic hand muscles (Andreisek et al., 2006).

5.1.3 Radial nerve

Radial tunnel syndrome (also known as posterior interosseous nerve syndrome or supinator (SP) muscle syndrome) is caused by entrapment or compression of the deep branch of the radial nerve, as it passes under the tendinous arch of the supinator muscle (arcade of Frohse). The posterior interosseous nerve supplies the extensor carpi ulnaris (ECU) muscle and the digital extensor muscles. The most consistent symptoms are deep aching pain in the forearm, pain radiation to the neck and shoulder, a sense of heaviness of the affected arm and an inability to sleep on the affected side (Rinker et al., 2004). Frequent causes of this syndrome are trauma, tumours, bursitis and cysts. Differential diagnoses include lateral epicondylitis (tennis elbow) and cervical radiculopathy. Electrophysiological studies are not useful in confirming the diagnosis, because the results are often normal or equivocal and no well-established criteria for diagnosis exist. MRI is useful to screen for a mass lesion compressing the posterior interosseous nerve. MRI may also detect denervation signals in the muscles supplied by the posterior interosseous nerve. Ferdinand and colleagues retrospectively studied 25 patients who were clinically suspected of having radial tunnel syndrome (Ferdinand et al., 2006). The most common MRI finding was denervation edema within the muscles innervated by the posterior interosseous nerve, most frequently within the SP (44%) and less frequently within the proximal forearm extensor muscles (12%). Seven patients (28%) showed evidence of a mass effect along the course of the posterior interosseous nerve, including thickening of the leading edge of the extensor carpi radialis brevis, prominent recurrent radial vessels, a schwannoma and a bicipitoradial bursa.

Case Presentation: Posterior interosseus nerve palsy

A 57-year-old male farmer noticed weakness of the right fingers after harvesting rice. Neurological examination revealed isolated finger extensor weakness 2/5 MRC scale with no sensory deficits. Deep tendon reflexes were normal. A painless mass was palpable in the right proximal forearm. The EMG showed active neurogenic change in the right extensor digitorum communis muscle. An MRI study detected a cystic lesion in the proximal forearm (Fig. 1a, arrow). The T2 high signal was observed in the radial-innervated muscles distal to the extensor carpi radialis brevis (ECRB) muscle (SP, ECU, extensor digitorum [ED], extensor digitorum minimi and abductor pollicis longus [APL] muscles in Fig. 1a, 1b, arrowheads). The signal was normal in the ECRB and brachioradialis (BR) muscles, which are innervated by branches of the radial nerve proximal to the posterior interosseous nerve. The pattern of the denervated muscles was compatible with the diagnosis of posterior interosseous nerve palsy caused by compression around the radial tunnel.

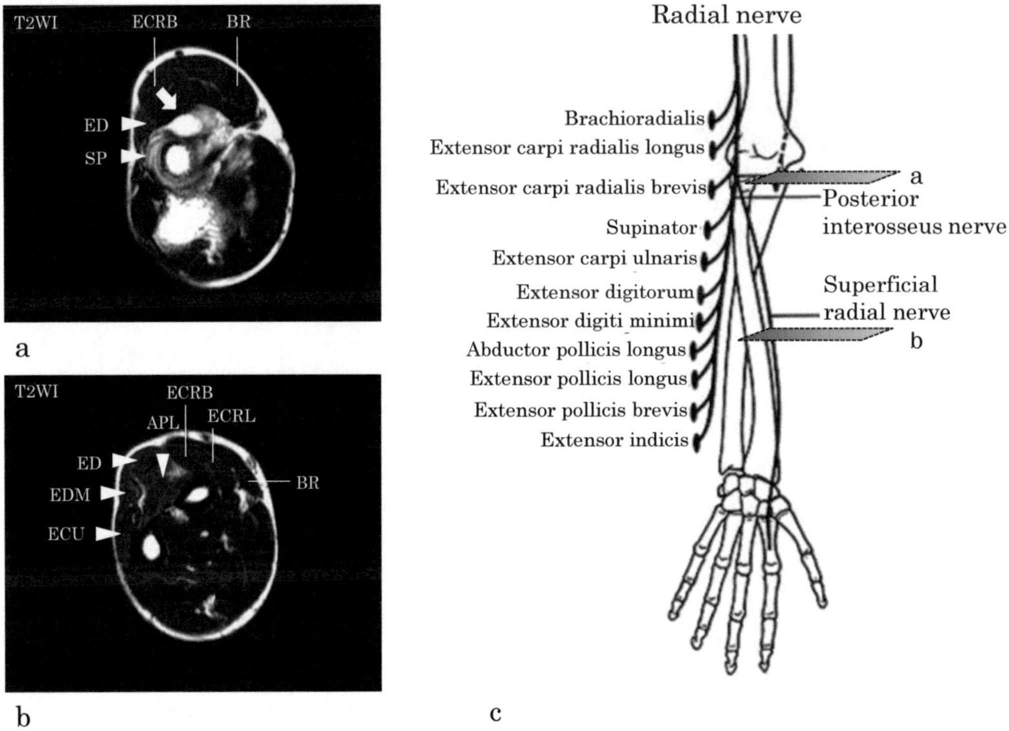

Abbreviations: abductor pollicis longus (APL), brachioradialis (BR), extensor carpi radialis brevis (ECRB), extensor carpi radialis longus (ECRL), extensor carpi ulnaris (ECU), extensor digitorum (ED), extensor digitorum minimi (EDM), supinator (SP).

Fig. 1. A case of radial tunnel syndrome caused by a cystic mass. (a, b) Axial T2-weighted MRI of the right forearm. (c) Schema of the radial nerve branches. The planes designated a and b in (c) correspond to the axial slice positions of (a) and (b), respectively.

5.1.4 Common peroneal nerve

Common peroneal nerve palsy is the most common mononeuropathy in the lower extremities. Its major cause is trauma, such as compression or stretch at the fibular neck, where the nerve is superficial and vulnerable to injury. The common peroneal nerve bifurcates into the superficial and deep peroneal nerves below the fibular neck. The superficial peroneal nerve supplies the peroneus longus (PL) and brevis muscles, and the deep peroneal nerve supplies the tibialis anterior (TA), extensor digitorum longus (EDL) and extensor hallucis longus muscles. Because both superficial and deep branches of the peroneal nerve innervate foot dorsiflexor muscles, foot drop is caused by damage to either branch. MRI may indicate specific sites of peroneal nerve damage: denervation limited in the anterior compartment (TA and EDL) or lateral compartment (PL) muscles indicates damage of the deep or superficial peroneal nerve, respectively. Involvement of the muscles in both anterior and lateral compartments (TA, EDL and PL) indicates a more proximal lesion of the common peroneal nerve. MRI may also be useful to detect mass lesions, such as ganglion, synovial cyst and osseous mass in a non-traumatic peroneal nerve (Iverson, 2005; Kim et al., 2007). The patterns of muscle denervation observed on MRI may also help distinguish peroneal nerve palsy from sciatic nerve palsy, L5 radiculopathy and lumbosacral plexopathy (Bendszus and Koltzenburg, 2001; Bendszus et al., 2003; see also section 5.2).

Case Presentation

Case 1: Common peroneal nerve palsy
A 21-year-old woman developed left foot weakness during the course of treatment for fulminant myocarditis in the intensive care unit. Neurological examination revealed weakness of left foot dorsiflexion 2/5 (MRC scale) and a tingling sensation was distributed on the left lateral leg and dorsal foot. MRI showed a high intensity signal in the TA, EDL and PL with STIR sequence (Fig. 2a), supporting the diagnosis of common peroneal nerve palsy.

Case 2: Tibial nerve palsy
A 52-year-old man, with a history of a left tibia fracture at the age of six, was referred to our hospital for the evaluation of his frequent stumbling. Neurological examination revealed weakness of plantar flexion and atrophy of the calf muscles on the left leg. MRI showed an increased T1 signal in the lateral and medial heads of the gastrocnemius (GC), soleus and tibialis posterior (TP) muscles (Fig. 2b). The MRI findings are compatible with the diagnosis of tibial mononeuropathy associated with tibial fracture.

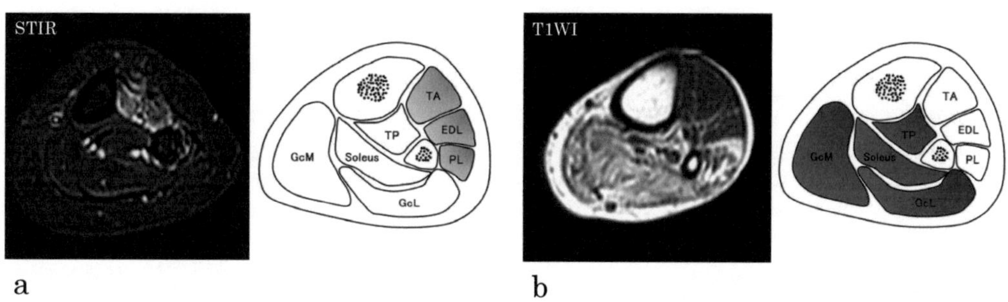

Abbreviations: extensor digitorum longus (EDL), gastrocnemius lateral head (GcL), gastrocnemius medial head (GcM), peroneus longus (PL), tibialis anterior (TA), tibialis posterior (TP).

Fig. 2. (a) Compression neuropathy of the common peroneal nerve. Axial MRI of the proximal part of the left leg with STIR sequence. (b) Tibial nerve palsy associated with tibia fracture. Axial T1-weighted MRI of the middle part of the left leg.

5.1.5 Sciatic nerve

The above two cases exemplify damages in the tibial and peroneal nerves (section 5.1.4), both of which are branches of the sciatic nerve. More proximal damage in the sciatic nerve may additionally involve the hamstring muscles. Causes of sciatic nerve neuropathy include trauma (e.g. dislocation of the hip joint and pelvic fracture), compression (e.g. tumour and metastatic lesions) and iatrogenic injury (e.g. in association with total hip replacement and intramuscular injection). Piriformis syndrome refers to compression of the sciatic nerve by the piriformis muscle. It induces sciatic pain and numbness in the buttocks, typically without weakness. The diagnosis of piriformis syndrome is often challenging because of limited sensitivity and specificity of physical signs and the absence of electrodiagnostic criteria. Filler and colleagues demonstrated that unilateral T2 high intensity of the sciatic nerve at the sciatic notch and asymmetry of the piriformis muscle on the MRI are the findings specific to piriformis syndrome (Filler et al., 2005). No abnormalities of the sciatic-innervated muscles are seen on the MRI. Accurate diagnosis of piriformis syndrome is important because it may lead to surgical treatment for pain relief.

5.1.6 Femoral nerve

Causes of femoral neuropathy include compression (e.g. retroperitoneal haemorrhage often from excessive anticoagulation), stretch injuries (e.g. prolonged lithotomy position), surgical procedures (e.g. hip replacement), direct injuries (inguinal surgery and wounds), radiation injury, ischemia (common iliac artery occlusion) and diabetic amyotrophy (Kuntzer et al., 1997). MRI is useful for the evaluation of mass lesions compressing the femoral nerve (Seijo-Martinez et al., 2003; Stuplich et al., 2005). In case of radiation injury, MRI may show local fibrosis constricting the femoral nerve (Nogués et al., 1998). Femoral neuropathy presents, often acutely, with thigh weakness and numbness. Femoral nerve supplies the psoas major, iliacus, pectineus, sartorius and quadriceps femoris muscles. Muscles involved may vary, depending on the level of the nerve lesion. MRI has a potential to detect denervation signals in these muscles (Nogués et al., 1998; Carter et al., 1995).

5.2 Radiculopathy

Clinical symptoms of radiculopathy are characterized by pain and radiating paresthesia along the affected dermatomes and motor weakness of the affected myotomes. The common causes of radiculopathy are structural lesions, such as herniated disk, bony impingement from spondylosis and mass lesions, such as epidural abscess and metastatic tumour to the spine. Radiculopathy may also be caused by non-structural lesions, such as carcionomatous or lymphomatous meningitis, borreliosis and herpes zoster infection.

MRI is widely used to identify structural lesions causing radiculopathy. Bone and disk diseases most frequently affect the cervical (C4–8) and lumbosacral (L3–S1) segments. MRI findings of foraminal impingement and nerve root compression directly support the diagnosis of radiculopathy. MRI is also useful for visualization of the denervated muscles to confirm the involved myotomes. For example, MRI for patients with subacute lumbar radiculopathy may show a high STIR signal in the muscles of the affected root level, with which needle EMG findings of acute denervation closely correlate (Carter et al., 1997).

Foot drop is a typical situation in which MRI is useful for diagnosis. When foot drop is caused by L5 radiculopathy, MRI may reveal denervation signals in the anterior compartment muscles (TA, EDL and PL) and the TP muscle. A peroneal mononeuropathy may also cause weakness of the anterior compartment muscles (see also the section 5.1.4), but TP would not be involved because it is innervated by the tibial nerve. Thus, whether TP muscle is involved or not has a key diagnostic value in foot drop (Bendszus and Koltzenburg, 2001).

Case Presentation

Case 1: S1 radiculopathy

A 75-year-old man has been conservatively treated for lumbago, sciatica and intermittent claudication, caused by lumbar canal stenosis associated with intervertebral disk hernia at L4/5 and L5/S1 levels. Neurological examination revealed weakness of the left GC muscle with absent ankle jerk. Active neurogenic EMG changes and increased STIR signals were observed in the soleus and GC muscles (Fig. 3a), supporting the diagnosis of S1 radiculopathy.

Case 2: L5-S1 polyradiculopathy

A 53-year-old man experienced progressive weakness of the left lower extremity. He had a past history of lumbar spondylosis, which was surgically treated at the age 49. MRI showed high STIR signals in the muscles of L5 and S1 myotomes (TA, EDL, PL, TP, soleus and GC, Fig. 3b).

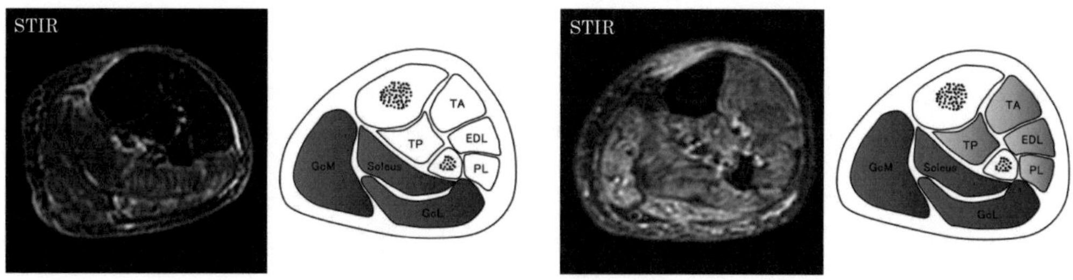

a b

Abbreviations: extensor digitorum longus (EDL), gastrocnemius lateral head (GcL), gastrocnemius medial head (GcM), peroneus longus (PL), tibialis anterior (TA), tibialis posterior (TP).

Fig. 3. Axial MRI (STIR) of the leg in two patients with S1 radiculopathy (a) and L5+S1 polyradiculopathy (b).

5.3 Polyneuropathy

Polyneuropathy is characterized by a distal symmetrical distribution of sensory motor deficits. Sensory loss occurs in a glove and stocking distribution, and motor weakness begins in the distal limbs. There are many causes of polyneuropathy, including nutritional deficiencies, immunological conditions, systemic metabolic disorders, toxins and hereditary disorders. The distal dominant distribution of the sensory motor symptoms may reflect a length-dependent process of dying-back axonopathy. Or it may reflect a demyelinating process, which also shows a length-dependent pattern because longer fibres have a higher probability of conduction block due to demyelination. Recent MRI studies have demonstrated the length-dependent pattern or centripetal progression of muscle denervation in both acquired (Andersen et al., 2004; Andreassen et al., 2009) and hereditary (Gallardo et al., 2006; Chung et al., 2008) forms of polyneuropathy.

Diabetic patients commonly develop sensory polyneuropathy with distal pain and sensory loss. Diabetic polyneuropathy also leads to denervation and loss of distal muscles. Andersen and colleagues estimated muscle volumes in patients with long-term diabetic polyneuropathy by using a stereological determination method based on cross-sectional T1-weighted MRI (Andersen et al., 2004). The volume of the intrinsic foot muscles was halved in diabetic patients with chronic neuropathy, in comparison with that of diabetic patients without neuropathy. The foot muscle volume was closely related to the compound muscle action potentials (CMAPs) of the peroneal nerve. Muscle atrophy occurs early in the feet and progresses steadily in the lower legs.

Distal dominant denervation also occurs in hereditary forms of polyneuropathy. Charcot-Marie-Tooth (CMT) disease is a pathologically and genetically heterogeneous polyneuropathy, divided into demyelinating type (e.g. CMT 1A) and axonal type (e.g. CMT 2A). Both CMT 1A and 2A are characterized by distal muscular atrophy and patients with minimal phenotype may show fatty infiltration limited to intrinsic foot muscles on T1-weighted MRI (Berciano et al., 2010). This finding supports the notion that pes cavus, a cardinal manifestation of CMT, is associated with selective denervation of intrinsic foot muscles. Afterwards, weakness in the more proximal muscles progresses with variable severity. Interestingly, CMT 1A patients show denervation predominantly in the muscles supplied by the peroneal nerve: muscles in the anterior and lateral compartments show selective fatty infiltration with relative preservation of the posterior compartment muscles (Price et al., 1993; Gallardo et al., 2006; Chung et al, 2008). By contrast, in most of the late-onset CMT 2A patients, MRI shows preferential involvement of the soleus muscle with relatively spared deep posterior compartment muscles. The thigh muscles may also be involved during the advanced stage of CMT. A T1-weighted signal may be stronger on the distal side of the vastus lateralis and medialis muscles on coronal images (Chung et al., 2008; Berciano et al., 2010). In addition to T1 high signals that reflect fatty infiltration, T2 high signals and Gd enhancement were also reported in both CMT 1A and 2A patients (Gallardo et al., 2005; Chung et al., 2008). Because T2 prolongation and Gd enhancement are usually observed in acutely denervated muscles, it is difficult to interpret these findings in a chronic disorder with minimal clinical progression over decades. It might indicate subclinical active denervation, but future studies are needed to better understand the muscle MRI findings in CMT.

Case Presentation: CMT type 2

A 41-year-old man, who gradually developed gait disturbance since adolescence, was referred to our hospital for neurological evaluation. One of his uncles has similar gait disturbance. On neurological examination, he had distal-dominant weakness of the lower extremities and sensory loss in a glove and stocking distribution. A nerve conduction study showed decreased CMAP and sensory nerve action potential amplitudes with preserved conduction velocities in all examined nerves, indicating sensory motor axonal polyneuropathy. Clinical diagnosis of CMT type 2 was made. On coronal T2-weighted MRI, the GC muscle showed a high intensity signal with distal accentuation (arrowheads in Fig. 4a). A T1-weighted MRI showed fatty infiltration of the anterior, lateral and superficial posterior compartment muscles (Fig. 4b).

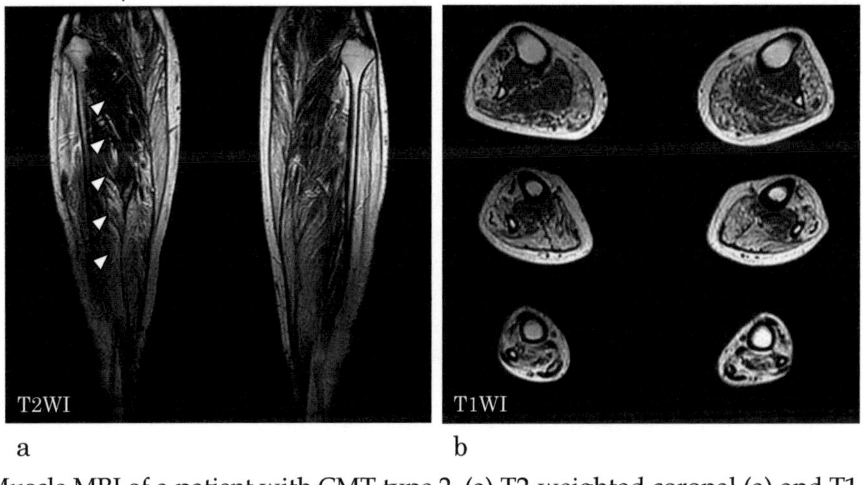

Fig. 4. Muscle MRI of a patient with CMT type 2. (a) T2-weighted coronal (a) and T1-weighted axial (b) MRI of legs.

5.4 Mononeuropathy multiplex

Mononeuropathy multiplex is a clinical syndrome characterized by an asymmetric, stepwise progression of sensory motor deficits involving more than one peripheral or cranial nerve. Mononeuropathy multiplex is often associated with systemic or non-systemic vasculitis, including polyarteritis nodosa, rheumatoid arthritis, systemic lupus erythematosus, Churg-Strauss syndrome and Wegener's granulomatosis. The common peroneal nerve is affected in 75% of patients with vasculitic neuropathy, causing a painful foot drop.

Multifocal motor neuropathy (MMN) and multifocal acquired demyelinating sensory and motor neuropathy (MADSAM, or Lewis-Sumner syndrome) also show the clinical pattern of mononeuropathy multiplex, with electrophysiological evidence of demyelination and conduction block. Brachial plexus of MMN patients is known to show swelling and an increased signal on T2-weighted MRI (van Es et al., 1997). In a few cases, the high intensity signal has been shown to co-localize with conduction block (Parry, 1996). The Gd enhancement effect of the swollen nerve roots has also been described in MMN (Kaji et al., 1993; Perry, 1996). On the other hand, little is known about the muscle MRI findings in MMN. An example case of MMN presented below showed an increased T1 signal in the muscles associated with the nerves with conduction block.

Case Presentation: MMN

A 59-year old man gradually developed clumsiness of the right hand over 10 years. On neurological examination, he had asymmetric weakness of the upper limbs, especially bilateral intrinsic hand muscles and the right extensor muscles. Severe atrophy was present in the bilateral thenar, hypothenar and right brachioradialis muscles (Fig. 5a). There was no sensory deficit and all deep tendon reflexes were absent. Nerve conduction studies revealed multiple conduction blocks. Radial-innervated muscles showed marked atrophy with (SP, ECU, APL; arrowheads in Fig. 5b, c) or without (ED, ECRB, BR; arrows in Fig. 5b, c) signal change on T1-weighted MRI.

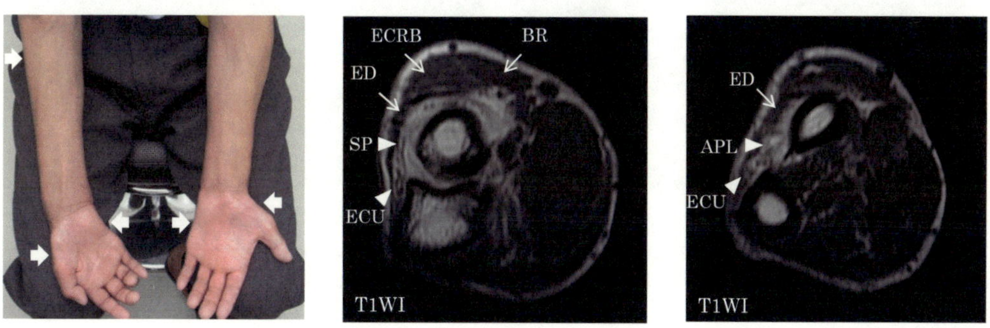

a b c

Abbreviations: abductor pollicis longus (APL), brachioradialis (BR), extensor carpi radialis brevis (ECRB), extensor carpi ulnaris (ECU), extensor digitorum (ED), supinator (SP).

Fig. 5. A case of multifocal motor neuropathy. (a) Muscle atrophy in the bilateral thenar, hypothenar and right brachioradialis muscles. (b, c) Axial T1-weighted muscle MRI of the right forearm.

5.5 Plexopathy

Brachial plexopathy causes pain, paresthesia and motor weakness in the distribution of nerve roots C5 to Th1. Common causes of brachial plexopathy include trauma, neoplastic infiltration, neuralgic amyotrophy, delayed radiation injury and thoracic outlet syndrome. Bilbey et al. showed that MRI is 63% sensitive and 100% specific in demonstrating the abnormality of the brachial plexus in a diverse patient population (Bilbey et al., 1994). When plexopathy is caused by a mass lesion, MRI can often determine whether the mass is intrinsic or extrinsic to the plexus. MRI is also useful for characterizing neoplastic processes (e.g. nerve sheath tumours, metastases, direct extension of non-neurogenic primary tumour and lymphoma) and benign processes (e.g. fibromatosis, lipoma, myositis ossificans, ganglioneuroma, hemangioma and lymphangioma) (Bowen and Seidenwurm, 2008).

Lumbosacral plexopathy is a relatively rare clinical entity that induces sensory motor deficits in the distribution of L1 to S3 segments, causing weakness and sensory loss in the territories of the obturator, femoral, gluteal (motor only), peroneal and tibial nerves. Common causes of lumbosacral plexopathy include trauma (e.g. pelvic fracture), diabetic amyotrophy, retroperitoneal haemorrhage, tumours and inflammation.

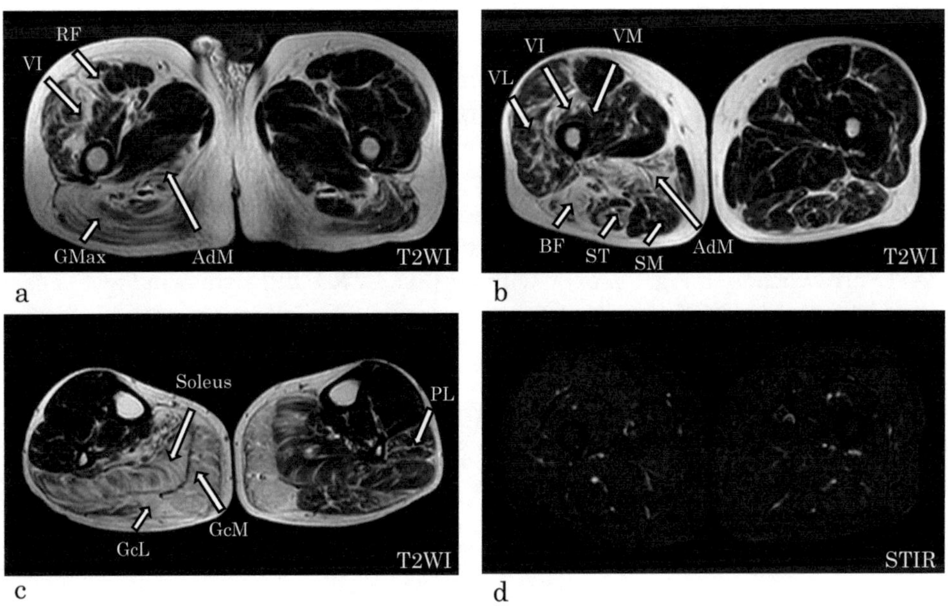

Abbreviations: adductor magnus (AdM), biceps femoris (BF), gastrocnemius lateral head (GcL), gastrocnemius medial head (GcM), gluteus maximus (GMax), peloneus longus (PL), rectus femoris (RF), semimenbranosus (SM), semitendinosus (ST), vastus intermedius (VI), vastus lateralis (VL), vastus medialis (VM).

Fig. 6. Post-irradiation lumbosacral pexopathy in a 50-year-old man. (a-c) Axial T2-weighted MRI of the hip (a), thigh (b) and leg (c). (d) STIR images of the thigh.

Muscle MRI findings of plexopathy have not been established yet. Several studies report muscle MRI findings in neuralgic amyotrophy, also known as Parsonage-Turner syndrome (Gaskin and Helms, 2006; Scalf et al., 2007). The most typical finding of neuralgic amyotrophy is diffuse high signal intensity on T2-weighted images involving one or more muscles innervated by the brachial plexus. T1-weighted images may also show atrophy of the affected muscles. The supraspinatus and infraspinatus muscles, both innervated by the suprascapular nerve, are most frequently affected (>80%). Less frequently involved are the axillary-innervated deltoid and teres minor muscles. MRI has an advantage in that it can exclude other causes of shoulder pain, such as rotator cuff tear, impingement syndrome or labral tear.

Case Presentation: Post-irradiation lumbosacral plexopathy

A 50-year-old man gradually developed weakness of the bilateral legs over 10 years. He had a history of suprasellar germinoma at the age of 24, which went into complete remission after radiation and chemotherapy. On neurological examination, he showed weakness of the bilateral legs without sensory deficits. Needle EMG showed chronic neurogenic changes and myokimic discharges in the leg muscles, which supported the diagnosis of radiation-induced delayed lumbosacral plexopathy.

T1- and T2-weighted MRI showed an asymmetric high intensity signal in the hip, thigh and calf muscles (arrows in Fig. 6a-c). The involved muscles showed isointensity signals on STIR images (Fig. 6d). Taken together, the MRI study was compatible with the idea of chronic-stage denervation in the distribution of lumbosacral plexopathy.

6. Conclusion

We reviewed the clinical utility of muscle MRI on a variety of peripheral nerve disorders. MRI has reasonable sensitivity for detecting denervated muscles. Future improvement of scan sequences and availability of higher field scanners would make the sensitivity even higher. Yet, its disease specificity is limited and MRI plays a complementary role in the diagnosis of peripheral nerve disorders.

7. References

Andersen H.; Gjerstad M.D. and Jakobsen J. (2004). Atrophy of foot muscles: a measure of diabetic neuropathy. *Diabetes Care*, Vol.27, No.10, (October 2004), pp. 2382-2385

Andreassen C.S.; Jakobsen J.; Ringgaard S.; Ejskjaer N. and Andersen H. (2009). Accelerated atrophy of lower leg and foot muscles--a follow-up study of long-term diabetic polyneuropathy using magnetic resonance imaging (MRI). *Diabetologia*, Vol.52, No.6, (January 2009), pp. 1182-1191

Andreisek G.; Crook D.W.; Burg D.; Marincek B. and Weishaupt D. (2006). Peripheral neuropathies of the median, radial and ulnar nerves: MR imaging features. *Radiographics*, Vol.26, No.5, (September-October 2006), pp. 1267-1287

Berciano J.; Gallardo E.; García A.; Ramón C.; Infante J. and Combarros O. (2010). Clinical progression in Charcot-Marie-Tooth disease type 1A duplication: clinico-electrophysiological and MRI longitudinal study of a family. *J Neurol*, Vol.257, No.10, (October 2010), pp. 1633-1641

Bendszus M. and Koltzenburg M. (2001). Visualization of denervated muscle by gadolinium-enhanced MRI. *Neurology*. Vol.57, No.9, (November 2001), pp. 1709-1711

Bendszus M.; Koltzenburg M.; Wessig C.; Solymosi L. (2002). Sequential MR imaging of denervated muscle: experimental study. *Am J Neuroradiol*, Vol.23, No.8, (September 2002), pp. 1427-1431

Bendszus M.; Wessig C.; Reiners K.; Bartsch A.J.; Solymosi L. and Koltzenberg M. (2003). MR imaging in the differential diagnosis of neurogenic foot drop. *Am J Neuroradiol*, Vol.24, No.7, (August 2003), pp. 1283-1289

Bilbey J.H.; Lamond R.G. and Mattrey R.F. (1994). MR imaging of disorders of the brachial plexus. *J Magn Reson Imaging*, Vol.4, No.1. (January-February 1994), pp. 13-18

Bowen B.C. and Seidenwurm D.J. (2008). Plexopathy. *Am J Neuroradiol*, Vol.29, No.2, (February 2008), pp.400-402

Carter G.T. and Fritz R.C. (1997). Electromyographic and lower extremity short time to inversion recovery magnetic resonance imaging findings in lumbar radiculopathy. *Muscle Nerve*, Vol.20, No.9, (September 1997) pp. 1191-1193

Carter G.T.; McDonald C.M.; Chan T.T. and Margherita A.J. (1995). Isolated femoral mononeuropathy to the vastus lateralis: EMG and MRI findings. *Muscle Nerve*, Vol.18, No.3, (March 1995), pp. 341-344

Chung K.W.; Suh B.C.; Shy M.E.; Cho S.Y.; Yoo J.H.; Park S.W.; Moon H.; Park K.D.; Choi K.G.; Kim S.; Kim S.B.; Shim D.S.; Kim S.M.; Sunwoo I.N. and Choi B.O. (2008). Different clinical and magnetic resonance imaging features between Charcot-Marie-Tooth disease type 1A and 2A. *Neuromuscul Disord*, Vol.18, No.8, (August 2008), pp. 610-618

Donovan A.; Rosenberg Z.S. and Cavalcanti C.F. (2010) MR imaging of entrapment neuropathies of the lower extremity. Part 2. The knee, leg, ankle and foot. *Radiographics*, Vol.30, No.4, (July-August 2010), pp. 1001-1019

Ferdinand B.D.; Rosenberg Z.S.; Schweitzer M.E.; Stuchin S.A.; Jazrawi L.M.; Lenzo S.R.; Meislin R.J. and Kiprovski K. MR imaging features of radial tunnel syndrome: initial experience. *Radiology*, Vol.240, No.1, (July 2006), pp. 161-168

Filler A.G.; Haynes J.; Jordan S.E.; Prager J.; Villablanca J.P.; Farahani K.; McBride D.Q.; Tsuruda J.S.; Morisoli B.; Batzdorf U. and Johnson J.P. (2005). Sciatica of non-disc origin and piriformis syndrome: diagnosis by magnetic resonance neurography and interventional magnetic resonance imaging with outcome study of resulting treatment. *J Neurosurg Spine*, Vol.2, No.2, (February 2005), pp. 99-115

Filler A.G.; Howe F.A.; Hayes C.E.; Kliot M.; Winn H.R.; Bell B.A.; Griffiths J.R. and Tsuruda J.S. (1993). Magnetic resonance neurography. *Lancet*, Vol.341, No.8846, (March 1993), pp. 659-661

Fleckenstein J.L.; Watumull D.; Conner K.E.; Ezaki M.; Greenlee R.G.Jr.;Bryan W.W.; Chason D.P.; Parkey R.W.; Peshock R.M. and Purdy P.D. (1993). Denervated human skeletal muscle: MR imaging evaluation. *Radiology*, Vol.187, No.1, (April 1993), pp. 213-218

Gallardo E.; García A.; Combarros O. and Berciano J. (2006). Charcot-Marie-Tooth disease type 1A duplication: spectrum of clinical and magnetic resonance imaging features in leg and foot muscles. *Brain*, Vol.129, No.2, (February 2006), pp. 426-437

Gaskin C.M. and Helms C.A. (2006). Parsonage-Turner syndrome: MR imaging findings and clinical information of 27 patients. *Radiology*, Vol.240, No.2, (August 2006), pp. 501-507

Grainger A.J.; Campbell R.S. and Stothard J. (1998). Anterior interosseous nerve syndrome: appearance at MR imaging in three cases. *Radiology*, Vol.208, No.2, (August 1998), pp. 381-384

Grant G.A.; Britz G.W.; Goodkin R.; Jarvik J.G.; Maravilla K. and Kliot M. (2002). The utility of magnetic resonance imaging in evaluating peripheral nerve disorders. *Muscle Nerve*, Vol.25, No.3, (March 2002), pp. 314-331

Gyftopoulos S.; Rosenberg Z.S. and Petchprapa C. (2010). Increased MR signal intensity in the pronator quadratus muscle: does it always indicate anterior interosseous neuropathy? *Am J Roentgenol*, Vol.194, No.2, (February 2010), pp. 490-493

Hayashi Y.; Ikata T.; Takai H.; Takata S.; Ishikawa M.; Sogabe T. and Koga K. (1997). Effect of peripheral nerve injury on nuclear magnetic resonance relaxation times of rat skeletal muscle. *Invest Radiol*, Vol.32, No.3, pp. 135-139

Hazlewood C.F.; Chang D.C.; Nichols B.L. and Woessner D.E. (1974). Nuclear magnetic resonance transverse relaxation times of water protons in skeletal muscle. *Biophys J*, Vol. 14, No.8, (August 1974), pp. 582-606

Hof J.J.; Kliot M.; Slimp J. and Haynor D.R. (2008). What's new in MRI of peripheral nerve entrapment? *Neurosurg Clin N Am* , Vol.14, No.4, (October 2008), pp. 583-595

Horch R.E.; Allmann K.H.; Laubenberger J.; Langer M. and Stark G.B. (1997). Median nerve compression can be detected by magnetic resonance imaging of the carpal tunnel. *Neurosurgery*, Vol.41, No.1, (July 1997), pp. 76-82

Iverson D.J. (2005). MRI detection of cysts of the knee causing common peroneal neuropathy. *Neurology*, Vol.65, No.11, (December 2005), pp. 1829-1831

Jarvik J.G.; Yuen E.; Haynor D.R.; Bradley C.M.; Fulton-Kehoe D.; Smith-Weller T.; Wu R.; Kliot M.; Kraft G.; Wang L.; Erlich V.; Heagerty P.J. and Franklin G.M. (2002). MR nerve imaging in a prospective cohort of patients with suspected carpal tunnel syndrome. *Neurology*, Vol.58, No.11, (June 2002), pp. 1597-1602

Jonas D.; Conrad B.; Von Einsiedel H.G. and Bischoff C. (2000). Correlation between quantitative EMG and muscle MRI in patients with axonal neuropathy. *Muscle Nerve*, Vol.23, No.8, (August 2000), pp. 1265-1269

Kaji R.; Oka N.; Tsuji T.; Mezaki T.; Nishio T.; Akiguchi I. and Kimura J. (1993). Pathological findings at the site of conduction block in multifocal motor neuropathy. *Ann Neurol*, Vol.33, No.2, (February 1993), pp. 152-158

Kamath S.; Venkatanarasimha N.; Walsh M.A and Hughes P.M. (2008). MRI appearance of muscle denervation. *Skeletal Radiol*, Vol.37, No.5, (May 2008), pp. 397-404

Kato H.; Hirayama T.; Minami A.; Iwasaki N. and Hirachi K. (2002). Cubital tunnel syndrome associated with medial elbow Ganglia and osteoarthritis of the elbow. *J Bone Joint Surg Am*, Vol.84-A, No.8, (August 2002), pp. 1413-1419

Kikuchi Y.; Nakamura T.; Takayama S.; Horiuchi Y. and Toyama Y. (2003). MR imaging in the diagnosis of denervated and reinnervated skeletal muscles: experimental study in rats. *Radiology*, Vol.229, No.3, (December 2003), pp. 861-867

Kim J.Y.; Ihn Y.K.; Kim J.S.; Chun K.A.; Sung M.S. and Cho K.H. (2007). Non-traumatic peroneal nerve palsy: MRI findings. *Clin Radiol*, Vol.62, No.1, (January 2007), pp. 58-64

Kim S.J.; Hong S.H.; Jun W.S.; Choi J.Y.; Myung J.S.; Jacobson J.A.; Lee J.W.; Choi J.A.; Kan and H.S. (2011). MR imaging mapping of skeletal muscle denervation in entrapment and compressive neuropathies. *Radiographics*, Vol.31, No.2, (March-April 2011), pp. 319-332

Koltzenburg M.; Bendszus M. (2004). Imaging of peripheral nerve lesions. *Curr Opin Neurol*, Vol.17, No.5, (October 2004), pp. 621-626

Kuntzer T.; van Melle G. and Regli F. (1997). Clinical and prognostic features in unilateral femoral neuropathies. *Muscle Nerve*, Vol.20, No.2, (February 1997), pp. 205-211.

Lisle D.A.; Johnstone S.A. (2007). Usefulness of muscle denervation as an MRI sign of peripheral nerve pathology. *Australas Radiol*, Vol.51, No.6, (December 2007), pp. 516-526

McDonald C.M.; Carter G.T.; Fritz R.C.; Anderson M.W.; Abresch R.T. and Kilmer D.D. (2000). Magnetic resonance imaging of denervated muscle: comparison to electromyography. *Muscle Nerve*, Vol.23, No.9, (September 2000), pp. 1431-1434

Mesgarzadeh M.; Schneck C.D.; Bonakdarpour A.; Mitra A. and Conaway D. (1989) Carpal tunnel: MR imaging. Part II. Carpal tunnel syndrome. *Radiology*, Vol.171, No.3, (June 1989), pp. 749-754.

Nogués M.A.; Salas E.; Martínez A. and Romero C. (1998). Unilateral femoral neuropathy. *Muscle Nerve*, Vol.21, No.1, (January 1998), pp. 126-127

Parry GJ. (1996). AAEM case report #30: multifocal motor neuropathy. *Muscle Nerve*, Vol.19, No.3, pp. 269-276

Pearce C.; Feinberg J. and Wolfe S.W. (2009). Ulnar neuropathy at the wrist. *HSSJ*, Vol.5, No.2, (September 2009), pp. 180-183

Petchprapa C.N.; Rosenberg Z.S.; Sconfienza L.M.; Cavalcanti C.F.; Vieira R.L. and Zember J.S. (2010). MR imaging of entrapment neuropathies of the lower extremity. Part 1. The pelvis and hip. *Radiographics*, Vol.30, No.4, (July-August 2010), pp. 983-1000

Polak J.F.; Jolesz F.A. and Adams D.F. (1988). Magnetic resonance imaging of skeletal muscle. Prolongation of T1 and T2 subsequent to denervation. *Invest Radiol*, Vol.23, No.5, (May 1988), pp. 365-369

Price A.E.; Maisel R. and Drennan J.C. Computed tomographic analysis of pes cavus. (1993). *J Pediatr Orthop*, Vol.13, No.5, (September 1993), pp. 646-653

Rinker B.; Effron C.R. and Beasley R.W. (2004). Proximal radial compression neuropathy. *Ann Plast Surg*, Vol.52, No.2, (February 2004), pp. 174-180

Rosenberg Z.S.; Beltran J.; Cheung Y.Y.; Ro S.Y.; Green S.M. and Lenzo S.R. (1993). The elbow: MR features of nerve disorders. *Radiology*, Vol.188, No.1, (July 1993), pp. 235-240

Sallomi D.; Janzen D.L.; Munk P.L.; Connell D.G. and Tirman P.F. (1998). Muscle denervation patterns in upper limb nerve injuries: MR imaging findings and anatomic basis. *Am J Roentgenol*, Vol.171, No.3, (September 1998), pp. 779-784

Scalf R.E.; Wenger D.E.; Frick M.A.; Mandrekar J.N. and Adkins M.C. (2007). MRI findings of 26 patients with Parsonage-Turner syndrome. *Am J Roentgenol,* Vol.189, No.1, (July 2007), pp. W39-44

Seijo-Martínez M.; Castro del Río M.; Fontoira E. and Fontoira M. (2003). Acute femoral neuropathy secondary to an iliacus muscle hematoma. *J Neurol Sci,* Vol.209, No.1-2, (May 2003), pp. 119-122

Shabas D.; Gerard G. and Rossi D. (1987). Magnetic resonance imaging examination of denervated muscle. *Comput Radiol,* Vol.11, No.1, (January-February 1987), pp. 9-13

Spratt J.D.; Stanley A.J.; Grainger A.J.; Hide I.G. and Campbell R.S. (2002). The role of diagnostic radiology in compressive and entrapment neuropathies. *Eur Radiol,* Vol.12, No.9, (September 2002), pp. 2352-2364

Stoll G.; Bendszus M.; Perez J. and Pham M. (2009). Magnetic resonance imaging of the peripheral nervous system. *J Neurol,* Vol.256, No.7, (July, 2009), pp. 1043-1051

Stuplich M.; Hottinger A.F.; Stoupis C. and Sturzenegger M. (2005). Combined femoral and obturator neuropathy caused by synovial cyst of the hip. *Muscle Nerve,* Vol.32, No.4, (October 2005), pp. 552-554

Takahara T.; Hendrikse J.; Yamashita T.; Mali W.P.; Kwee T.C. Imai Y. and Luijten P.R. (2008). Diffusion-weighted MR neurography of the brachial plexus: feasibility study. *Radiology,* Vol.249, No.2, (November 2008), pp. 653-660

Thawait S.K.; Wang K.; Subhawong T.K.; Williams E.H.; Hashemi S.S.; Machado A.J.; Thawait G.K.; Soldatos T.; Carrino J.A. and Chhabra A. (2011). Peripheral nerve surgery: the role of high-resolution MR neurography. *Am J Neuroradiol,* (April 2011), [Epub ahead of print], DOI 10.3174/ajnr.A2465

Tsujii M.; Hirata H.; Morita A. and Uchida A. (2009). Palmar bowing of the flexor retinaculum on wrist MRI correlates with subjective reports of pain in carpal tunnel syndrome. J *Magn Reson Imaging,* Vol.29, No.5, (May 2009), pp. 1102-1105

Uetani M.; Hayashi K.; Matsunaga N.; Imamura K. and Ito N. (1993). Denervated skeletal muscle: MR imaging. Work in progress. *Radiology.* Vol. 189, No.2, (November 1993), pp. 511-515

Van Es H.W.; Van den Berg L.H.; Franssen H.; Witkamp T.D.; Ramos L.M.; Notermans N.C.; Feldberg M.A. and Wokke J.H. (1997). Magnetic resonance imaging of the brachial plexus in patients with multifocal motor neuropathy. *Neurology,* Vol.48, No.5, (May 1997), pp. 1218-1224

Wessig C.; Koltzenburg M.; Reiners K.; Solymosi L. and Bendszus M. (2004). MRI of peripheral nerve degeneration and regeneration: correlation with electrophysiology and histology. *Exp Neurol,* Vol.188, No.1, (July 2004), pp. 171-177

West G.A.; Haynor D.R.; Goodkin R.; Tsuruda J.S.; Bronstein A.D.; Kraft G.; Winter T. and Kliot M. (1994). Magnetic resonance imaging signal changes in denervated muscles after peripheral nerve injury. *Neurosurgery,* Vol.35, No.6, (December 1994), pp. 1077-1086

Zhang Z.; Song L.; Meng Q.; Li Z.; Pan B.; Yang Z. and Pei Z. (2009). Morphological analysis in patients with sciatica: a magnetic resonance imaging study using three-dimensional high-resolution diffusion-weighted magnetic resonance neurography techniques. *Spine*, Vol.34, No.7, (April 2009), pp. E245-250

5

Blink Reflex Alterations in Various Polyneuropathies

Figen Guney
Department of Neurology, Selçuk University, Meram Medical Faculty Konya, Turkey

1. Introduction

An eyelid closure in response to some stimulus is a blink reflex (BR), which is normally isolated. In humans and primates, the closing is bilateral while in other animals, mostly those with eyes set laterally, the closure is frequently unilateral. In clinical practice, a BR is characteristically provoked by light corneal or eyelash touching or glabellar tapping. The British physician Overrend first elicited the blink reflex by tapping one side of the forehead. Kugelberg analysed the blink reflex electromyographically by electrically stimulating the supraorbital nerve. Since the original description of the blink reflex 100 years ago the study of this reflex has given understanding the central and peripheral mechanisms of the trigeminofacial pathways in normal and different disorder. Stimulation of the supraorbital nerve, a distal branch of the ophtalmic division of the trigeminal nerve , is the common technique in clinical neurophysiology to obtain a BR (Figure 1). Characteristically, an electrical stimulus on the supraorbital nerve induces two recordable responses in the orbicularis oculi muscles: an early one R1, ipsilateral to the stimulated side, and a later one, R2, which is bilaterally expressed. R2 response ipsilateral to the stimulus is frequently cited as R2i, and the R2c is the one obtained on the contralateral side. R1 component of BR has a rather stable latency. R2 typically shows relative variable latencies and larger magnitudes than R1 and its threshold is lower. R2 component is responsible for the eyelid closure of the blink. It has been observed that common motor unit potentials contribute to the buildup of both responses, that is, the same orbicularis oculi motor unit is depolarized after the stimulation at times corresponding to the latencies of R1 and R2 responses, the latter presumably in a repetitive reverberating pattern. Both response are cutaneous and nociceptive in origin. The classical findings, indicative of such a lesion are an afferent defect with prolonged latencies of R1, ipsilateral R2 and contralateral R2. The efferent type pattern occurs also with intraaxial lateral pontine lesions involving the pons at the trigeminal entrance zone. In facial nerve lesions there is a delay in the reflex latency only on the affected side, regardless of the side of stimulation. Such abnormalities were found in Bell's palsy or other lesions of the facial nerve.

2. Discussion

Generalized polyneuropathy may induce bilateral abnormalities of the trigeminal reflex. Blink reflex alterations were first described in large series of patients with polyneuropathy in 1982 by Kimura. He analyzed the blink reflex obtained from the patients with Guillain-Barre syndrome (GBS), chronic inflammatory polyneuropathy (CIPN), Fisher syndrome (FS), hereditary motor and sensory neuropathy (HMSN) Types I and II, diabetic polyneuropathy. The patients with diabetic polyneuropathy were selected as having maturity-onset diabetes with diffuse symmetrical neuropathy. None had renal complications, mononeuropathy, distinctly asymmetrical features, dysautonomia, or predominantly proximal weakness. In GBS, CIPN, and HMSN Type I, R1 responses were either absent or delayed in a majority of patients. The incidence of abnormality was considerably less in DPN. In FS, the direct and R1 responses were normal in all except for 1 patient who had peripheral palsy associated with delayed R1 on the affected side. In HMSN Type II, the studies were normal in all except for 1 patient who had an absent R1 on one side. The average latencies of the much lesser degree in DPN, and were normal in FS and HMSN Type II. The latency ratio of R1 to the direct response showed a mild increase in GBS, a moderate decrease in CIPN and HMSN Type I and a mild decrease in DPN. In GBS, the latency ratio of R1 to direct response is increased slightly, indicating more proximal involvement of the facial nerve, provided, trigeminal nerve is relatively intact. This ratio is decreased significantly in CIPN and DPN, as migh be expected from a distally prominent involvement in a chronic neuropathic process. Although latencies of R2 were commonly within the normal range when analysed individually, the average value was greater significantly in the neuropathies than in the controls. In normal subjects, R2 begins clearly after R1. This distinction became unclear in some patients with demyelinating neuropathy, in which R1 was temporally dispersed. However, the ipsilateral and contralateral R2 were of nearly identical latency in neuropathy. Thus, a simultaneously recorded contralateral R2 helped to identify that the apparent initial portion of the ipsilateral response contained a delayed R1 continuous with R2. Abnormalities of the blink reflex and direct response generally were well correlated with slowing of motor nerve conduction velocities. A marked delay in latency of R1 and the direct response offers conclusive evidence that the facial nerve is severely involved in some polyneuropathies. This is expected in GBS, which is associated characteristically with facial weakness, but not in HMSN Type I, in which weakness of the facial muscle, if any, is clinically very subtle. The blink reflex abnormalities in CIPN are similar to those in GBS, but, interestingly, studies are normal in FS unless associated with facial nerve palsy. Analogous to a bimodal distribution of motor nerve conduction velocities in HMSN, the latency of direct and R1 responses usually are prolonged in Type I and normal in Type II.

Blink reflex provides clinically useful information in the assessment of the cranial nerves in polyneuropathies. The blink reflex reflects the integrity of the afferent and efferent pathways, including the proximal segment of the facial nerve. Thus, the latency of R1 represents the conduction time along the trigeminal and facial nerves and pontine relay. R2 is less reliable for this purpose because of inherent latency variability from one trial to the next. Furthermore, the latency of R2 reflect excitability of interneurons and synaptic transmission in addition to axonal conduction.

Polo et al. found that in patients with polyneuritis cranialis which is Guillain Barre syndrome's rare varient both R1 and R2 components of blink reflex were absent. Five months later blink reflex could be elicited, the R1 latency was significantly increased.

Neau et al. have studied blink reflex in 50 patients with Guillain-Barre polyradiculitis. They detected bilateral lenghtening of the early and late reflex responses of the blink reflex with unilateral or bilateral increase of motor facial latency. The blink reflex showed various abnormalities in slightly more than one third of the cases of polyradiculoneuritis presenting no clinical signs of facial involvement, thus constituting subclinical lesional evidence of the reflex arc.

Abnormalities of blink reflexes have been reported in acute inflammatory demyelinating polyneuropathy (AIDP). Ropper et al. examined blink reflex in AIDP within 21 days of symptom onset. In that study, it was documented that 46% of patients with AIDP exihibited abnormality of blink reflexes, 96% of these patients exhibited facial weakness. In addition, R1 onset latency correlated positively with prolonged median nerve distal motor latency. One study has examined the blink reflex abnormalities in AIDP within 10 days of symptom onset. Abnormalities of blink reflexes, absent or prolonged ipsilateral R1 and R2 responses and contralateral R2 responses, were noted in 16 of 31 patients (52%) tested. Abnormalities of R1 component (51%) were slightly more frequent than abnormalities of the R2 component (48%). In those patients with abnormalities of blink reflexes, facial weakness was evident in 11 (69%) patients. This would suggest that blink reflexes, might be abnormal in some AIDP patients with apparently normal facial strength, and hence should be performed systematically if AIDP was suspected. Furthermore, abnormalities of blink reflexes also correlated positively with prolonged mean summated distal motor latency in this study, suggesting that in early AIDP, distal demyelination occurs in parallel in many nerves. These abnormalities of blink reflexes most likely represent demyelination in either the facial and/or the trigeminal nerves, reflecting the multifocal nature of demyelination in AIDP.

Cruccu et al. made blink reflex study in 14 patients with chronic inflammatory demyelinating polyneuropathy (CIDP), in 23 patients with severe distal sensory or sensorymotor form of diabetic polyneuropathy, and in 12 patients with mild diabetic polyneuropathy. Recordings of the blink reflexes showed abnormal R1 blink reflex, and on 7/29 an abnormal R2. Recording of the blink reflexes showed on 11/29 sides an abnormal R1 blink reflex, and on 7/29 an abnormal R2 in patients with chronic inflammatory demyelinating polyneuropathy. The mean R1 and R2 latencies were slightly longer than control values. R1 blink reflex was abnormal on 8/43 sides and R2 on 3/43 in patients with severe diabetic polyneuropathy. On one side of 1 patient the R1 and R2 delays originated from the facial-nerve reflex efferents. They examined 20 sides in 12 patients with mild diabetic polyneuropathy. They detected only the latency of R1, which might reflect the sum of mild trigeminal and facial abnormalities, was slightly longer than control values. In patients with CIDP, the motor and sensory nerves were affected symmetrically. The long delays in the latency of R1 were probably due to demyelination in the facial, supraorbital nerves. Even the absent responses did not necessarily imply axonal loss. In diabetic patients, the abnormalities had a far more irregular distribution. The supraorbital R1 was affected unilaterally in several patients. The mean R1 latency was only slightly longer in the severe than in the mild neuropathy group. Individual patients had relatively small delays, compatible with slightly longer synaptic times due to the defect of spatial summation entailed by axonal loss.

Kokubun et al. examined 20 patients with CIDP using blink reflex. All patients had symptomatic motor and sensory neuropathies for more than 2 months, and demyelinating polyneuropathy was diagnosed by conventional nerve conduction studies. The latency of the R1 response was prolonged on the left side in 16 of 20 patients and on the right in 16 patients. Only 3 patients had a normal R1 response bilaterally. The ipsilateral R2 response was abnormal on the left in 8 patients and on the right in 7, but was normal bilaterally in 10 patients. The contralateral R2 response was prolonged on the left in 8 patients and on the right in 3, could not be evoked in 2 patients, and was normal bilaterally in 11. The latencies of the R1, and R2 responses in CIDP patients were significantly prolonged compared with those of normal subjects. The prevalence of subclinical facial neuropathy in their CIDP patients was high; an abnormal direct response was observed bilaterally in 10(50%) and unilaterally in 2 patients (10%). However, none of the patients showed unilateral trigeminal nerve involvement, based on the result of the blink reflex. The R1 and R2 latencies were prolonged and the responses were not evoked bilaterally in 4 patients, perhaps because of trigeminal nerve or brainstem involvement in addition to bilateral facial nerve involvement. Bilateral or unilateral prolongation of R1 latency alone was observed in 10 patients. This result may be due to some defect in the pons (5). Only one patient's R1 latency was within the normal range bilaterally; however R2 latency was markedly increased. This patient possibly had medullary involvement in addition to trigeminal or facial nerve involvement. Kokobun's study results suggested that involvement of trigeminal and facial nerves probably occurred early during the onset of CIDP because there was no correlation between clinical disability or disease duration, and direct or R1 response. The study of the blink reflex was used widely and it was an established test. Although their study had certain limitations, the direct response and the blink reflex are useful for functional evaluation of trigeminal and facial nerves in patients with CIDP, especially since the data has indicated a lack of correlation between clinical features and electrophysiological detections in CIDP patients.

Varela et al. reported an 83 year-old-woman with a remote history of localized melanoma and breast carcinoma (treated with resection without chemothreapy or radiation in the early 1980s), but no history of systemic medical disease such as diabetes, who presented with a 2-month history of progressive tongue and perioral numbness and difficulty sipping liquids, in 2009. She described a decrease in sensation and occasional "tingling" mostly involving the perioral region but occasionally throughout the face. She denied diplopia, ptosis, or other cranial nerve symptoms and had no limb weakness or sensory loss, apart from intermittent numbness in her hands that would awaken her intermittently at night. Neurologic examination demonstrated mild weakness (Medical research Council grade 4) of her orbicularis oculi, orbicularis oris, and frontalis and a mild decreased pinprick sensation in her feet bilaterally. Reflexes were present but mildly reduced diffusely. On routine nerve conduction studies, only median motor distal latencies were prolonged,& conduction velocities slowed in the forearm, but there was no abnormal temporal dispersion or conduction block. Median sensory responses were absent bilaterally. Blink reflex study demonstrated prolonged R1 and R2 latencies bilaterally. Cerebrospinal fluid demonstrated an elevated protein of 87 mg/dl. Patient was diagnosed as chronic inflammatory demyelination neuropathy, prednisone (60 mg daily) was initiated after intravenous immunoglobulin teratment. One month after initation of prednisone, her symptoms and examination improved, prolonged latencies were detected on blink reflex study leading to the diagnosis of demyelinating neuropathy. Therefore, blink reflex study is useful in helping to confirm selected cases of suspected CIDP.

Ogawara et al. reported a case of anti-GQ1b antibody syndrome. The patient had symptoms and signs suggesting both peripheral lesions i.e. asymmetric ophthalmoplegia, facial diplegia, upper limb weakness, areflexia and central lesions i.e. drowsiness, and hemisensory loss. The anti-GQ1b antibody titres were very high. Extensive electrophysiologic studies supported the involvement of both peripheral and central nervous systems. The coexistence of central and peripheral components refutes the idea of simple relationship between Bickerstaff encephalitis and purely central involvement, or between Fisher syndrome and a simple peripheral neuropathy. Published reports have described cases of Fisher syndrome associated with evidence of brainstem or cerebellar lesions on MRI and indicated that central components were occasionally associated with Fisher syndrome. Magnetic resonance imaging of the brain T1- and T2- weighted images showed no abnormalities. R1 responses were small with normal latency (9.1 ms), in this patient's blink reflex study. The R2 responses were not elicited on either side. Absence of R2 despite detectable R1 after repeated trials raised the possibility of central abnormality. Therefore, blink reflex study is useful in differentiating the diagnosis from Bickerstaff encephalitis, too.

Urban et al. examined both electromyographical investigation and blink reflex study in 40 patients with diaetes mellitus. Compared with age related normal values, the patient group showed abnormal nerve conductions to the sural nerve (absent sensory nerve action potential in 33%, reduced amplitude in 17.9%, reduced sensory conduction velocity in 33.3%), the peroneal nerve (reduced motor conduction velocity in 28.5%, reduced amplitude in 26%), the median motor fibers (reduced motor conduction velocity in 7.7%) and the median sensory fibers (abolished the sensory nerve action potential in 5%, reduced sensory conduction velocity in 18%, reduced amplitude in 51%). Nerve conduction studies confirmed sensory or sensorimotor polyneuropathy in all 24 of the clinically affected patients. Urban et al. detected significantly prolonged R1 latency concluding that subclinical facial and trigeminal nerve involvement is not unusual in diabetes mellitus although it is significantly less frequent than the involvement of limb nerves. Nazliel et al. showed abnormal blink reflex responses in 55% of 20 diabetic patients with polyneuropathy. They detected prolonged R2i and R2c latencies but R1 values in diabetic patients with polyneuropathy did not differ sigificantly from those of normal controls. Guney et al. studied 95 diabetic patients and found bilateral significantly increased R1 and R2i and R2c latencies in diabetic patients with polyneuropathy (Figure 2). And as an interesting result, R1 values in diabetic patients without polyneuropathy did not differ significantly from normal controls. These results suggest R1 is mainly conducted by exteroceptive, medium thick myelinated A-beta fibres, whereas R2 is predominantly conveyed by the nociceptive, thin myelinated A-delta fibers. As a result of these studies, there is no surprise sparing of R1 in diabetic patients without clinical or subclinical neuropathy. The reflex arc of R1 has its central representation in main trigeminal nucleus of the pons, its circuit bases in an olygosynaptic organisation with three neurons, respectively on the Gasser's ganglion, the trigeminal principal nucleus and the facial nucleus, and at least one interneuron between two latter structures, as reported by Trontelj and Tamai et al. It is not completely known if these interneuron's location is on the multisynaptic way of R2 in man. For R2 response, the central way is multisynaptic. Holstege et al. postulated that blink premotor area located at the pontine and medullary tegmental fields projecting into the blink motoneuronal pool would probably be involved in R2 blink reflex component. Prolongation to Gasser's ganglion, throughout the tractus spinalis trigeminalis reached the second-order neurons located on the nucleus spinalis trigeminalis. From here, a long interneuronal ascending system connected to the ipsilateral and contralateral facial nuclei. This multisynaptic pathway included the lateral propriobulbar system of the reticular formation, lying medial to the trigeminal spinal nucleus. A bilateral delayed R2i and R2c response in all diabetic patients with or without polyneuropathy indicates interneuron subclinical dysfunction in the low brainstem reticular formation.

Four published works on blink reflex in chronic renal failure were found. In one 47 patients undergoing hemodialysis, 24 showed clinical or electromyographical evidence of peripheral neuropathy, and in 13 patients abnormal early R1 blink response was noted. In another, there was a 64% coincidence of abnormal peroneal nerve conduction and R1 blink reflex abnormalities (9/15 patients); delayed blink responses with simultaneous reduced conduction velocity in the median nerve were only found in four cases (29%). In the third study there were no reports of conduction studies of the peripheral nerves. Resende et al. studied blink reflex in 20 non-diabetic adult males who had chronic renal failure. They detected abnormal blink reflex in 10 (50%) patients and axonal sensorymotor peripheral neuropathy in 8 (80%) of these 10. They detected a bilateral delayed early R1 response, and this indicated bilateral dysfunction of the trigeminal and/or facial nerve, elongation at limit in R2i, and R2c latencies, and this was indicative of interneuron subclinical dysfunction in low brainstem reticular formation. Late response abnormalities in the blink reflex suggest subclinical brainstem dysfuncion in chronic renal failure with this study.

Ishpekova et al. studied blink reflex in 27 patients with hereditary motor and sensory neuropathy. In these patients , they detected three components (R1, R2 and R3) of blink reflex instead of usual two which are recordable in normal subjects on the side ipsilateral to the stimulation. On the contralateral side the latter two components (R2 an R3) were present. The responses were distinct in all patients and their mean latencies were prolonged in comparison with those of healthy subjects. An unusual three component blink reflex was observed in the HMSN patients. R3 component appeared to be distinct temporally from R2. It could only be evoked by strong electrical pulses and had a latency about 50 ms longer than R2 in healthy subjects. R1 latency was increased 2.5 times over normal values. Latencies of R2 and R3 components were prolonged in these patients. The medium thick myelinated A-beta fibres were mainly responsible for R1 component, whereas R2 was mediated by the nociceptive thin myelinated A-delta fibres. The cutaneous A-beta and nociceptive A-delta fibres contributed to the generation of the very late component R3. Identical changes of R2 and R3 components in HMSN patients supported the conclusion that the reflex arc for R2 and R3 uses the same brain stem pathways.

Charcot-Marie-Tooth (CMT) is the most frequent inherited neuropathy. X-linked CMT (CMTX) is the second most frequent form after CMT1A, with a frequency about 20%. Signs of CNS involvement have been reported in a few CMTX patients. Moreover, the use of modern imaging and electrophysiological methods has provided evidence of occasional subclinical CNS involvement in some patients with CMT. Zambelis et al. studied blink reflex in all members of X-linked Charcot-Marie-Tooth family (seven probands; 4 male and 3 female) . Blink reflex showed bilaterally prolonged R1 and R2 responses in four symtomatic patients with normal distal latency of the facial nerve. This is supporting electrophysiological evidence of subclinical involvement of central nervous system in CMTX neuropathy.

Table 1 summarizes blink reflex alterations in various polyneuropathies.

	R1 (latency)	R2i (latency)	R2c (latency)
Diabetic polyneuropathy	**Delayed**	**Delayed**	**Delayed**
Uremic neuropathy	**Delayed**	**Delayed**	**Delayed**
GBS	**Delayed**	**Delayed**	**Delayed**
CIDP	**Delayed**	**Delayed**	**Delayed**
Fisher syndrome	**Normal**	**Normal**	**Normal**
Polyneuritis cranialis	**Absent**	**Absent**	**Absent**
AntiGQ1b antibody syndrome	**Normal**	**Absent**	**Absent**
HMSN	**Delayed**	**Delayed**	**Delayed**

Table 1. Blink reflex alterations in various polyneuropathies.

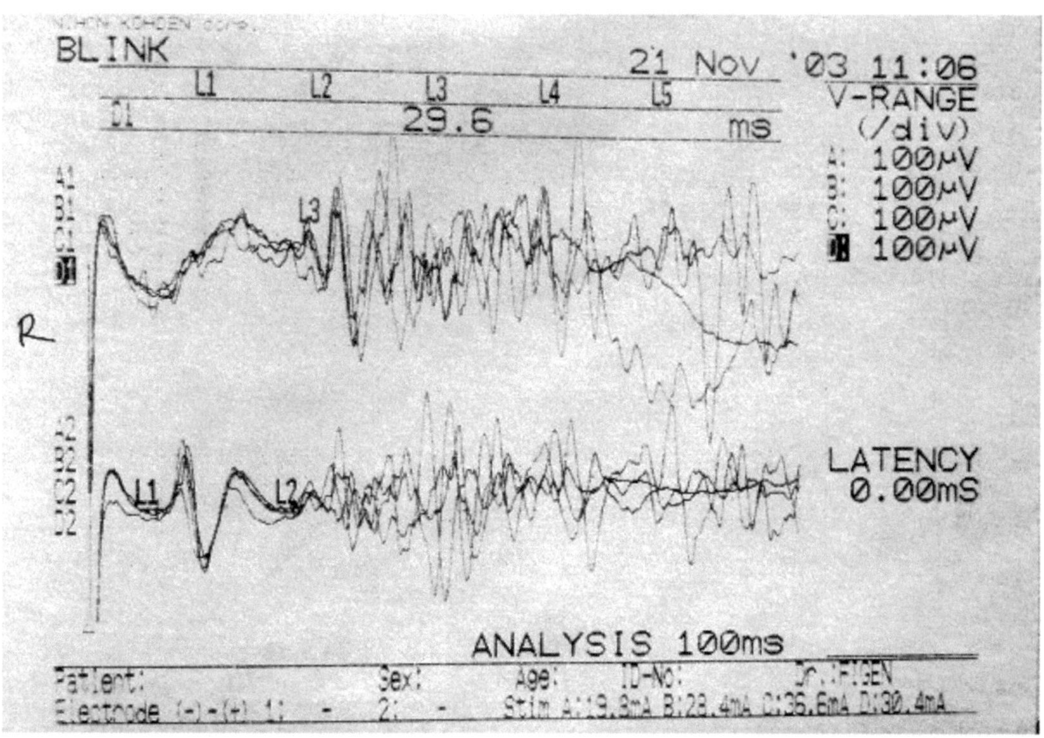

Fig. 1. Blink reflex in normal subject.

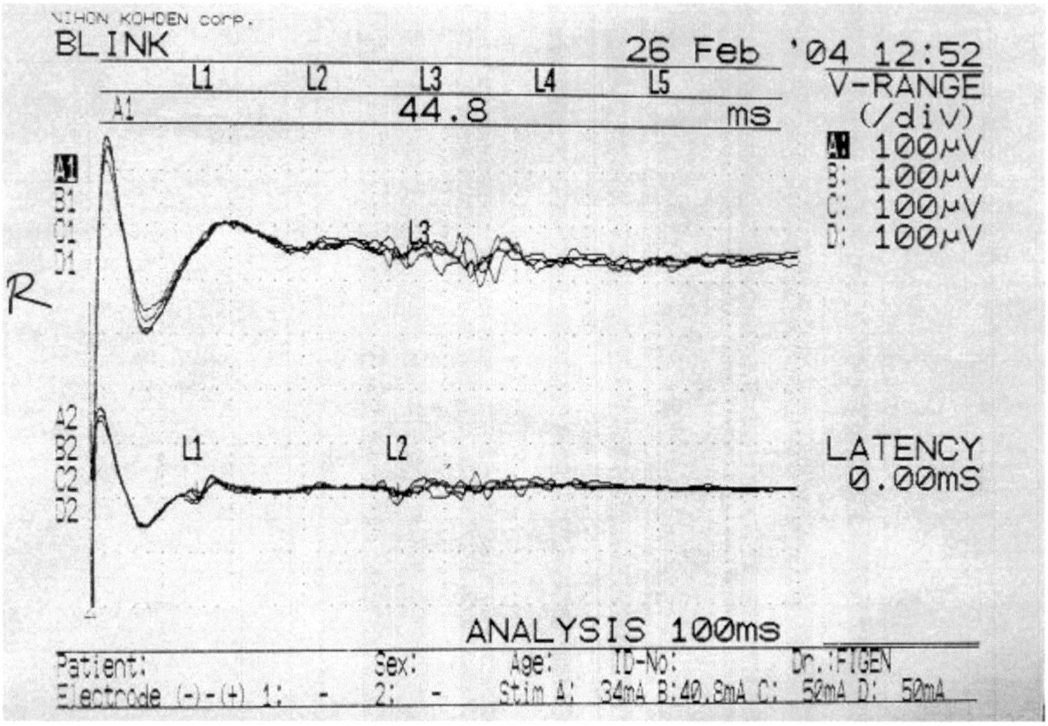

Fig. 2. Increased R1, R2i and R2c latencies in diabetic patient with polyneuropathy.

3. Conclusion

Finally blink reflex can be useful tool for detection of clinically silent intraaxial brainstem functional abnormalities or extraaxial lesions patients with polyneuropathy.

4. References

[1] Overend W. Preliminary note on a new cranial reflex. Lancet 1896; 1:619.
[2] Kugelberg E. Facial reflexes. Brain 1952; 75: 385-396.
[3] Kimura J. Conduction abnormalities of the facial and rigeminal nerves in polyneuropathy. Muscle Nerve 1982; 5: 149-154.
[4] Sanes JN, Ison JR. Conditions that affect the thresholds of the eyeblink reflex in human. J Neurol Neurosurg Psychiatry 1982; 45:543-9.
[5] Shahani BT, Young RR. Human orbicularis oculi reflexes. Neurology 1972; 22:149-54.
[6] Snow BJ, Frith RW. The relationship of eyelid movement to the ik reflex. J Neurol Sci 1989; 91: 179-89.
[7] Dengler R, Rechl F, Struppler A. Recruitment of single motor units in the human blink reflex. Neuroscience Lett 1982; 34: 301-5.
[8] Hiraoka M, Shimamura M. Neural mechanisms of the corneal blinking reflex in cat. Brain Res 1977; 125: 265-75.
[9] Esteban A. A neurophysiological approach to brainstem reflexes. Blink reflex. Neurophysiol Clin 1999; 29: 7-38.

[10] Polo A, Manganotti P, Zanette G, Grandis D. Polyneuritis cranialis: clinical and electrophysiological findings. J Neurol Neurosurg Psych 1992; 55: 398-400.
[11] Neau JP, Gil R, Boissonnot L, Lefevre JP. The blink reflex and stimulus detection by the facial nerve in 50 cases of Guillain Barre polyradiculitis. Acta Neurol Belg 1987; 87(1):12
[12] Ropper AH, Wijdicks EF, Shahani BT. Electrodiagnostic abnormalities in 113 consecutive patients with Guillain-Barre syndrome. Arch Neurol 1990; 47:881-7.
[13] Vucic S, Cairns KD, Black KR, Chong PST, Cros D. Neurophysiologic findings in early acute inflammatory demyelinating polyradiculoneuropathy. Clin Neurophysiol 2004; 115: 2329-2335.
[14] Cruccu G, Agostino R, Inghiller M, Innocenti P, Romaniello A, Manfredi M. Mandibular nerve involvement in diabetic polyneuropathy and chronic inflammatory demyelinating polyneuropathy. Muscle Nerve 1998; 21: 1673-1679.
[15] Kokubun N, Hirata K. Neurophysiological evaluation of trigeminal and facial nerves in patients with chronic inflammatory demyelinating polyneuropathy. Muscle Nerve 2007; 35: 203-207.
[16] Varela H, Rubin DI. Facial and trigeminal neuropathies as the initial manifestation of chronic inflammatory demyelinating polyradiculopathy. J Clin Neuromuscul Dis 2009; 10: 194-98.
[17] Ogawara K, Kuwabara S, Yuki N. Fisher syndrome or Bickerstaff brainstem encephalitis? Anti-GQ1b IgG antibody syndrome involving both the peripheral and central nervous systems. Muscle Nerve 2002; 26: 845-49.
[18] Urban PP, Forst T, Lenfers M, Koehler J, Connemann BJ, Beyer J. Incidence of subclinical trigeminal and facial nerve involvement in diabetes mellitus. Electromyogr Clin Neurophysiol 1999; 39: 267-72.
[19] Nazliel B, Yetkin I, Irkec C, Kocer B. Blink reflex abnormalities in diabetes mellitus. Diabetes Metab Res Rev 2001; 17: 396-400.
[20] Guney F, Demir O, Gonen MS. Blink reflex alterations in diabetic patients with or without polyneuropathy. Int J Neurosci 2008; 118(9): 1287-98.
[21] Trontelj MA, Trontelj JV. Reflex arc of the first component of the human blink reflex: a simgle motoneuron study. J Neurol Neurosurg Psychiatry 1978; 41: 538-47.
[22] Tamai Y, Iwamoto M, Tsujimoto T. Patway of the blink reflex in the brainstem of the cat: interneurons between the trigeminal nuclei and the facial nucleus. Brain Res 1986; 380: 19-25. Holstege G, Van Ham JJ, Tan J. Afferent projections to the orbicularis oculi motoneuronal cell group: An autoradiographic tracing study in the cat. Brain Res 1986; 374: 306-320.
[23] Schneider C. Le reflexe de clignement dans quelques polyneuropathies. Electrodiag Ther 1979; 16(1): 41-6.
[24] Strenge H. The blink reflex in chronic renal failure. J Neurol 1980; 222: 205-14.
[25] Stamboulis E, Scarpalezos S, Malliara-Loulakaki S, Voudiklari S, Koutra E. Blink reflex in patients submitted to chronic periodical hemodialysis. Electromyo Clin Neurophysiol 1987; 27: 19-23.
[26] Resende LAL, Caramori JCT, Kimaid PAT, Barretti P. Blink reflex in end-stage-renal disease patients undergoing hemodialysis. J Electromyogr Kinesiol 2002; 12: 159-63.

[27] Ishpekova BA, Christova LG, Alexandrov AS, Thomas PK. The electrophysiological profile of hereditary motor and sensory neuropathy-Lom. J Neurosurg Psychiatry 2005; 76: 875-78.
[28] Ellrich J, Hopf HC. The R3 component of the blink reflex: normative data and application in spinal lesions. Electroencephalogr Clin Neurophysiol 1996; 101: 349-54.
[29] Rossi B, Risaliti R, Rossi A. The R3 component of the blink reflex in man: a reflex response induced by activation of high threshold cutaneous afferents. Electroencephalogr Clin Neurophysiol 1989; 73: 334-40.
[30] Ellrich J, Bromm B, Hopf HC. Pain-evoked blink reflex. Muscle Nerve 1997; 20: 265-70.
[31] Ellrich J, Katsarava Z, Przywara S, Kaube H. Is the R3 component of the human blink reflex nociceptive in origin? Pain 2001; 91: 389-95.
[32] Zambelis T, Panas M, Kokotis P, Karadima G, Kararizou E, Karandreas N. Central motor and sensory pathway involvement in an X-linked Charcot-Marie-Tooth family. Acta neurol Belg 2008; 108: 44-47.
[33] Aramideh M, Ongerboer De Visser BW. Brainstem reflexes: Electrodiagnostic techniques, physiology, normative data, and clinical applications. Muscle Nerve 2002; 26:14-30.

Part 3

Clinical Manifestations of Peripheral Neuropathies

6

Polyneuropathy and Balance

Kathrine Jáuregui-Renaud
Instituto Mexicano del Seguro Social
México

1. Introduction

Equilibrium or balance is a complex skill, which describes the dynamics of the control of posture in preventing falling. It is required for maintaining a position, remaining stable while moving from one position to another, as well as for performing activities and moving freely; it also serves to maintain bodily orientation to the environment. From a biomechanical perspective, balance can be defined as the ability to maintain or return the body's centre of gravity within the limits of stability that are determined by the base of support (i.e., the area of the feet) (Horak, 1987).

During upright stance, body movements and external perturbations apply continuous torques, if balance is to be maintained, those perturbations must be opposed by coordinated motor responses. To maintain balance, it is required to choose appropriate responses to each perturbation, to modify these responses on the basis of sensory input and, finally, to produce the needed muscular contractions (Era et al., 1996). Reflex movements regulate muscle force; whereas automatic reactions (stretch reflex-based movements) resist possible disturbances. Patients with polyneuropathy often have a deteriorated proprioception and/or motor function, which may imply deficits on postural control and gait, with an increased risk of falling.

2. Postural control

Postural control has been defined as the control of the body's position in space for the purposes of balance and orientation (Shumway-Cook & Woollacott, 2000a), with variable attention requirements that depend on the task (Shumway-Cook & Woollacott, 2000b; Teasdale & Simoneau, 2001).

2.1 Posture

Postural control and its adaptation to the environment is based on background postural tone and on postural reactions (De Kleijn, 1923; Magnus, 1924), assisted by sensory feedback of mainly labyrinthine, visual, proprioceptive and cutaneous origin. Studies of normal stance have found the most rapid postural reactions to be a class of motor activities mediated primarily by inputs derived from the forces and motions of the feet upon the support surface (Nashner, 1977), foot sole and ankle muscle inputs contribute jointly to posture regulation (Kavounoudias et al., 2001). Locations of the centre of gravity close to the borders of limits of stability correspond to the region where balance cannot be maintained without moving the feet (Horak et al., 1989).

A stance position that provides good stability is maintained mainly by ankle torque; when segmental oscillation is allowed to minimize the effect of perturbations, hip mechanisms are mainly used instead of ankle mechanisms (Figure 1). Postural tone is predominantly observed at the extensor muscles that counteract the effect of gravity and depends on the motor responses, particularly the integrity of the myotatic reflex loop, tonic labyrinthine reflexes and neck and lumbar reflexes. However, there are also supporting reactions and placing reactions (tactile, visual and vestibular), which adapt the activity of the postural muscles of the limbs to their function of body support.
Sensory information from multiple sources is crucial for the neural control of body orientation and body stabilization. Unsteadiness can be detected very early by proprioceptive sensory systems responding to motion and muscle stretch at the ankle, knee and trunk, as well as by head linear and angular accelerations sensed by the vestibular system (Allum et al., 1993), while visual inputs appear to primarily influence later stabilizing reactions to the initial balance corrections (Allum, 1985; Allum et al., 1993).

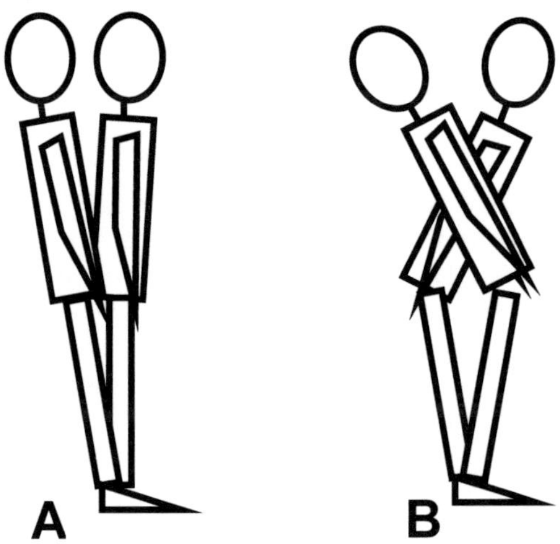

Fig. 1. Use of the ankle torque (A) or the hip (B), in order to maintain the centre of mass within the limits of stability.

The multiple sensory inputs may have an additive effect, without implying that the relative contributions of all sensory modalities have to be equivalent. Evidence support that the major contributor to balance control during quiet upright stance may be proprioceptive inputs (Allum et al., 1993; Horak et al., 1990). In the case of sensory conflict the nervous system may select one input that becomes dominant. However, a combined deficit of vestibular and somatosensory input may preclude adjustments to postural control (Aranda-Moreno et al., 2009).
Since balance perturbations cause stretch responses at the ankle, knee, hip and neck joints, balance corrections imply the interaction among several proprioceptive inputs (Allum et al., 1993). Once balance corrections are triggered it is generally accepted that a confluence of proprioceptive and vestibular modulation to the basic centrally initiated template of activity establishes the amplitude pattern of the muscle response synergy (Diener et al., 1988; Forssberg & Hirschfeld, 1994; Horak et al., 1994). Evidence suggests that somatosensory

information from the legs may be utilized for both, direct sensory feedback and use of prior experience in scaling the magnitude of automatic postural responses (Inglis et al., 1994).
Postural sway results in different but consistent patterns of discharge from muscle spindles, Golgi tendon organs and cutaneous receptors (Aniss et al., 1990). A number of different receptors in the legs and feet may provide the afferent information for the proprioceptive reflex but, because of the complex structure and dynamics of these receptors they don't transmit pure movement or torque information.
Disruption of somatosensory information from the feet only, by ischemic block at the ankle, results in normal muscle response latencies, but increased hip sway in response to support surface translations (Horak et al,. 1990). However, when the ischemic block is applied at the level of the thigh, which also blocks proprioceptive information from the muscles of the lower leg, body sway increases even more (Diener et al. 1984a).In standing humans, there is a notable attenuation of postural sway at frequencies above 1 Hz; sway may appear at this frequency when afferents from the leg muscles and feet are blocked with ischemia (Diener et al., 1984a; Mauritz & Dietz, 1980); proprioceptive reflex response to sway may also contribute significantly to stability at these frequencies (Fitzpatrick et al., 1992; Oppenheim et al., 1999). Also, significant attenuation is due to low-pass filtering by the body's inertia and the short-range visco-elastic stiffness of the ankles and leg muscles (Allum & Buidingen, 1979; Nashner, 1976).
The attention requirements for postural control vary depending on the postural task (Teasdale & Simoneau, 2001), the age of the individual and their balance abilities (Camicioli, 1997; Kerr, 1985; Woollacott, 2002). Even in young adults, postural control is demanding of attention; however not all cognitive tasks affect postural control in the same way, balance tasks may disrupt spatial but not nonspatial memory performance (Kerr et al., 1985). In both healthy and older adults with balance impairment, studies using dual task paradigms to examine attention requirements of balance control when performing a secondary task suggest that these are important contributions to instability, depending not only on the complexity of the task, but also on the type of the second task being performed (Camicioli et al., 1997; Woollacott & Shumway-Cook, 2002).

2.2 Gait

Human walking requires neural and muscular coordinated actions with adequate skeletal function; the generation and regulation of walking involve all levels of neural substrates, as well as an adequate function of several effectors. Walking differs from standing balance in that the centre of mass constantly moves beyond the base of support, and in fact the support leg can do little to alter this motion (Winter & Scott, 1991).
The gait cycle is divided into stance and swing phases:
STANCE PHASE:
- initial contact,
- loading response,
- mid stance,
- terminal stance,
- pre-swing.

SWING PHASE:
- initial,
- mid,
- terminal swing.

During initiation and termination of gait, ankle and hip mechanisms control the trajectory of the centre of pressure to ensure the desired acceleration and deceleration of the centre of mass; shifts of the centre of pressure are controlled by the hip abductors/adductors and the ankle plantar dorsi-flexors (Winter, 1995).
The control of placement of the swing foot can be used to stabilize balance by manipulating the redirection of the centre of mass that occurs as the foot contacts the ground (Townsend, 1985) (Figure 2). Besides peripheral inputs and proprioceptive reflexes processed in the spinal cord, the cerebellum, basal ganglia, and cortical mechanisms contribute to the motor control necessary for normal gait (Dietz, 2001).

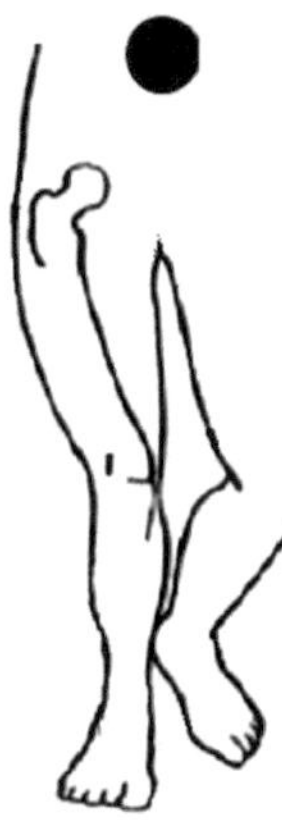

Fig. 2. Position of the center of mass.

3. Evaluation of postural control

3.1 Clinical history

Effective assessment of balance requires an understanding of the many systems underlying postural control. To assess a history of instability or walking difficulty, the clinician should evaluate the affected movements and circumstances in which they occur, as well as any other associated symptoms about postural control, motor control, muscular force, sensory deficiency and balance, including limitations imposed by pain, by restriction of joint range of motion and by muscle strength.
A history of falls is common in patients with disorders of balance and gait. If the occurrence of fall(s) is identified, it is important to investigate the circumstances in which each fall occurred, such as the environment (eg. environmental light) and the specific situation at the moment of falling (eg. activity & movement). Spontaneous falls are frequent in patients with sensory deficit (eg. sensory ataxia), who usually report unsteadiness that may be exacerbated under circumstances in which the visual information is reduced (eg. while walking in the dark).

3.2 Balance examination

In order to evaluate balance, a neurological examination is required. A proper evaluation should contain an examination of motor and sensory function, including: spinal column, joints with their range of motion, muscle tone and strength, reflex responses, proprioception, primary sensation as well as higher order aspects of sensation. Additional care should be taken to observe the postural control and gait, and to identify vestibular disorders.

The postural control during upright stance has to be observed, including the width of the stance, the symmetry/balance at the level of the joints and the trunk posture, during at least the following conditions: with the eyes open, with the eyes closed, while standing with the feet together, while balancing on the two legs and while standing on foam. Additionally, the reaction to push gently the patient while standing will provide information on postural reflexes. Patients with a sensory deficit usually show a wide base of support while standing, and they also have difficulties on maintaining balance when closing their eyes. This finding can easily be observed during Romberg´s test.

To evaluate gait, a sensory-motor evaluation should be performed, as well as a postural and skeletal examination (Thompson & Marsden, 1996). While observational gait assessment is relatively subjective in nature, instrumented gait assessment is restricted by the fact that it is laboratory based (Toro et al., 2003).

During observation of walking it is important to analyse the initiation, stepping and the associated movements. The initiation of walking requires a complex interaction of postural changes which could be affected by several factors; during stepping, at least the speed of walking, the rhythm and the length of each stride have to be evaluated; the synergy of the associated mobility of the trunk, arms and head can be helpful to identify a problem. In patients with somatosensory deficit the patient may guide the movement by vision and hit the floor with the heel.

A neuro-otological evaluation may detect vestibular deficiencies, which could be compounding polyneuropathy (eg. diabetic patients) or may have a different origin (central or peripheral). A detailed evaluation of long tracts, cranial nerves, motor control, the eyes and the ears should be performed. The evaluation of eye movements may include (Leigh & Zee, 1991): the inspection of the eyes as the patient keeps the head stationary and fixes upon a distant point to observe spontaneous eye movements (eg. spontaneous nystagmus), the range of movements in the plane of each pair of extra-ocular muscles, the eye convergence, the fast eye movements guided by visual stimuli (saccades), the slow eye movements guided by visual stimuli (smooth pursuit), the opto-kinetic response, the eye movement response to passive head movement and the eye movements during and after postural changes.

When spontaneous nystagmus is observed, it is classified according to the position of the eyes in which it is observed (Figure 3) and according to the direction of the fast phase: horizontal (right/left), vertical (up/down) or torsional (clockwise/ counter-clockwise).

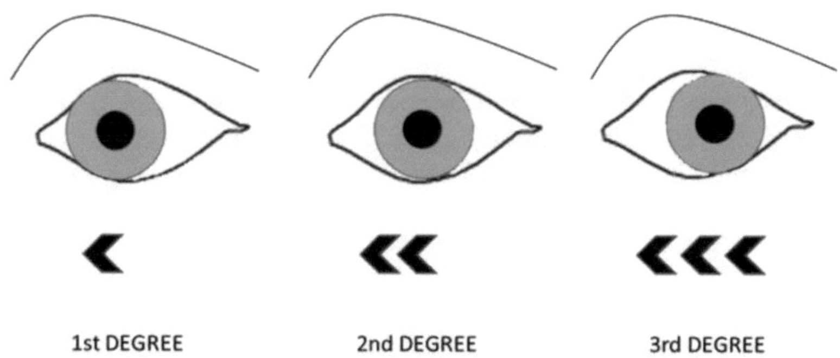

Fig. 3. Classification of horizontal spontaneous nystagmus: 1st degree when present only with gaze deviation in the fast phase direction, 2nd degree when present in primary gaze, and 3rd when it is evident even during gaze deviation in the direction opposite to the fast phase direction.

When it is not possible to identify slow and fast phases, it is a pendular nystagmus of central origin. To evaluate small eye movements or prevent visual fixation, the nystagmus can be observed during observation of the retina by ophthalmoscopy. However, in interpreting the findings during ophthalmoscopic examination, it should be noted that because the retina is behind the centre of rotation of the eye, the direction of the eye movement is the opposite of that observed by viewing the front of the eyes. When postural changes, such as the Hallpike manoeuvre, elicit postural nystagmus, the characteristics of its presentation suggest a peripheral or a central origin: a peripheral vestibular origin is consistent with a latent period, adaptation and fatigability, with accompanying vertigo.

To evaluate the vestibular system and its relationships with other sensory inputs and the oculo-motor system, specific tests have to be performed, including eye movement recordings and vestibular reflexes. There are several tests that require high technology equipment. However, the simplest test that can be applied with minimal technology is the bi-thermal caloric testing at 30°C and 44°C, to analyse the oculo-motor response to labyrinth stimulation by thermic changes.

When measuring balance, different aspects can be considered: neurophysiological recordings of the electric potentials due to muscle activation, kinematics concerned with movement itself and kinetics, which is concerned with the forces and the moments of forces that are developed during movements. Posturography platforms are used to record kinetic data. The analysis of the centre of pressure is used to assess the ability of a subject to maintain a stable stance over a period of time, while standing on the force platform (wearing a safety harness). Although it is difficult to unravel the vestibular, visual and somatosensory influence on balance, posturography platforms allow the general evaluation of the interactions between vestibulo-spinal and proprioceptive reflexes for balance control, and the influence of vision. The simplest method to record postural sway uses a force plate. These devices measure the position of the centre of force, according to the feet pressure on the surface of support, which is a good estimate of the position of the centre of mass during upright stance. Unfortunately, static force plates do not yield controlled stimulus-response measures.

To overcome the limitations of static force platforms, several moving force platforms have been designed. These devices can maintain a constant angle between the foot and lower leg and the movement of the visual enclosure of the platform can be coupled to the body sway.

Dynamic posturography is useful in the assessment of the equilibrium performance in patients with polyneuropathy. It has been proposed as a tool for the follow-up, to follow course of the balance deficit related to the disorder (Jáuregui-Renaud et al., 1998; Vrethem et al., 1991). In short, dynamic posturography uses a computer-controlled movable platform and movable visual surrounding; the platform and visual surrounding are either stable or moving, referenced to the patient, creating a disturbed proprioceptive and visual input (Nashner & Peters, 1990) (Figure 4). The test protocols usually include a sensory organization protocol, a motor control protocol and adaptation protocols.

Gait analysis includes the measurement of joint kinematics (concerned with movement itself), and kinetics (concerned with the forces developed during movements); other measurements commonly made are electromyography, oxygen consumption and foot pressures. Neurophysiological recordings are used to analyse the involvement of specific muscles or muscle groups during movement and the latency of their activation; a recording is made of the generation and propagation of action potentials in nerve and muscle cells.

Kinematics can be evaluated by opto-electric methods, among them is the use of opto-electric imaging systems to record the movements of body segments and their directions; another option is to track the position of the body segments by measuring the positions of light-emitting markers.

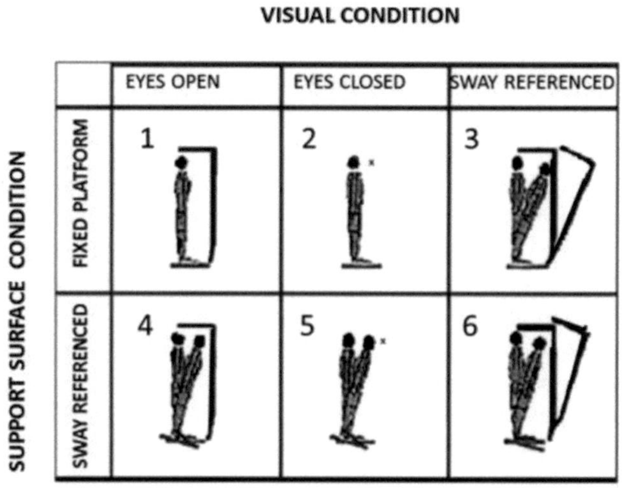

Fig. 4. Sensory conditions of Dynamic Posturography (Nashner & Peters, 1990): 1. Eyes open with fixed surrounding and fixed support. 2. Eyes closed with fixed support. 3. Sway-referenced surrounding with fixed support. 4. Eyes open with fixed surrounding and sway-referenced support. 5. Eyes closed with sway-referenced support. 6. Sway-referenced surrounding with sway-referenced support.

Research investigating human gait has traditionally focused on kinematic variables (eg, joint angles, stride length, walking velocity). Power is the kinetic variable that reflects the rate of work performed at a given joint (Mueller et al., 1994). It can be calculated by taking the product of the moment and the joint angular power; it will be positive when the moment and the angular velocity have the same direction. A positive power usually indicates that the muscle is generating mechanical energy (concentric contraction).A negative power usually indicates that the muscle is absorbing mechanical energy (eccentric contraction) Although muscle power varies during walking, the power generated by the plantar flexors at push-off is typically the largest power burst recorded during the gait cycle (Minor et al., 1994).

Other methods to evaluate balance include standardized scales and clinical tests. Functionally directed balance tests are typically dynamic tests that measure a person's ability to maintain balance as the subject walks or performs tasks to simulate the actions of daily activities and work. The choice of a clinical tool needs to reflect the purpose for which the tool is to be applied. If the purpose is to screen for high-risk populations, a tool is needed that is quick and easy to apply, yet has good sensitivity and specificity. If the purpose is to reduce risk, the tool needs to reliably identify remediable risk factors on which interventions can be focused.

Among the functional balance scores and performance scales are the "Get up and go test" (Podsiadlo & Richardson, 1991), the Berg's Balance Scale (1992) and the Tinetti scale (1986).

Although these scores and scales do not give specific information about the origin of balance impairment, they are useful to evaluate and follow-up deficits that are evident on circumstances of daily life. There are also a number of fall-risk assessment tools available with some evidence to support their use in predicting risk of falls (Scott et al., 2007).
On the basis of predictive values of 70% or higher for both sensitivity and specificity of the instrument (Olivier et al., 2004; Perell et al., 2001), some tools tested with predictive validity are the 5 min walk, the five-step test and the Functional Reach (Wang et al., 2005), the Mobility Fall Chart (Lundin-Olsson et al., 2000) and the evidence based risk assessment tool (Olivier et al., 1997).
To interpret the results of any balance evaluation, several factors have to be considered. Regardless of the technique of measurement used, standing body sway has been generally shown to increase with age, with an increased dependence on vision (Colledge et al., 1994; Poulain & Giraudet, 2008). Deterioration in balance function clearly starts at relatively young ages and further accelerates from about 60 years upwards; males tend to have more pronounced sway than females, and the difference increases in the older age groups (Era et al., 2006). Evidence suggests that body weight may also have an influence on postural stability, particularly when vision is not available (Cruz-Gómez et al., 2011).
Among other factors, in patients with polyneuropathy, adaptive compensation to changes in biomechanical factors and vice versa may complicate evaluation of the source of balance impairment. Plantar ulceration is the most common consequence of the loss of sensation in the lower extremities, patients with diabetes may have limited joint mobility of the feet independent from peripheral neuropathy (Shinabarger, 1987), as well as visual deficiency related to retinopathy.

4. Postural control and gait of patients with polyneuropathy

Intact balance is required to maintain postural stability as well to assure safe mobility during activities of daily life. Maintaining balance encompasses the acts of maintaining, achieving or restoring the body center of mass relative to the limits of stability, which are given by the base of support (Pollock, 2000). Reduced somatosensory information from the lower limbs in human beings alters the ability both, to trigger postural responses to perturbations in stance and to scale the magnitude of the response to the magnitude of the perturbation (Diener et al., 1984b; Horak et al.,1990; Jáuregui-Renaud et al., 1998) (Figure 5). Performance on clinical balance tests is associated with electrophysiological and clinical measures of neuropathy (Goldberg et al., 2008).
Subjects with severe neuropathy are significantly less stable than normal subjects and patients without neuropathy (Oppenheim et al., 1999). Patients with polyneuropathy exhibit decreased stability while standing and walking (Boucher et al., 1995; Richardson et al., 1992; Simoneau et al., 1994), as well as when subjected to dynamic balance conditions (Bloem et al., 2000; Inglis et al., 1994). Evidence suggests that the role of peripheral sensory information in postural control may differ depending both, on the postural control task and on the quality of the sensory information available (Inglis et al., 1994). Compared to healthy age/sex matched controls, in patients with severe peripheral neuropathy without known origin, visual and vestibular input cannot fully compensate for the impairment in proprioception, with progressive deterioration of balance (Jáuregui-Renaud et al., 1998) (Figure 6).

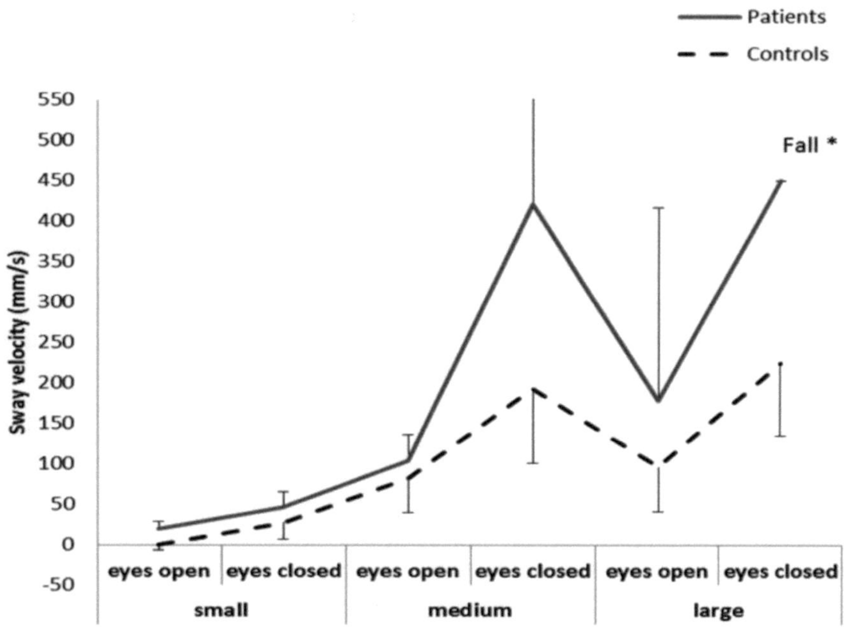

Fig. 5. Mean and standard deviation of the mean of sway velocity of 14 patients with polyneuropathy of unknown origin and 14 age/sex matched healthy controls, during responses to small, medium and large anterior-posterior translations of the support surface fashion (Jáuregui-Renaud 1998). (*) During the large translations with eyes closed 13/14 patients fell.

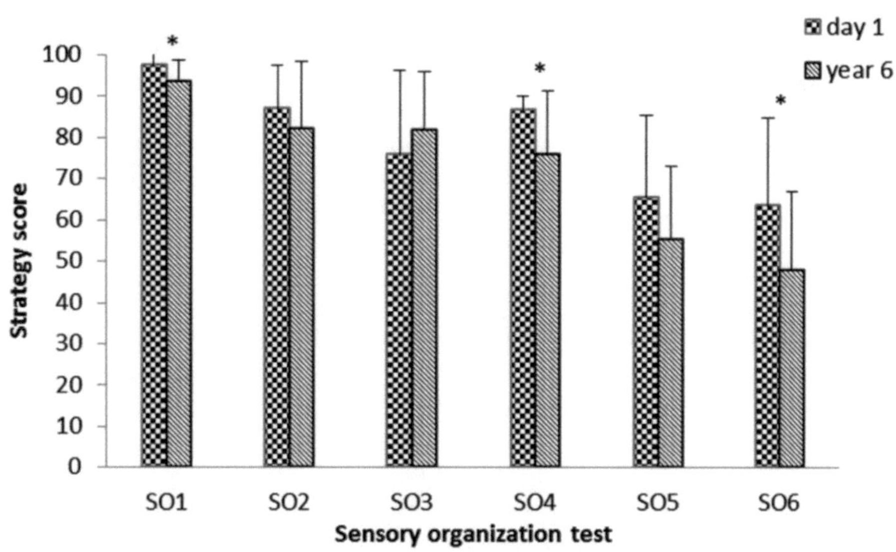

Fig. 6. Mean and standard deviation of the mean of the strategy scores, related to the amount of shear forces generated, during the six sensory organization conditions of dynamic posturography, of 14 patients with polyneuropathy of unknown origin during a 6 year follow-up (Jáuregui-Renaud 1998). (* $p<0.05$)

A frequent source of polyneuropathy is diabetes mellitus; its clinical characteristics make it a unique neurophysiological model to study balance problems related to polyneuropathy. Peripheral diabetic neuropathy is initially characterized by a reduction in somesthesic sensitivity due to the sensitive nerve damage.

The prevalence of sensory ataxia in diabetic patients ranges from 10% to 90% depending on screening protocol and criteria to define neuropathy (Vinik et al., 2000). With the progression of the diabetic neuropathy, motor nerves are damaged. In neuropathic patients, the peroneal nerve and the sural nerve frequently present abnormalities in electrophysiological tests (Dyck et al., 1985). However, the frequency of balance symptoms in diabetic patients is related to both the time elapsed since the diabetes was diagnosed and the history of peripheral neuropathy and retinopathy (Jáuregui-Renaud et al., 2009), and the bio-mechanical impairment caused by progression of foot complications has to be considered in addition to the instability caused by neuropathy (Kanade et al., 2008).

During posturography, compared to patients without neuropathy, patients with diabetic polyneuropathty may show: larger area of sway and speed of sway (Boucher et al., 1995; Uccioli et al., 1995), as well as larger center of pressure range (Simoneau et al., 1994) and increased oscillation at 0.5-1 Hz (Oppenheim et al., 1999). In this group of patients, the standing balance area of sway may predict functional gait (Manor & Li, 2009).

Although patients with diabetic sensory neuropathy may show a normal distal-to-proximal dorsal muscle activation pattern in response to backward support surface translation, their electromyography onset latencies may be delayed by 20-30 ms at all segments when compared with age-matched control subjects (Meyer et al., 2004). The consistency in delays at all segments, despite the fact that diabetic neuropathy is more severe in distal limb segments than in proximal leg segments and the trunk, suggests that slowed sensory conduction in the lower legs results in the late onset of an otherwise intact, centrally programmed response (Meyer et al., 2004).

The most effective gait allows a person to move over a variety of terrains safely and with minimal effort. In neuropathic gait, there is a longer support phase related to a flexor dysfunction of the tibialis anterior during the flat foot phase and also to a typical delay of the recruitment of tibialis anterior, peroneus brevis and longus and soleus (Mueller et al., 1994; Abboud et al., 2000). Polyneuropathy modifies the amount and the quality of the information necessary to motor control. Consequently, there is an increase in instability during gait (Richardson et al., 1992). The gait velocity, step length, amplitude of ankle movement, ankle moments of force, power and anterior-posterior ground reaction force variables are smaller in diabetic patients with polyneuropathy, compared to control subjects (Mueller et al. 1994). This group of patients may show decreased ankle plantar-flexor strength and ankle mobility compared with age-matched controls, as well as increased frontal plane motion at the ankle (Katoulis et al., 1997). The use of dual force platforms has also shown that ankle evertor/ invertor motor activities are impaired (Lafond et al., 2004). These deficits appear to contribute to the limited ankle motion, ankle moments, ankle power, stride length, and velocity during walking. Also, reaction times while walking may be higher for diabetic neuropathic patients than for control subjects (Courtemanche et al., 1996).

Diabetic patients with polyneuropathy may show greater hip moments and power than ankle moments and power during terminal stance, opposite to the pattern shown by control subjects (Minor et al., 1994); they appear to pull their leg forward using hip flexor muscles rather than pushing the leg forward using plantar flexor muscles.

During gait, the motor system will generate motor responses according to the mechanical loads received by the foot in order to attenuate the load in this initial contact. In diabetic patients with polyneuropathy, the study of the plantar pressure distribution and electromyographic activity of tibialis anterior, peroneus brevis, peroneus longus and soleus muscles during gait, have shown that all these muscles present an important delay in their recruitment (Abboud et al., 2000).The feet of the diabetic patients contact the ground in mid-stance earlier than what has been verified for healthy subjects, and the forefoot keeps longer contact with the ground during stance phase and presents higher peak pressure in comparison with other plantar areas (Abboud et al., 2000).

The tibialis anterior has a fundamental role in the initial contact phase of gait. Its function is to reduce the initial shock of the forefoot during the flat foot phase (Winter & Scott, 1991). In patients with polyneuropathy, if a delay in the tibialis anterior activation occurs, the shock attenuation mechanism will fail, and higher loads on the forefoot are generated, with an alteration in the contribution of the ankle (Sacco & Amadio, 2003).

Older women with polyneuropathy may walk reasonably stable on flat surfaces with good lighting, but their gait speed under these ideal circumstances is somewhat slower than needed in the community for crossing streets; under ideal conditions they are able to regulate their gait to a similar degree as healthy women of similar age, but at the cost of speed and efficiency. In addition, when the environment is challenging, the gait speed of this group of patients may be severely reduced (Richardson et al., 2004).

5. Polyneuropathy and falls

A fall is often defined as inadvertently coming to rest on the ground, floor or other lower level, excluding intentional change in position to rest in furniture, wall or other objects (World Health Organization, 2007). Falls occur as a result of complex interactions among demographic, physical and behavioural risk factors. Risk factors have been identified and categorized as intrinsic or extrinsic factors: intrinsic factors include demographic and biological factors, while extrinsic factors encompass environmental and behavioural factors (WHO, 2007).

Gait and balance problems are the most frequently cited cause of falling in all age and gender groups, but women have a higher percentage of falls than men (Talbot et al., 2005). In older people, falls are a risk factor for disability and may account for 40% of all injury deaths (Rubinstein, 2006). While approximately one in three older people fall each year, this proportion varies depending on the country and the target population studied (WHO, 2007). In this age group, the majority of falls occur while walking on a level surface during ordinary daily activities in the absence of hazardous behaviour (Talbot et al., 2005; Niino et al, 2000).

During physical examination of older patients, peripheral neurologic deficits are commonly found. Among the causes are: diabetes mellitus, alcoholism, nutritional deficiencies, malignancies, and autoimmune diseases. When somato-sensation is affected (eg. neuropathy or after anaesthesia) a decline in control of balance may occur, associated with an increased risk of falling (Simoneau et al., 1994; Van Deursen & Simoneau 1999). However, quantifying the somatosensory loss cannot fully predict falls. Evidence support that older persons with polyneuropathy are at a markedly increased risk for injurious falls (Cavanah et al., 1992; Richardson et al., 1992).

Epidemiological surveys have established that a reduction of leg proprioception is a risk factor for falls in the elderly (Lord et al., 1996; Richardson & Hurvitz., 1995). Even with vision, the postural stability of neuropathic patients is impaired and may put them at higher risk of falling when performing challenging daily tasks (Boucher et al., 1995).

A study focused to investigate if polyneuropathy could be just a marker for a comorbidity (e.g., central nervous system dysfunction) as the true cause of falls, have shown that polyneuropathy is a true risk factor for falls in the elderly (Richardson & Hurvitz 2005). In this group of patients, loss of plantar sensation may be an important contributor to the dynamic balance deficits and increased risk of falls (Meyer et al., 2004). Cavanagh et al. (1992) reported that patients with diabetes and peripheral neuropathy were 15 times more likely to report an injury (fall, fracture, sprained ankle, or cuts and bruises) during walking or standing, compared to subjects in a control group of patients with diabetes but no peripheral neuropathy.

The ability to re-weight sensory information depending on the sensory context is important for maintaining stability when an individual moves from one sensory context to another, such as a flat walking surface to an uneven surface or a well-lit sidewalk to a dimly lit garden. Individuals with peripheral vestibular loss or somatosensory loss from neuropathy are limited in their ability to re-weight postural sensory dependence (Jáuregui-Renaud et al., 1998; Agrawal et al., 2010) and thus, they are at risk of falling in particular sensory contexts. Older patients with peripheral neuropathy have a high rate of falls associated with walking on irregular surfaces (DeMott et al., 2007). Compared to healthy subjects, patients with diabetes and peripheral neuropathy may show poorer balance during standing in diminished light compared to full light and no light conditions (Petrofsky et al., 2006).

However, peripheral neuropathy and retinopathy may not completely account for the measures of physical performance significantly associated with increased risk for falling (Shwartz et al, 2008). Subjects with lower extremity weakness, usually measured by knee extension, ankle dorsiflexion, and chair stands, have a 1.8-fold increased risk of falling and three-fold risk for recurrent falls (Moreland et al., 2004). Among other risk factors, the occurrence of falls may be significantly associated with a best-corrected Snellen visual acuity of less than 6/12 (Kuang et al, 2008), the use of four or more prescription medications (Tinetti et al., 2003; Huang et al., 2009) and foot deformities (Cavanah et al., 1992; WHO, 2007). In addition, fear of falling and poor physical performance commonly occurs after falls (Tinetti et al., 1994). One of the major consequences of fear of falling is the restriction and avoidance of activities, which results in muscle atrophy and loss of strength, especially in the lower extremities, and may also be predictive for future falls (Maki et al., 1991; Delbaere et al., 2004).

In order to modify the risk of falling a multidisciplinary approach is required; some of the modifiable or preventable risk factors may include: balance and gait deficits, psychological factors like fear of falling, polypharmacy, lower extremity impairments and environmental threats. However, crucial to the success of any intervention is changing the beliefs, attitudes and behaviour of both, the people/community and the health/ social care professionals.

The World Health Organization Model for Prevention of Falls is built around three pillars (WHO, 2007):

1. building awareness of the importance of falls prevention and treatment;
2. improving the assessment of individual, environmental and societal factors that increase the likelihood of falls; and
3. facilitating the design and implementation of culturally-appropriated evidence based interventions that will significantly reduce the number of falls.

Health professionals, particularly those who take care of patients with polyneuropathy, have a critical opportunity to identify individual risk factors for falling and to identify the best evidence to select the most appropriate evaluations and interventions needed for the prevention and treatment of falls.

6. Conclusions

Balance encompasses the acts of maintaining, achieving and restoring the body centre of mass relative to the limits of stability, in preventing falling.

Postural stability is dependent upon integration of signals from the somatosensory, visual and vestibular systems, with central integration, to generate motor responses.

Assessment of balance requires an understanding of the many systems underlying postural control. To evaluate balance, a neurological examination is required, including motor and sensory function, as well as postural control and gait. Measures of standing balance may be performed using neurophysiological recordings of the electric potentials due to muscle activation, kinematics concerned with movement itself and kinetics.

The analysis of the centre of pressure during upright stance is used to assess the ability of a subject to maintain a stable stance over a period of time. The simplest method to record postural sway uses a force plate to measure the position of the centre of force, according to the feet pressure on the surface of support (Static posturography). To further evaluate the control of posture, moving force platforms and visual surroundings have been designed to modify the somatosensory and visual inputs (Dynamic posturography). Gait analysis may include the measurement of joint kinematics and kinetics, electromyography, oxygen consumption and foot pressures Other methods to evaluate dynamic balance include standardized scales, which are usually directed to measure a person's ability to maintain balance while performing tasks to simulate the actions of daily activities.

Polyneuropathy modify the amount and the quality of the sensorial information that is necessary for motor control, with increased instability during both, upright stance and gait. Compared to healthy controls, in patients with severe peripheral neuropathy, visual and vestibular input may not fully compensate for the impairment in proprioception, with progressive deterioration of balance. During posturography, patients with diabetic polyneuropathty may show an increase of both the area of sway and the speed of sway, as well as an increased sway at medium - high frequencies. In this group of patients, gait may also be deficient, even under ideal circumstances (level surface with good lighting).

Spontaneous falls are frequent in patients with sensory deficit, who usually report unsteadiness that may be exacerbated under circumstances in which the visual information is reduced. In patients with peripheral polyneuropathy, reduced somatosensory information from the lower limbs also deteriorate the ability to produce adequate postural responses to perturbations in stance.

Gait and balance problems are the most frequently cited cause of falling in all age and gender groups, and polyneuropathy is a risk factor for falls in the elderly. Individuals with somatosensory loss from neuropathy are limited in their ability to re-weight postural sensory inputs and, they are at risk of falling particularly in challenging contexts. However, several factors may account for the measures of physical performance significantly associated with increased risk for falling, such as foot deformities, deficient visual acuity, polypharmacy and fear of falling.

The health care providers, who take care of patients with polyneuropathy, have a critical role to play in identifying individual risk factors for falling and selecting appropriate interventions for the prevention and treatment of falls.

7. References

Abboud, R.J., Rowley, D.I., Newton, R.W. (2000). Lower limb muscle dysfunction may contribute to foot ulceration in diabetic patients. *Clinical Biomechanics (Bristol, Avon)*, Vol. 15,No. 1, (January 2000), pp. (37-45), ISSN 0268-0033

Agrawal, Y., Carey, J., Della, Santina. C., Schubert, M., Minor, L.B. (2010). Diabetes, Vestibular Dysfunction, and Falls: Analyses From the National Health and Nutrition Examination Survey. *Otology & Neurotology*, Vol.31,No. 9,(December 2010), pp. (1445-1450), ISSN 1531-7129

Allum, J.H., Budingen, H.J. (1979). Coupled stretch reflexes in ankle muscles: an evaluation of the contributions of active muscle mechanisms to human posture stability. *Progress in Brain Research*, Vol. 50, No. 1, (n.d. 1979), pp. (185-195), ISSN 0079-6123

Allum, J.H., Honegger, F., Schicks, H. (1993). Vestibular and proprioceptive modulation of postural synergies in normal subjects. *Journal of Vestibular Research: Equilibrium & Orientation*, Vol. 3, No. 1, (Spring 1993), pp. (59-85). ISSN 0957-4271

Aniss, A.M., Diener, H.C., Hore, J., Burke, D., Gandevia, S.C. (1990). Reflex activation of muscle spindles in human pretibial muscles during standing. *Journal of Neurophysiology*, Vol. 64, No. 2, (August 1990), pp. (671-679), ISSN 0022-3077

Aranda-Moreno, C., Meza, A., Rodriguez, R., Mantilla, M.T., Jáuregui-Renaud, K. (2009). Diabetic polyneuropathy may increase the handicap related to vestibular disease. *Archives of Medical Research*, Vol 40, No. 3, (April 2009), pp. (180-185), ISSN 0188-4409

Berg, K.O., Wood-Dauphinee, S.L., Williams, J.I., Maki, B.E. (1992). Measuring balance in the elderly: validation of an instrument. *Canadian Journal of Public Health*, Vol. 83, Suppl 2, (July-August 1992), pp. (S7-S11), ISSN 0008-4263

Bloem, B.R., Allum, J.H., Carpenter, M.G., Honegger, F. (2000). Is lower leg proprioception essential for triggering human automatic postural responses? *Experimental Brain Research*, Vol. 130, No. 3, (February 2000), pp. (375-391), ISSN 0014-4819

Boucher, P., Teasdale, N., Courtemanche, R., Bard, C., Fleury, M. (1995). Postural stability in diabetic polyneuropathy. *Diabetes Care*, Vol. 18, No. 5, (May 1995), pp. (638-645), ISSN 0149-5992

Camicioli, R., Howieson, D., Lehman, S. (1997). Talking while walking: the effect of a dual task in ageing and Alzheimer's disease. *Neurology*, Vol. 48, No. 4 (April 1997), pp. (955-958), ISSN 0028-3878

Cavanagh, P.R., Derr, J.A., Ulbrecht, J.S., Maser, R.E., Orchard, T.J. (1992). Problems with gait and posture in neuropathic patients with insulin- dependent diabetes mellitus. *Diabetic Medicine*, Vol. 9, No, 5, (June 1992), pp. (469-474), ISSN 0742-3071

Colledge, N.R., Cantley, P., Peaston, I., Brash, H., Lewi,s S., Wilson, J.A. (1994). Aging and balance: the measurement of spontanaeous sway by posturography. *Gerontology*, Vol. 40, No. 5, (1994), pp. (273-278). ISSN 0734-0664

Courtemanche, R., Teasdale, N., Boucher, P., Fleury, M., Lajoie, Y, Bard C. (1996). Gait problems in diabetic neuropathic patients. *Archives of Physical Medicine and Rehabilitation*, Vol. 77, No. 9, (September 1996), pp. (849-855), ISSN 0003-9993

Cruz-Gómez, N.S., Plascencia, G., Villanueva-Padrón, L.A., Jáuregui-Renaud, K. (2011) Influence of obesity and gender on the postural stability during upright stance. Obesity Facts, Vol. 4, No. 3, (June 2011), pp. (212-217), ISSN 1662-4025

De Kleijn, A. Experimental physiology of eth labyrinth. (1923). *Journal of Laryngology and Otology*, Vol. 38, No. 12, (December 1923), pp. (646-663), ISSN 0022-2151

Delbaere, K., Crombez, G., Vanderstraeten, G., Willems, T., Cambier, D. (2004). Fear-related avoidance of activities, falls and physical frailty. A prospective community-based cohort study. *Age and Ageing*, Vol. 33, No. 4, (July 2004), pp. (368-373), ISSN 0002-0729

DeMott, T.K., Richardson, J.K., Thies, S.B., Ashton-Miller, J.A. (2007). Falls and gait characteristics among older persons with peripheral neuropathy. *American Journal of Physical Medicine and Rehabilitation*, Vol. 86, No. 2, (February 2007), pp. (125-132), ISSN 0894-9115

Diener, H.C., Dichgans, J., Guschlbauer, B., Mau, H.(1984a). The significance of proprioception on postural stabilization as assessed by ischemia. *Brain Research*, Vol. 296, No. 1, (March 1984), pp. (103-109), ISSN 0006 8993

Diener, H.C., Dichgans, J., Bootz, F., Bacher, M. (1984b). Early stabilization of human posture after a sudden disturbance: influence of rate and amplitude of displacement. *Experimental Brain Research*, Vol. 56, No. 1, (August 1984), pp. (126-134), ISSN 0014-4819

Diener, H.C., Horak, F.B., Nashner, L.M. (1988). Influence of stimulus parameters on human postural responses. *Journal of Neurophysiology*, Vol. 59, No. 6, (June 1988), pp. (1888-1905) ISSN 0022-3077

Dietz, V. Physiology of human gait: neural processes. (2001). *Advances in Neurology* 2001;Vol. 87, (n.d. 2001), pp. (53–61), ISSN 0091-3952

Dyck, P.J., Karnes, J.L., Daube, J., O'Brien, P., Service, F.J. (1985). Clinical and neuropathological criteria for the diagnosis and staging of diabetic polyneuropathy. *Brain*, Vol. 108, Pt. 4, (December 1985), pp. (861–880), ISSN 0006-8950

Era, P., Schroll, M., Ytting, H., Gause-Nilsson, I., Heikkinen, E., Steen, B. (1996). Postural balance and its sensory - motor correlates in 75-year-old men and women: A cross-national comparative study. *Journals of Gerontology. Series A, Biological Sciences and Medical Sciences*, Vol. 51, No. 2, (March 1996), pp. (M53 -M63), ISSN 1079-5006

Era, P., Sainio, P., Koskinen, S., Haavisto, P., Vaara, M., Aromaa, A. (2006). Postural balance in a random sample of 7,979 subjects aged 30 years and over. *Gerontology*, Vol. 52, No. 4 (2006), pp. (204-213), ISSN 0304-324X

Fitzpatrick, R.C., Gorman, R.B., Burke, D., Gandevia, S.C. (1992). Postural Proprioceptive Reflexes In Standing Human Subjects: Bandwidth of response and transmission characteristics. *Journal of Physiology*, Vol. 458, (December 1992), pp. (69-83). ISSN 0022-3751

Forssberg, H., Hirschfeld, H. Postural adjustments in sitting humans following external perturbations: muscle activity and kinematics. (1994). *Experimental Brain Research*, Vol. 97, No. 3, (January 1994), pp. (515–527), ISSN 0014-4819

Goldberg, A., Russell, J.W., Alexander, N.B. Standing Balance and Trunk Position Sense in Impaired Glucose Tolerance (IGT)-Related Peripheral Neuropathy, (2008). *Journal of the Neurological Sciences*, Vol. 270, No. 1-2, (July 2008), pp. (165 -171), ISSN 0022-510X

Horak, F.B. (1987). Clinical measurement of postural control in adults. (1987). *Physical Therapy*, Vol. 67, No. 12, (Dec1987), pp. (1881-1885), ISSN 0031-902

Horak, F.B., Shupert, C.L., Mirka, A. (1989). Components of postural sway dyscontrol in the elderly: a review. Neurobiology of Aging, Vol. 10, No. 6, (November-December 1989), pp. (727-738), ISSN 0197-4580

Horak, F.B., Nashner, L.M., Diener, H.C. (1990). Postural strategies associated with somatosensory and vestibular loss. *Experimental Brain Research,* Vol. 82, No. 1, (August 1990), pp. (167-177), ISSN 0014-4819

Horak, F.B., Shupert, C.L., Dietz, V., Horstmann, G. (1994). Vestibular and somatosensory contributions to responses to head and body displacements in stance. *Experimental Brain Research,* Vol 100, No. 1, (July 1994), pp. (93-106), ISSN 0014-4819

Huang, E.S., Karter, A.J., Danielson, K., Warton, E.M., Ahmed, A.T. (2010). The Association Between the Number of Prescription Medications and Incident Falls in a Multi-ethnic Population of Adult Type-2 Diabetes Patients: The Diabetes and Aging Study. *Journal of General Internal Medicine,* Vol. 25, No. 2; (February 2010), pp. (141-146), ISSN 0884-8734

Inglis, J.T., Horak, F.B., Shupert, Ch.L., Jones-Rycewicz, C. (1994). The importance of somatosensory information in triggering and scaling automatic postural responses in humans. *Experimental Brain Research,* Vol. 101, No. 1, (September 1994), pp. (159-164), ISSN 0014-4819

Jáuregui-Renaud, K., Kovacsovics, B., Vrethem, M., Odjvist L.M., Ledin, T. (1998). Dynamic and Randomized perturbed posturography in the follow-up of patients with polyneuropathy. *Archives of Medical Research,* Vol. 29, No. 1, (Spring 1998), pp. (39-44), ISSN 0188-4409

Jáuregui-Renaud, K., Sánchez, B.M., Ibarra-Olmos, A., González-Barcena, D. (2009). Neuro-otologic symptoms in patients with type 2 diabetes mellitus. *Diabetes Research and Clinical Practice,* Vol 84, No. 3, (June 2009), pp. (e45-47). ISSN 0168-8227

Kanade, R.V., Van Deursen, R.W., Harding, K.G., Price, P.E. (2008). Investigation of standing balance in patients with diabetic neuropathy at different stages of foot complications. *Clinical Biomechanics (Bristol, Avon),* Vol. 23, No. 9 (November 2008), pp. (1183-1191), ISSN 0268-0033

Katoulis, E.C., Ebdon-Parry, M., Lanshammar, H., Vileikyte, L., Kulkarni, J., Boulton, A.J.M. 1997 Gait abnormalities in diabetic neuropathy. *Diabetes Care, Vol.* 20, No. 12, (December 1997), pp. (1904-1907), ISSN 0149-5992

Kavounoudias, A., Roll, R., Roll, JP. Foot sole and ankle muscle inputs contribute jointly to human erect posture regulation. *Journal of Physiology,* Vol. 5532, Pt. 3, (May 2001), pp. (869-878), ISSN 0022-3751

Kerr, B., Condon, S.M., McDonald, L.A. (1985). Cognitive spatial processing and the regulation of posture. *Journal of Experimental Psychology. Human Perception and Performance,* Vol. 11, No. 5, (October 1985), pp. (617-622), ISSN 0096-1523

Kuang, T.M., Tsai, S.Y., Hsu, W.M,, Cheng, C.Y., Liu, J.H., Chou, P. (2008). Visual Impairment and Falls in the Elderly: The Shihpai Eye Study. Journal of the Chinese Medical Association, Vol. 71, No. 9, (September 2008) pp. (467-472), ISSN 1726-4901

Lafond, D., Corriveau, H., Prince, F. (2004). Postural control mechanisms during quiet standing in patients with diabetic sensory neuropathy. *Diabetes Care,* Vol. 27, No. 1, (January 2004), pp. (8173-178), ISSN 0149-5992

Leigh, J.R., Zee, D.S. (1991). *The Neurology of eye movements*, F.A. Davis Company, ISBN 0 8036 5528 2, Philadelphia, United States of America

Lord, S.R., Lloyd, D.G., Li, S.K. (1996). Sensori-motor function, gait patterns and falls in community-dwelling women. *Age and Ageing*, Vol. 25, No. 4, (July 1996), pp. (292-299), ISSN 0002-0729

Lundin-Olsson, L., Nyberg, L., Gustafson, Y. (2000). The mobility interaction fall chart. *Physiotherapy Research International*, Vol. 5, No. 3, (n.d. 2000), pp. (190–201), ISSN 1358-2267

Magnus, R. (1924). *Körperstellung*. Springer, Berlin, Germany

Maki, B.E., Holliday, P.J., Topper, A.K. (1991). Fear of falling and postural performance in the elderly. *Journal of Gerontology*, Vol. 46, No. 4, (July 1991), pp. (M123-131), ISSN 0022-1422

Manor, B., Li, L. (2009). Characteristics of functional gait among people with and without peripheral neuropathy. *Gait & Posture*, Vol. 30, No. 2, (August 2009), pp. (253-256), ISSN 0966-6362

Mauritz, K. H., Dietz, V. (1980). Characteristics of postural instability induced by ischaemic blocking of leg afferents. *Experimental Brain Research*, Vol. 38, No. 1, (January 1980), pp. 117-119, ISSN 0014-4819

Meyer, P.F., Oddsson, L.I., De Luca, C.J. (2004). Reduced plantar sensitivity alters postural responses to lateral perturbations of balance. *Experimental Brain Research*, Vol 157, No. 4, (August 2004), pp. (526-536), ISSN 0014-4819

Moreland, J.D., Richardson, J.A., Goldsmith, C.H., Clase, C.M. (2004). Muscle weakness and falls in older adults: a systematic review and meta-analysis. *Journal of the American Geriatrics Society*, Vol. 52, No. 7, (July 2004), pp. (1121-1129), ISSN 0002-8614

Mueller, M.J., Minor, S.D., Sahrmann, A.S., Schaaf, J.A., Strube, M.J. (1994). Differences in the gait characteristics of patients with diabetes and peripheral neuropathy compared with age-matched controls. *Physical Therapy*, Vol. 74, No. 4, (April 1994), pp. (299-313), ISSN 0031-9023

Nashner, L.M. (1976). Adapting reflexes controlling the human posture. *Experimental Brain Research*, Vol. 26, No. 1, (Aug 1976), pp. (59 -72), ISSN 0014-4819

Nashner L.M. (1977). Fixed patterns of rapid postural responses among leg muscles during stance. *Experimental Brain Research*, Vol. 30, No. 1, (October 1977), pp. (13-24), ISSN 0014-4819

Nashner, L.M., Peters, J.F. (1990). Dynamic posturography in the diagnosis and management of dizziness and balance disorders. *Neurologic Clinics*, Vol. 8, No. 2, (May 1990), pp. (331-349), ISSN 0733-8619

Niino, N., Tsuzuku, S., Ando, F., Shimokata, H. (2000). Frequencies and circumstances of falls in the National Institute for Longevity Sciences, Longitudinal Study of Aging (NILS-LSA). *Journal of Epidemiology*, Vol. 10, Suppl. 1, (April 2000), pp. (S90 -S94), ISSN 0917-5040

Oliver, D., Britton, M., Seed, P., Martin, F.C., Hopper, A.H. (1997) Development and evaluation of evidence based risk assessment tool (STRATIFY) to predict which elderly inpatients will fall: case-control and cohort studies. *British Medical Journal*, Vol. 315, No. 7115, pp. (1049-1053), ISSN 0007-1447

Oliver, D., Daly, F., Martin, F.C., McMurdo, M.E. (2004). Risk factors and risk assessment tools for falls in hospital in-patients: a systematic review. *Age and Ageing*, Vol. 33, No. 2, (March 2004), pp. (122-130), ISSN 0002-0729

Oppenheim, U., Kohen-Raz, R., Alex, D., Kohen-Raz, A., Azarya, M. (1999). Postural characteristics of diabetic Neuropathy. *Diabetes*, Vol. 22, No. 2, (February 1999), pp. (328-332), ISSN 0012-1797

Perell, K.L., Nelson, A., Goldman, R.L., Luther, S.L., Prieto-Lewis, N., Rubenstein, L.Z. (2001). Fall risk assessment measures: an analytic review. *Journals of Gerontology. Series A, Biological Sciences and Medical Sciences*, Vol. 56, No. 12, (December 2001), pp. (M761-766), ISSN 1079 5006

Petrofsky, J.S., Cuneo, M., Lee, S., Johnson, E., Lohman, E. (2006). Correlation between gait and balance in people with and without Type 2 diabetes in normal and subdued light. *Medical Science Monitor*, Vol. 12, No. 7, (July 2006), pp. (CR273-281), ISSN 1234-1010

Podsiadlo, D., Richardson, S. (1991). The timed "Up & Go": a test of basic functional mobility for frail elderly persons. *Journal of the American Geriatric Society*, Vol. 39, No. 2, (February 1991), pp. (142-148), ISSN 0002-8614

Pollock, A., Durward, B.R., Rowe, P.J., Paul, J.P. (2000). What is balance? Clinical Rehabilitation, Vol. 14, No. 4, (August 2000), pp. (402-406), ISSN 0269-2155

Poulain, I., Giraudet, G. (2008). Age-related changes of visual contribution in posture control. *Gait & Posture* Vol. 27, No. 1, (January 2008), pp. (1-7), ISSN 0966-6362

Richardson, J.K., Ching, C., Hurvitz, E.A. (1992) The relationship between electromyographically documented peripheral neuropathy and falls. *Journal of the American Geriatric Society*, Vol. 40, No. 10, (October 1992), pp. (1008-1112), ISSN 0002-8614

Richardson, J.K., Hurvitz, E.A. (1995). Peripheral Neuropathy: A True Risk Factor for Falls. *Journals of Gerontology. Series A, Biological Sciences and Medical Sciences*, Vol. 50, No. 4, (July 1995), pp. (M211-215), ISSN 1079 5006

Richardson, J.K., Thies, S.B., DeMott, T.K., Ashton-Miller, J.A. (2004). A comparison of gait characteristics between older women with and without peripheral neuropathy in standard and challenging environments. *Journal of the American Geriatric Society*, vol. 52, No. 9, (September 2004), pp. (1532–1537), ISSN ISSN 0002-8614

Rubenstein, L.Z. (2006). Falls in older people: epidemiology, risk factors and strategies for prevention. *Age and Ageing*, Vol. 35, Suppl 2, (September 2006), pp. (ii37-41), ISSN 0002-0729

Sacco, I.C.N., Amadio, A.C. (2003). Influence of the diabetic neuropathy on the behavior of electromyographic and sensorial responses in treadmill gait. *Clinical Biomechanics (Bristol, Avon)*, Vol. 18, No. 5, (June 2003) pp. (426-434), ISSN 0268-0033

Scott, V., Votova, K., Scanlan, A., Close, J . (2007). Multifactorial and functional mobility assessment tools for fall risk among older adults in community, home-support, long-term and acute care settings. *Age and Ageing*, Vol. 36, No. 2, (March 2007), pp. 130–139), ISSN 0002-0729

Schwartz, A.V., Vittinghoff, E., Sellmeyer, D.E., Feingold, K.R., de Rekeneire. N., Strotmeyer, E.S., Shorr, R.I., Shinabarger, N.I. (1987). Limited joint motility in adults with diabetes mellitus. *Physical Therapy*, Vol. 67, No. 2, (February 1987), pp. (215-218), ISSN 0031-9023

Shumway-Cook, A., Woollacott, M. (2000a). *Motor Control: Theory and Practical Applications* (2nd edition), MD: Lippincott, Williams and Wilkins, ISBN 1-60831-018-3, Baltimore, Unites States of America

Shumway-Cook, A., Woollacott, M. (2000b). Attentional demands and postural control: the effect of sensory context. *Journals of Gerontology. Series A, Biological Sciences and Medical Sciences*, Vol 55, No. 1, (January 2000), pp.(M10-16), ISSN 1079 5006

Simoneau, G.G., Ulbrecht, J.S., Der, J.A., Becker, M.B., Cavanagh, P.R. (1994). Postural Instability in Patients with Diabetic Sensory Neuropathy. *Diabetes Care* , Vol. 17, No. 12, (December 1994), pp. (1411-1421), ISSN 0149-5992

Talbot, L.A., Musiol, R.J., Witham, E.K., Metter, E. J. (2005). Falls in young, middle-aged and older community dwelling adults: perceived cause, environmental factors and injury. *BMC Public Health* 2005,5:86 doi:10.1186/1471-2458-5-86, ISSN 1471-2458

Teasdale, N., Simoneau, M. (2001). Attentional demands for postural control: the effects of ageing and sensory reintegration. *Gait & Posture*, Vol 14, No. 3, (December 2001), pp. (203-210), ISSN 0966-6362

Thompson, P.D. , Mardsen, C.D. (1996). Clinical Neurological assessment of balance and gait disorders. In: *Clinical Disorders of Balance, Posture and Gait.* Bronstein A.M., Brandt T., Woollacott M. pp. (79-84), Arnold, ISBN 0 340 60145 0, London, England

Tinetti ME. (1986). Performance-oriented assessment of mobility problems in elderly patients. *Journal of the American Geriatric Society*, Vol. 34, No. 2, (February 1986), pp. (119-126), ISSN 0002-8614

Tinetti, M.E., Medes de Leon, C.F., Doucette, J.T., Baker, D.I. (1994). Fear of falling and fall-related efficacy in relationship to functioning among community-living elders. *J Gerontology*, Vol. 49, No. 3, (May 1994), pp. (M140–147), ISSN 0022-1422

Tinetti, M.E. (2003). Clinical practice. Preventing falls in elderly persons. *New England Journal of Medicine*, Vol. 348, No. 1, (January 2003), pp. (42-49), ISSN 0028-4793

Toro, B., Nester, C.J., Farren, P.C. (2003). The status of gait assessment among physiotherapists in the United Kingdom. *Archives of Physical Medicine and Rehabilitation*, Vol. 84, No. 12, (December 2003), pp. (1878-1884), ISSN 0003-9993

Townsend, M.A. (1985). Biped gait stabilization via foot placement. *Journal of Biomechanics*, Vol. 18, No. 1, (n.d. 1985), pp. (21-38), ISSN 0021-9290

Uccioli, L., Giacomini, P., Monticone, G., Magrin,i A., Durols, A., Bruno, E., Parist, L., Di Girolamo, S., Menzinger. G. (1995). Body sway in diabetic neuropathy. *Diabetes Care*, Vol 18, No. 3, (March 1995), pp. (339-344), ISSN 0149-5992

Van Deursen, R.W., Simoneau, G.G. (1999). Foot and ankle sensory neuropathy, proprioception, and postural stability. *Journal of Orthopedic and Sports Physical Therapy*, Vol. 29, No. 12, (December 1999), pp. (718-726), ISSN 0190-6011

Vinik, A.I., Park, T.S., Stansberry, K.B., Pittenger, G.I. (2000). Diabetes neuropathies. *Diabetologia*, Vol. 43, No. 8, (August 2000), pp. (957-973), ISSN 0012-186X

Vrethem, M., Ledin, T., Ernerudh, J., Odkvist, L.M., Holmgren, H., Moller, C. (1991). Correlation between dynamic posturography, clinical investigation and neurography in patients with polyneuropathy. *ORL Journal for Otorhinolaryngology and its Related Specialities*, Vol. 53, No. 5, (n.d. 1991) , pp. (294-298), ISSN 0301-1569

Wang, C.Y., Olson, S.L., Protas, E.J. (2005). Physical-performance tests to evaluate mobility disability in community-dwelling elders. *Journal of Aging and Physical Activity*, Vol 13, No. 2, (April 2005), pp. (184-197), ISSN 1063-8652

World Health Organization. (2007). *A Global report on falls prevention. Epidemiology of falls.* World Health Organization, Retrieved from <http://www.who.int/ageing/publications/Falls_prevention7March.pdf>

Winter, D.A., Scott, S.H. (1991).Technique for interpretation of electromyography for concentric and eccentric contractions in gait. *Journal of Electromyography and Kinesiology*, Vol. 1, No. 4, (December 1991), pp. (263-269), ISSN 1050-6411

Winter, D.A. (1995). Human balance and posture control during standing and walking *Gait & Posture*, Vol 3, No. 4, (December 1995), pp. (193-214), ISSN 0966-6362

Woollacott, M., Shumway-Cook, A. (2002). Attention and the control of posture and gait: a review of an emerging area of research. *Gait & Posture*, vol 16, No. 1, (August 2002), pp. (1-14), ISSN 0966-6362

7

Clinical Cases in Pediatric Peripheral Neuropathy

Leigh Maria Ramos-Platt
Children's Hospital of Los Angeles, University of Southern California
USA

1. Introduction

There are many challenges to diagnosing peripheral neuropathy in children. While the symptoms are similar to those in adults, young children and those with developmental delays pose difficulties in extracting the appropriate history and performing a consistent and careful neurological examination. Neuropathic processes that present in childhood can be divided into those that are progressive and those that will tend improve over time. While there are exceptions, children with the latter category are those that fall into the acquired neuropathies such as vitamin deficiencies, toxicities, some immune mediated, and focal mononeuropathies. Those in the progressive category include the neuropathies that are hereditary/genetic in nature such as the heterogenous group of Hereditary Sensory Motor Neuropathies and some immune mediated neuropathies. In general, when the neuropathies of this group present earlier in childhood, the course and prognosis is worse than if they were to present in adolescence and adulthood. There are exceptions to this as some children who initially present as floppy infants due to a congenital neuropathy with respiratory difficulties can attain the ability to walk independently.

A lot of the entities discussed in this chapter have been discussed in others that are dedicated to their specific mechanisms. What this chapter will try to achieve is to discuss the pediatric presentations of these disorders and to highlight, if present, differences between the adult and pediatric presentations of neuropathies. While this chapter will touch on the pathophysiology, electrodiagnostic findings, and laboratory findings, it will not try to duplicate these areas of discussion found in other chapters of this book. The intent of this chapter is to discuss pediatric presentations of peripheral neuropathy in the context of clinical cases to allow the reader to consider these diagnoses in children.

A mention of performing electrodiagnostic testing is essential in any chapter discussing peripheral neuropathy. The evaluation of weakness often employs using nerve conduction studies and electromyograms. In young children and especially in those who have developmental delays, this can be difficult. In this author's experience, performing these electrodiagnostic studies in children is more time consuming. Frequent coaching and coaxing is often needed. Without sedation available, many studies are truncated due to tolerance, inability to cooperate, and inability to follow commands. A child life specialist can be valuable in utilizing distraction techniques. Certified Child Life Specialists have been used in various clinical settings to help ease the anxiety associated with procedures (McGee, 2003). Also, use of a local anesthetic cream such as topical lidocaine may be helpful in reducing the amount of discomfort. While most diagnoses can be supported by obtaining 2 motor nerves with F-waves, 2 sensory nerves, and needle examination in one proximal and one distal muscle, some patients will require a more complete study under sedation. It is in this author's opinion that the ability to perform sedated EMGs should be available in facilities that performs these studies on children.

2. Case #1

History: A previously healthy 12 year old boy first started to notice difficulties with tripping while walking. Over the following week, his conditioned worsened and by the time he presented to the emergency room, on day 8 of symptoms, he had difficulty walking. On further questioning, he had a sore throat and runny nose approximately 2 weeks prior to the onset of symptoms.
Examination highlights: 3/5 strength in his anterior tibialis and gastrocnemius muscles bilaterally. Weakness was symmetrical. Hip girdle muscles were nearly normal as was upper extremity strength. Remarkable on his examination were trace to absent reflexes out of proportion to his degree of weakness.
Studies: CT of the head was negative. LP demonstrated a protein of 105 mg/dL with 3 WBC/hpf and no RBCs. CSF glucose was 58 mg/dL (65% of his peripheral glucose). MRI of the brain was normal. MRI of the spine demonstrated enhancing caudal equina roots.

Study	Findings
Right Median Motor CMAP	normal
Right Tibial Motor CMAP	normal
Right Radial Sensory SNAP	normal
Right Sural Sensory SNAP	normal
Right Median F-wave	Normal duration, 40% persistence
Right Tibial Motor F-wave	Normal duration, <20% persistence

EMG/NCV Findings

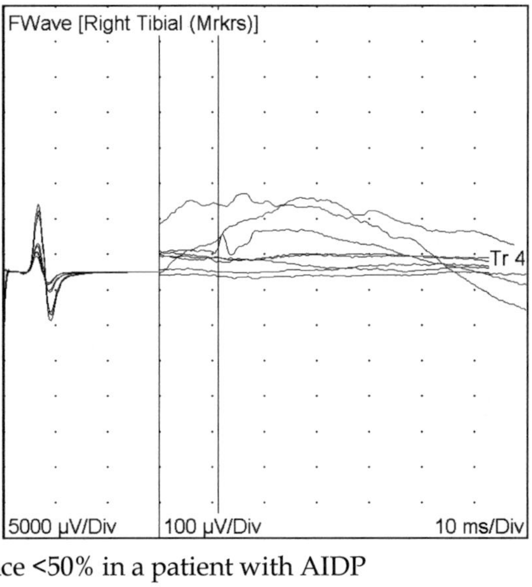

Fig. 1. F-wave persistence <50% in a patient with AIDP

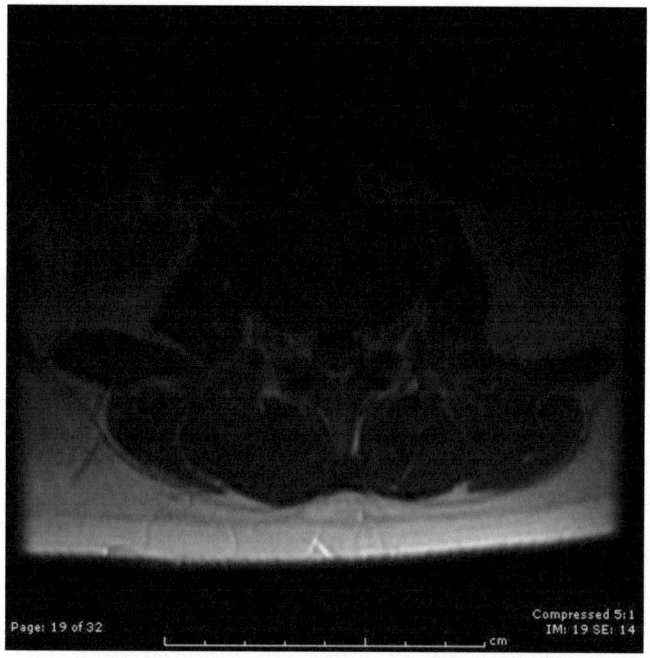

Fig. 2. Enhancing nerve roots of the cauda equine in a patient with AIDP

Clinical Course: The patient received a 5 day course of IVIG (0.4 grams/kg/day) for a total dose of 2 grams/kg. He started to improve on day 3 of treatment. After 4 weeks in the inpatient rehabilitation service, he was discharged home, able to walk, climb stairs, and play basketball.

Diagnosis: Acute Inflammatory Demyelinating Polyradiculoneuropathy (AIDP) also known as the Guillain Barre Syndrome (GBS).

Discussion: In a child that presents with classic ascending paralysis and loss of reflexes, it is important to evaluate for AIDP (Simmons, 2010). The diagnosis of AIDP is mainly clinical with supporting information gathered from laboratory, neurophysiological, and radiological studies. There is little in the differential diagnosis with this history but acute cord lesions should be excluded especially if there is a history of bowel and bladder difficulties. Sensory changes can occur in AIDP. Motor symptoms predominate (Kuwabara, 2004). However, a recent study in adults reported that approximately 70% of AIDP patients had decreased superficial or deep sensation in distal extremities (Kuwabara, 2004). Acute cord lesions tend to be more abrupt (such as an anterior spinal artery syndrome). Arterior spinal artery syndrome has dissociated sensory impairment and sphincter involvement (Servais, 2001). AIDP is difficult to distinguish from the first presentation of CIDP. Especially in younger children where examination can be difficult, other diagnoses to consider include myasthenia gravis (Markowitz, 2008), acute cerebellar ataxia, and other post-infectious disorders such as acute disseminated encephalomyelitis (ADEM). Diminished or absent reflexes, MRI findings, and prolongation F-waves would support AIDP. In this case, a lack of F-wave persistence was seen. Decreased F-wave persistence is seen with AIDP (Frasier, 1992). The lack of fatigueability in this patient would argue against myasthenia gravis. In addition, the majority of patients with myasthenia gravis present with bulbar signs (Andrews, 2003). In these situations, careful examination of DTRs is essential.

The case highlights the clinical features of AIDP: ascending paralysis, association with an inciting infection which is seen in 60-70% of cases, and diminished or absent reflexes. Progressive weakness is seen in more than one limb and progress rapidly over 4 weeks. The nadir is usually reached by 2 weeks. Typically, there is relative symmetry. Sphincters are usually spared but there can be an occasional patient with bladder dysfunction (Asbury, 1990; Cosi, 2006; Agrawal, 2007). A variation that must be mentioned is the Miller Fischer variant. This triad of symptoms includes ophthalmoplegia, ataxia, and areflexia (and an association with the Gq1b antibody (Mori, 2001).

Prolonged F-waves are among the first electrophysiological sign seen in this disease and are suggestive of proximal demyelination even when motor conduction studies are normal. Prolongation of distal latencies is also an early finding (Simmons, 2010). This can be seen in the first week of symptoms. Other features, which are seen later in the course (weeks) include conduction block on nerve conduction studies. 80% of patients who will be eventually diagnosed with AIDP will have abnormalities in their neurophysiological studies upon presentation. In one study, 96% will have abnormal motor responses within 3 weeks. It is also of value to note that 20% will not have abnormalities on their nerve conductions at the time of presentation thus re-enforcing that information gained from neurophysiological studies is supportinve but not diagnostic. Although mild sensory complaints can be an initial feature, approximately 70% can have abnormal sensory responses within 3 weeks of symptom onset. Nerve involvement can be patchy. (Asbury 1990).

Lumbar puncture is needed to exclude infection as well as to evaluate for albuminocytological disassociation which strongly supports the diagnosis of GBS/AIDP (Simmons, 2010). One of the most predictable and consistent early findings in AIDP is enhancement of the nerve roots of the cauda equina. This can be seen within the first 2 weeks of symtoms. Cauda equina root enhancement is 83% sensitive for Guillain Barre Syndrome and is seen in 95% of typical cases (Gorson, 1996).

There are electrophysiologic criteria for both AIDP and CIDP which includes conduction block in one of more nerves, prolonged late responses, prolonged distal latencies in two or more nerves, and conduction slowing in two or more nerves. Excellent discussions and tables are in various sources. One particularly helpful source is the textbook by Preston and Shapiro. For AIDP, at least one of the following (conduction slowing, prolonged late responses, prolonged distal latencies) in 2 or more nerves within the first 3 weeks of illness (Ho, 1997).

Like most other autoimmune diseases, the pathophysiology lies in molecular mimicry. An inciting infection results in production of antibodies that cross react with myelin components. In some cases, there is axonal involvement such as in those associated with campylobacter infection.

Treatment is not necessary in all cases. Both IVIG and Plasma Exchange are efficacious in the treatment of Guillain Barre Syndrome within 2 and 4 weeks of symptoms. Fewer complications are seen with IVIG. The combination of the two modalities in sequence is not recommended as an initial treatment. There is no benefit from treatment with corticosteroids (Hughes, 2003). An example dose for IVIG is 2 grams per kg and given as 0.4 gram to 1 gram per kg/day for 2 to 5 days. IVIG treatment can be associated with a reduced need for mechanical ventilation (Shanbag, 2003). IVIG treatment is also likely associated with a shorter time to independent ambulation in children (Shaher, 2003; Agrawal, 2007). An example of a plasma exchange schedule is 1 volume plasma exchange every other day for a total of 5 exchanges. Other aspects of treatment include surveillance for and treatment of associated autonomic dysfunction, pain, and respiratory compromise. Rehabilitation services are important in the overall care of a pediatric patient with AIDP.

Patients with preceding *c. jejuni* infection were more likely to have acute axonal neuropathy or axonal degeneration in association with AIDP. This subset of patients is associated with slower recovery, and generally, a worse outcome. Careful history of a preceding gastroenteritis 2-3 weeks before the symptoms of weakness would help in identifying if evaluation for past c. jejuni infection is warranted. In adult studies where c. jejuni infection was associated with the presentation of AIDP, the majority of patients recalled watery diarrhea and a smaller percentage recalled bloody diarrhea. Along with an association with c. jejuni infection, other poor prognostic factors include need for ventillatory support and confinement to a bed within 2 days of neuropathic symptom onset (rapid progression) (Rees, 1995). Also, patients with anti-GM1 antibodies can be associated with poorer prognosis (Van der berg, 1991).
Overall, prognosis is excellent with >80% of patients recovering the ability to ambulate (Simmons 2010). It should be cautioned that (50.00%) of patients who will be eventually diagnosed with CIDP were first diagnosed with AIDP. AIDP can recur in a small percentage of patients. It may also be the first presentation of other autoimmune disorders such as SLE (exceptionally rare, see below). Other associations with AIDP besides viral intections and c. jejuni infection include preceding surgery, vaccinations (although controversial), cancer, and multiple sclerosis (Asbury, 1990).

3. Case # 2

History: A previously healthy 6 year old boy presented with a 3 month history of progressive weakness. Over the course of 3 months, he lost the ability to walk independently.
Examination highlights: He had near normal strength in his bilateral proximal muscles and 4/5 strength distally. He had 2/5 strength in the anterior tibialis bilaterally and 4/5 strength in all remaining muscles. Sensation was preserved grossly. He had no elicitable reflexes.
Studies: Cerebral spinal fluid analysis demonstrated elevated protein at 100 mg/dL with no white blood cells and no red cells. Glucose was 60 mg/dL.

Study	Findings
Right Median CMAP	Slowed conduction 38 m/s; preserved amplitude
Left Median CMAP	Slowed conduction 35 m/s; preserved amplitude
Right Ulnar CMAP	Slowed conduction 32 m/s; conductions block with increased temporal dispersion of CMAP
Left Tibial CMAP	Slowed conduction 34 m/s; conduction block with increased temporal dispersion of CMAP
Left Peroneal CMAP	Slowed conduction 38 m/s; preserved amplitude
Left Radial SNAP	Normal conduction and amplitude of SNAP
Right Medial Plantar SNAP	Slowed conduction 35 m/s; preserved amplitude of SNAP
Left Medial Plantar SNAP	Slowed conduction 33 m/s; preserved amplitude of SNAP
EMG Right APB	Large amplitude, long duration, unstable complex MUAPs with decreased recruitment
EMG Right EDC	Large amplitude, long duration, unstable complex MUAPs with decreased recruitment
EMG Right anterior tibialis	Large amplitude, long duration, unstable complex MUAPs with decreased recruitment

EMG/NCV Findings

Clinical Course: He responded partially to IVIG. However, due to ongoing weakness despite a repeat course of IVIG, he was started on prednisone. Due to intolerance and side effects of prednisone (pathological factors, hepatitis, markedly elevated cholesterol levels), he was subsequently started on mycophenylate. 6 months after the initial diagnosis, he is able to walk independently but cannot run. He has trace reflexes. He continues to make improvement with immune suppression.

Diagnosis: Chronic Inflammatory Polyradiculoneuropathy

Discussion: In a child presenting with 3 months of progressive weakness, deciphering the timing and the progression of weakness is needed to aid with the differential diagnosis. AIDP is among the highest on the differential. Had the patient peaked in weakness, and what was presenting 3 months from the onset was improved, then AIDP is a possibility. However, this was not the case in this patient. Hereditary sensory motor neuropathies can also present as progressive weakness, and are a consideration in this patient. Making this diagnosis less likely is that the patient was normal prior to the start of symptoms. In addition, while patients with HSMN can present with elevated protein in the CSF, conduction block is characteristically not a feature. Conudction block is an indication of non-uniform slowing seen on NCV studies along with increased temporal dispersion. HSMN tends to have a more uniform slowing with a few exceptions. As will be discussed in a later section, children with HSMN typically have a history of delayed motor development.

Like in adults, CIDP in children is less likely to have an antecedent event (such as URI symptoms). An antecedent event can be recalled in 20-30% of patients with CIDP. Some studies report up to 57%; but still considerable less than with AIDP (Markowitz, 2008). CIDP presents as a symmetrical predominantly motor polyradiculoneuropathy affecting both proximal and distal muscle groups. Hyporeflexia or areflexia is seen. In adult patients, a predominantly distal course is seen in 17%. A predominantly sensory form is seen in 15% and asymmetry can be seen in just under 10% of patients. Cranial nerves can be involved in 5% of patients and CNS involvement is seen in 8% (Rotta, 2000). The overall course can be relapsing or chronic progressive (Rotta, 2000). The initial presentation in general is typically quite striking in children such as gait disturbance and weakness. Tremor and ataxia are also reported symptoms. This is in contrast to adults who may present with minor complaints such as subtle weakness, mild sensory disturbances or decreased dexterity. Like adults, approximately 50% of children will have sensory discturbances such as parasthesias at the time of diagnosis (Simmons, 1997). Symptoms must be present for at least eight weeks to fit the clinical criteria of CIDP. The incidence of patients younger than 20 diagnosed with CIDP is 0.48 per 100,000 (in contrast to CIDP in adults 1.9 per 100,000) (Markowitz, 2008).

Like with AIDP, neurophysiological studies are supportive of this diagnosis but not diagnostic (see below). Just under 10% of patients will have caudal root enhancement. Elevated protein in the CSF is seen but not all patients have this (Rotta, 2000).

Nearly all CIDP patients will respond to their first treatment within a week. Like adults with CIDP, children will fit electrodiagnostic criteria (Simmons, 1997). Treatment options include IVIG (initially 2 grams per kilogram divided into 4-5 days) with subsequent treatment up to 2 grams/kg every 3 weeks, steroids (prednisone, typically 1-2 mg per kg/day), plasmapharesis for refractory cases, and other immunosuppressive agents such as mycophenilate (Cellcept). Other immunosuppressive agents used include azathioprine, methotrexate, cyclosporine, and interferon therapies (Markowitz, 2008).

In this author's practice, in patients requiring prolonged immune suppression with a combination of medications, it is important to consider prophylaxis with trimethoprim sulfa. Regular evaluation of potential side effects of these medications and toxicity is essential in the care of patients with CIDP. Routine labs to consider include complete blood counts, chemistry profiles, liver profiles, levels of immunosuppressant agents and their toxic metabolites, lipid panel, vitamin D level, and lipase/amylase. The frequency of surveillance labs will be dictated by the patient's needs.

Prognosis for patients with CIDP is variable. Some patients remit after the first treatment and most patients have improvement after the first treatment. 60% of patients will respond to IVIG, 70% to steroids, 50% to plasma exchange, and 36% to cytotoxic agents. However, it is not well delineated which of the pediatric patients will have a course of frequent relapsing and partial remitting with treatment (Rotta, 2000). It must be highlighted that early treatment will provide the best opportunity for improvement. Pediatric patients tend to have more of a remitting-relapsing course and not typically have a progressive decline. Those patients that have a more insidious, slower onset are more likely to be associated with disease that is more difficult to treat. Pediatric patients with CIDP are less likely to need ventillatory support compared to those with AIDP, and adults with CIDP (although it has been reported). Long term treatment with IVIG has been demonstrated to be beneficial in patients with CIDP. Relapses can correlate with tapering of treatment (Simmons, 1997). Adults with an associated IgM monoglonal gammoathy and predominanrly sensory symptoms with or without serum anti-MAG antibodies have a poorer response to treatment. Further studies in children regarding positive antibody subsets are needed. One study comparing treatment of CIDP with high dose intermittent IV methylprednisolone demonstrated no difference in outcome between those treated with oral steroids and IVIG (Lopate, 2005). This study was in adults. Intermittent high dose IV methyprednisolone may be a lower cost, lower side effects treatment option. Further studies, particularly in children, are needed.

4. Case #3

History: A 7 year old boy did not start walking until he was 2 years of age. His parents report that although he has maintained the ability to walk, he has been tripping more as if he cannot pick up his feet. He cannot keep up with the other children when playing although cognitively, he is at grade level, if not advanced. His mother was able to play basketball and soccer in high school. She still helps with coaching their other children in soccer. Family history is notable for three of his father's siblings with muscular dystrophy. Two of his father's brothers died in their 30s after being wheelchair bound in their teens. His older sister is in her 50s and is wheelchair bound. His father is healthy. On his mother's side, multiple family members needed special shoes for their high arches. Although ambulatory into their 60s, several of his mother's relative had feet that started to turn in and toes to claw. One relative had to use a wheelchair.

Examination highlights: Negative Gower maneuver. Proximally, he has full strength. In his hands, he had 4/5 strength in his intraossei and FDI. Although he has full strength in the hip girdle muscles, he has 3/5 strength in the anterior tibialis and 4/5 strength in the gastrocnemius muscles bilaterally. He has absent reflexes and no fasciculations. His calves are thin and he has high arches in his lower extremities. He has a high steppage gait and bilateral foot drop. The patient has a pes cavus. His mother similarly has high arches and absent reflexes in the lower extremities. Strength is normal in her proximal muscles of her upper and lower extremities. She has minimal weakness in bilateral ankle dorsiflexion.

Study	Findings
Right Median CMAP	Prolonged distal latency >8 seconds Slowed conduction velocity <30 m/s Normal CMAP amplitude No conduction block
Right Ulnar CMAP	Prolonged distal latency >8 seconds Slowed conduction velocity <30 m/s Normal CMAP amplitude No conduction block
Left Tibial CMAP	Prolonged distal latency >8 seconds Slowed conduction velocity <30 m/s Normal CMAP amplitude No conduction block
Left Peroneal CMAP	Prolonged distal latency >8 seconds Slowed conduction velocity <30 m/s Normal CMAP amplitude No conduction block
Right Median SNAP	Slowed conduction velocity <40 m/s Normal SNAP amplitude
Right Radial SNAP	Slowed conduction velocity <40 m/s Normal SNAP amplitude
Left Sural SNAP	Slowed conduction velocity <35 m/s Normal SNAP amplitude
Left Medial Plantar SNAP	Slowed conduction velocity <35 m/s Normal SNAP amplitude
Mother's Right Median CMAP	Prolonged distal latency >8 seconds Slowed conduction velocity <30 m/s Normal CMAP amplitude No conduction block

EMG/NCV Findings

Other Studies: CPK is normal. Genetic testing confirms that the patient and his mother are positive for duplication in the PM22 gene.
Diagnosis: Hereditary Motor Sensory Neuropathy - CMT1a
Discussion: Especially in a young boy who presents with progressive weakness, the differential diagnosis must include muscular dystrophy such as a dystrophinopathy. In general, the distribution of weakness and the reflexes in comparison to the degree of weakness help to separate myopathic from neuropathic processes. In general, myopathic processes involve proximal muscles first and neuropathic processes involve distal muscles initially. Reflexes that are proportionate to the degree of weakness are consistent with a myopathic process and that are out of proportion (much less than expected) to the degree of weakness are consistent with a neuropathic process. A negative Gower's sign, normal CPK, and thin calves make a diagnosis of a dystrophinopathy not likely. A dystrophinopathy classically presents with a Gower maneuver, toe walking (rather than foot drop), large, firm (pseudohypertrophied calves), and markedly elevated CPK. What may be confusing is that the patient has uncles with muscular dystrophy. It should be observed that the uncles who were affected were paternal relatives. Although some sporadic occurrence can happen, the typical inheritance pattern for a dystrophinopathy (the most common type of muscular dystrophy in boys), is X-linked (maternally inherited).

Hereditary Sensory Motor Neuropathy is a heterogenous group of disorders affecting the peripheral nerves and affects 1:2500 people. It is characterized by atrophy in the distal extremities (anterior tibialis often affected early) and diminished or absent deep tendon reflexes. Associated features include a high steppage gait, impaired sensation, high arches of the feet, and pes cavus (Antonellis, 2003). It was first described in 1886 by the physicians whose names bear the eponym. Duplications in the PMP22 gene lead to the most common type of CMT, CMT1a (as is the case in our patient). This is located on chromosome 17 p11.2. CMT1b is associated with an abnormality mapping to chromosome 1 resulting in abnormal P0 protein (involved with the compaction of peripheral myelin) (Kulkens, 1993). What appears to be recurring a theme in the majority of demyelinating Charcot Marie Tooth Disease, is that they are the result of abnormal function in the Schwan cell.

In general, HSMN can be divided into demyelinating forms (designated as CMT 1) and axonal forms (designated as CMT 2). Nerve conduction studies can help with the distinction between the two. If the underlying process is predominantly a demyelinating abnormality, prolonged distal latencies and slowed conductions will be seen with relatively preserved amplitudes. If the underlying process is axonal, then conduction velocity will be relatively preserved, but CMAP and SNAP amplitudes will be small. NCS can also help with distinguishing HSMN from CIDP when the history may not be as clear. As described above, one of the electrodiagnostic features of CIDP is conduction block. In type 1 CMTs, slowing typically is uniform.

Symptoms of patients with CMT1 usually begin in childhood. Progression is generally slow but progressive. Symptoms include inability to keep up with other children, clumsiness, tripping, and foot drop (typically, the muscles of the anterior compartment of the legs are affected first and most noticeably). Reflexes tend to be trace at best but will most likely be absent.

It is not uncommon for the family history to have multiple relatives presenting with various degrees of weakness severity. The disease of most HSMN patients is inherited in an autosomal dominant pattern, although inheritance can also be autosomal recessive, X-linked, and sporadic. There are many mutations seen in X-linked CMT. However, these mutations are all associated with various Connexin 32 mutations (Cxn 32 is a gene responsible for encoding gap junctions, mapped to Xq13) (Oh, 1997). X-linked CMT is the second most frequent in the HSMN demeyelinating category. As with other X-linked disorders, males are much more affected than females with respect to clinical presentation as well as from a neurophysiological standpoint. However, as is the trend in patients with HSMN, there is a spectrum of clinical presentations. Most females with X-linked CMT are asymptomatic (Dubourg, 2001). As in this case, it is not uncommon for parents of affected children to be unaware that they are also affected; albeit to a lesser degree.

CMT2, the heterogenous group of disorders characterized by their predominantly axonal involvement also is autosomal dominant in inheritance (although, sporadic forms do occur). In the author's experience with children, this is much more of a rarity. The age of onset is older;- usually young adulthood. There are now 8 subtypes of CMT-2 (and designated as A-I) (NINDS, 2011). Molecular biology has allowed for the identification of the genes associated with these phenotypes including CMT2A associated with a mutation in KIF1B, CMT2B with the RAS-related GTP binding protein, CMT2E with the neurofilament light chain gene (NEFL), and a mutation in glycyl trNA synthase mapped to chromosome 7p in CMT 2D (Antonellis, 2003). CMT2F is characterized by a symmetrical distal limb weakness and subsequent atrophy. There are multiple genes that can be associated with this phenotype including one mapping to chromosome 7q11-q21. Other mutations in small heat shock protein 27 have been reported to cause this phenotype (Evgrafov, 2004).

Dejerine Sottas Disease is also known as CMT3 or HSMN 3. It presents in infancy and is a severe peripheral neuropathy. Nerve conduction studies demonstrate markedly slowed velocities, generally less than 12 m/s. CSF protein can be elevated. Inheritance can be dominant, recessive, or sporadic. Genes affected include the PMP22, P0, EGR2, and PRX. The same abnormality that causes CMT1a in one family member can be associated with DSD in another. Patients are slow to make motor milestones and some do eventually achieve the ability to walk.

The course of disease varies depending on the type of abnormality (hence the type of CMT). Families with the same mutation can have variable courses as do individual members within the same family, as seen in our case presentation.

There is no cure for CMT. Treatment of the patient is supportive. Braces may help with ambulation. Physical and occupation therapy ongoing will help to maintain function. Regular screening for scoliosis is important. Pulmonary function screening is also vital especially if there is scoliosis. There can be associated cardiac abnormalities including conduction abnormalities and filling defects. However, this is not in the majority of patients. Most patients with CMT have normal life expectancies. There is ongoing gene therapy research (NINDS 2011). High dose vitamin C was studied but was not found to be helpful in the majority of young patients (ages 12 to 25 years) with CMT1a. This same study also deemed that high dose vitamin C was found to be safe (Vehamme, 2009).

5. Case #4

History: A 16 year old left handed girl presents with a 6 month history of numbness in the left hand. She feels that her handwriting is mildly affected. There is no associated pain. She exercises on a regular basis but not more than an hour a day. Upon further questioning, the patient stated that during her 45 minute drives to and from school, she leans on her left elbow to text her friends.

Examination highlights: She has mild atrophy of the ADM and weakness in the interossei. There does not seem to be involvement of her Abductor Policis Brevis (APB). She has decreased sensation in the 4th and 5th digits. Only her left ulnar reflex was diminished.

Study	Findings
Right Median CMAP	Normal
Left Median CMAP	Normal
Right Ulnar CMAP	Normal
Left Ulnar CMAP	Normal at the wrist and segment from wrist to below elbow with a conduction velocity of 58 m/s. When stimulated above the elbow, conduction velocity diminishes to 33 m/s and drop in CMAP amplitude to 2.5 mV from 8.4 mV
Left Radial SNAP	Normal
Left Median SNAP	Normal
Left Ulnar SNAP	Normal

EMG/NCV

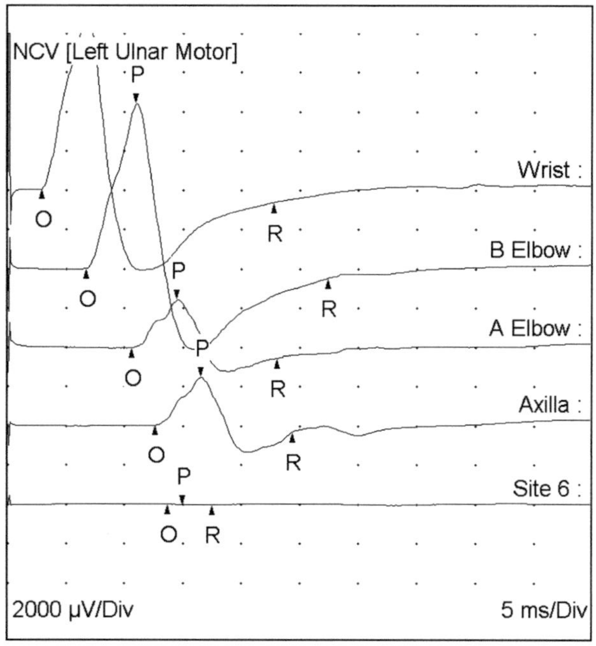

Fig. 3. Left ulnar CMAP

Diagnosis: left ulnar mononeuropathy in the segment across the elbow.

Discussion: A detailed discussion to separate a mononeuropathy, plexopahthy, and radiculopathy is beyond the scope of this chapter. These remain in the differential diagnosis in a child with numbness in the hand. Generally, in a lower brachial plexopathy (such as what is seen with thoracic outlet syndrome), there is involvement of the ABP (which is median nerve innervated). Pain is typically a prominent symptom. If a plexopathy is suspected, obtaining sensory nerve conductions of the medial and lateral antebrachial cutaneous nerves of the forearms bilaterally would be useful as these would be abnormal (typically of low amplitude) in lesions of the brachial plexus. If the patient had a radiculopathy of the C8 and T1 nerve roots, it would be expected that nerve conduction studies would be normal. Neck pain could also be present and as with a radiculopathy, there would be multiple nerve distribution involvement. In this patient, it is necessary to confirm that she has only a mononeuropathy and not a mononeuropathy multiplex or a more generalized neuropathic process. Differential diagnosis for a mononeuritis multiplex includes autoimmune disease (such as SLE), infections (such as Lyme disease), and diabetes mellitus.

In a 16 year old girl, connective tissue disease should be considered as a potential cause of peripheral neuropathy. A length-dependent predominantly axonal sensorimotor polyneuropathy or mononeuritis multiplex can be seen in pediatric patients with Systemic Lupus Erythmatosis (SLE). Vaso nevorum vasculitis, deposits of immune complexes, or damage to the neural tissue by antibodies against their components are proposed mechanisms. Because of the scarcity of published studies in the literature, treatment for the pediatric population is not well established. Limited published pediatric studies have reported response to steroids, azathioprine, and cyclophosphamide. Peripheral neuropathy associated with SLE tends to be concurrent with central nervous system disease. Gabapentin and Carbamazepine can be used for symptomatic (pain control) treatment (Harel, 2002).

Hereditary Neuropathy with Pressure Palsies (HNPP) is in the differential diagnosis of a child who presents with multiple episodes of painless focal neuropathies in common sites of entrapment such as the ulnar nerve at the elbow and the peroneal nerve at the fibular head. Like CMT1a, the abnormality is in the PMP22 gene. However, rather than a duplication, PMP22 deletions lead to the HNPP phenotype.

In an otherwise healthy child with no history of trauma, especially with a family history of nontraumatic mononeuropathies, benign tumors such as osteochondromas compressing individual nerves should be considered. Although uncommon, case series' have been published on osteochondromas causing mononeuropathies and mononeuropathy multiplex. These are treatable causes of focal neuropathies. In some patients, this is hereditary. In these patients with autosomal dominant hereditary osteochondromata, sarcomatous transformation can occur and thus careful attention must be paid to these patients (Levin, 1991). Compressive mononeuropathies are not as common in children compared to adults. In one series, non-traumatic causes of ulnar mononeuropathies fared better than traumatic causes at one year follow-up (83% vs 56% improved) (Jones, 1986; Jones, 1996). In another small study, 4/5 focal compressive peroneal neuropathies had good recovery (Jones, 1986).

6. Case #5

History: An 11 year old girl with a history of acute lymphoblastic leukemia is admitted to the intensive care unit for hypotension and respiratory distress secondary to sepsis from her indwelling central line. She had received vincristine as one of her chemotherapeutic agents. She is intubated, paralyzed, and on pressors. Over the next three weeks, her condition slowly improves, she is weaned off of pressors, sedation and neuromuscular blockade are lifted. Despite apparent alertness and responsiveness, she does not hit parameters for extubation. Much more, after the intensive care physicians are concerned that 3 days after neuromuscular blockade is stopped, the ICU physicians and nurses note that she does not move any extremity.

Examination highlights: She is able to open her eyes spontaneously. She will fix and track. Pupils are equally reactive to light. She will grimace (although intubated) with noxious stimuli. She does not move her extremities spontaneously, to gentle, or to noxious stimuli. She is areflexic.

Studies: Her complete blood count is significant for pancytopenia (ANC <1.5, H&H 9.7 and 30, and platelets of 112). Her electrolytes were normal. Her LFTs normalized. Coagulation profile was corrected as well. CSF was with normal cell count, glucose, and protein level.

An exact cause is difficult to pinpoint in this patient's weakness. This case was used to springboard into a the following discussion of possible contributing factors.

An AIDP presentation has been described as both a paraneoplastic phenomenon as well as associated with complications of chemotherapy (Reddy, 2003).

There are multiple considerations of the underlying cause of this patient's weakness. Two likely contributors are an acquired neuropathy from vincristine and critical care neuropathy. Other possibilities are AIDP and critical care myopathy. Evaluation of the CSF may be helpful in excluding AIDP as a potential cause. Regarding critical myopathy as a cause, it is not uncommon to have both a critical care neuropathy and myopathy in the same patient. The risk factors of critical care neuropathy do overlap with those of the myopathy. EMG findings may not be able to separate the two early in the course and the only definitive test is a muscle biopsy.

Study	Findings
Right Tibial CMAP	Normal distal latency Conduction velocity 38 m/s Amplitude <0.5 mV
Left Median CMAP	Normal distal latency Conduction velocity 45 m/s Amplitude <0.5 mV
Right Sural SNAP	Normal distal latency Conduction velocity 40 m/s Amplitude 2 uV
Left Radial SNAP	Normal distal latency Conduction velocity 48 m/s Amplitude 1.5 uV
Needle EMG Right Anterior Tibialis	fibrillation potentials and long duration, polymorphic MUAPs.

EMG/NCV findings

Chemotherapy induced neuropathy (CIN) generally are predominant sensory or sensorimotor in character, clinically and neurophysiologically. CIN can also affect the autonomic nervous system. Typically, CIN severity and permanence of symptoms depends on the agent, duration of treatment, and whether there is an underlying other cause of neuropathy (see below). Some agents (such as Taxol) have idiosyncratic neuropathy (there is no consistency of a threshold toxicity level) (Quasthoff, 2000).

Vincristine is one of the chemotherapeutic agents that can cause a peripheral neuropathy. The pattern is one of predominantly axonal. Typical presenting symptoms include paresthesias and diminished deep tendon reflexes. Although the neuropathy associated with vincristine is dose related, even at low therapeutic ranges, there is generally involvement of the peripheral nervous system. There is some ability for regeneration of damaged nerve fibers once the medication is stopped. In some patients who develop peripheral neuropathy as a side effect of chemotherapeutic agents, sometimes, their course can be completed with a lower dose of the agent (McLeod and Penny, 1969; Packer, 1994).

Another consideration in this patient would be quadriparesis as a result of vincristine given to a patient with an underlying hereditary neuropathy. Unusually rapidly developing severe vincristine associated neuropathy presenting with a flaccid quadriplegia resembling AIDP has been described in patients who also had an underlying hereditary neuropathy (Graf, 1996).

Cisplatin at a cumulative dose of 350mg/m^2 (although some report as little as 200 mg/m^2) has been demonstrated to be associated with a predominantly sensory neuropathy/neuronopathy that is characterized early as parasthesias, loss of vibratory sense and joint position sense, and absent ankle jerks. It tends to spare pain and temperature modalities (Reddy, 2003). Studies in adults have demonstrated accumulation of cisplatin in the dorsal root ganglia of patients undergoing this treatment (Thompson, 1984). Both Vincristine and Cisplatin (and other related platinum agents such as Carboplatin) may present after treatment has stopped (referred to as a coasting effect) (Quasthoff, 2000).

Thalidomide has been used to treat various inflammatory diseases in children and adolescents such as Crohn's and Bechet's Disease. Like some chemotherapeutic agents, the neuropathy course associated with Thalidomide is not predictable. Stopping this chemotherapeutic agent does not necessarily lead to resolution of CIN symptoms. In one study, after 4-6 years post cessation of Thalidomide, in those patients that had its associated neuropathy, only 25% had recovered completely (Strauss, 2000; Priolo, 2008).

There is no cure for CIN. Studies on prophylactic regimens to prevent its occurrence have not been fruitful so far. Alpha Lipoic Acid has been suggested as possibly helpful. Treatment of Chemotherapy induced neuropathy is symptomatic. Medications such as Gabapentin, Carbamazepine, and tricyclic anti-depressants have been used to treat CIN (Quastaff, 2000). However, there are some studies that contradict the helpfulness of tricyclic anti-depressants specifically for the neuropathic pain in CIN (Kautio, 2008; Wolf, 2008). Gabapentin and Carbamazepine have not been helpful either in more recent studies although Oxcarbazapine may (Wolf, 2008). Vitamin E may may be helpful in the prevention of Cisplatin associated CIN but further larger studies are needed to investigate its safety in chemotherapy patients (Wolf, 2008).

Critical Care neuropathy has been recognized more frequently in recent years. Much of the description has been in adult patients. However there are case reports and case series in the pediatric population. The presentation in children is similar to that in adults. The risk factors are also similar including sepsis (critical care neuropathy is typically seen 2-3 weeks after the onset of sepsis) and multiorgan failure. There are likely several mechanisms of injury resulting in critical care neuropathy. These include hypoperfusion of the peripheral nerves, ischemic injury leading to impairment of axonal transport, hyperglycemic injury to the peripheral nervous system, malnutrition leading to vitamin deficiency and consequently vitamin deficiency neuropathy, possible injury from antimicrobials (such as aminoglycosides and metronidazole which can also be associated with axonal polyneuropathies), and low albumin levels resulting in endoneural edema. Clinically, patients present with difficulty with extubation. Patients are reported to be either paraplegic or tetraplegic with hyporeflexia or areflexia (Petersen, 1999).

Neurophysiological studies are abnormal in 70% of patients and demonstrate a predominantly axonal polyneuropathy of the motor nerves. Sensory nerves are not spared. Both CMAPs an SNAPs have decreased amplitudes with significant slowing of conduction (Gutman, 1999). There is no direct treatment for critical illness neuropathy. Treatment is treating the underlying disease and supportive care. Unfortunately, recovery is prolonged and not as favorable compared to adults. A favorable outcome (complete recovery) is seen in approximately 50% of patients with critical care neuropathy (Petersen, 1999). Folate deficiency has been associated with peripheral neuropathy. Especially in children with brain tumors who also have seizures, consider older generation AEDs as a potential course/contributor to peripheral neuropathy symptoms if they are using these (Figueroa, 1990).

7. Case # 6

History: A 17 year old boy was referred to the EMG lab with a 3 month history of progressive weakness of his bilateral lower extremities with involvement of the right greater than the left. The specific question asked by the referring physician was whether the patient needed surgery. He complained of shooting pains down the right leg. His mother reports that he started having enuresis at this time. His pediatrician had ordered an MRI of his lumbosacral spine and this was "positive" for a small disc bulge at L5. At this time, his mother asked if this had anything to do with the medication that was given to him a week and a half prior to his presentation. His PMD was contacted. Faxed records revealed he had a hemoglobin A1c of 16.6%. He had been started on Metformin 1 1/2 weeks prior to his appointment in EMG lab.
Examination highlights: Significant weakness (3-4/5 strength) of the hip flexors, quadriceps, hip adductors, hip extensors, plantarflexion, and dorsiflexion. He was using 2 canes to walk that he borrowed from his grandmother. Although he did not complain of upper extremity weakness, he had 4+/5 strength in the interossei with the remainder of his upper extremity muscles having good strength. He had a positive Gower's sign.
Studies: Review of his outside films demonstrated a small central disc bulge at L5 but there was no compression of the roots and there were no abnormal cord signals.

Study	Findings
Left Peroneal CMAP	Distal Latency 6.30 ms CMAP Amplitude 2.2 mV Conduction Velocity 32.5 m/s
Right Peronal CMAP	Distal Latency 7.9 ms CMAP Amplitude 8.1 mV Conduction Velocity 36 m/s
Left Peroneal F-Wave	Prolonged
Right Peroneal F-wave	Prolonged
Needle EMG right anterior tibialis	Fibrillation potentials 2+ polyphasic MUAPS with increased duration
Needle EMG right gastrocnemius (medial)	Fibrillation potentials 2+ polyphasic MUAPS with increased duration
Needle EMG right lumbar paraspinal muscle	Fibrillation potentials 2+ polyphasic MUAPS with increased duration

EMG/NCV FIndings

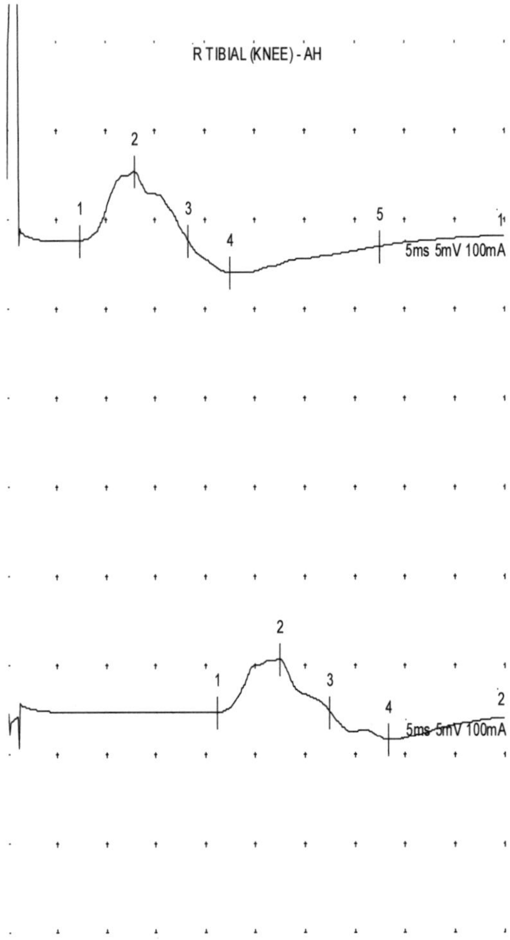

Fig. 4.

Diagnosis: diabetic peripheral neuropathy, diabetic amyotrophy.
Clinical Course: The patient was admitted from the EMG lab to the hospital. He was seen by an endocrine consult who determined that the patient had insulin dependent diabetes mellitus. LP performed demonstrated mildly elevated protein of 55 mg/dL. His CSF glucose was also elevated at 100 mg/dL. There were no abnormalities in the cell counts. He completed a course of IVIG (2 grams per kg divided over 5 days). He remained on the inpatient rehabilitation service for 2 weeks, By the time of his discharge, he was walking independently and his sugars were under control on a regimen that included the use of Lantus insulin. Although at follow-up 3 months later, he still had weakness in the hip flexors, quadriceps, hip abductors, hip adductors, hip extensors, anterior tibialis, and gastrocnemius muscles, there was an improvement to 4-4+/5 strength. He was then lost to follow-up when he turned 18 years of age.
Discussion: Diabetic neuropathy is present in approximately half of patients who have had the diagnosis for more than 5 years. Like adults, impaired glucose metabolism prior to the diagnosis of diabetes mellitus can affect nerve function. Hemoglobin A1c and glucose

tolerance tests can be helpful in diagnosing impaired glucose metabolism in patients that have normal random glucose levels (Nelson, 2006).

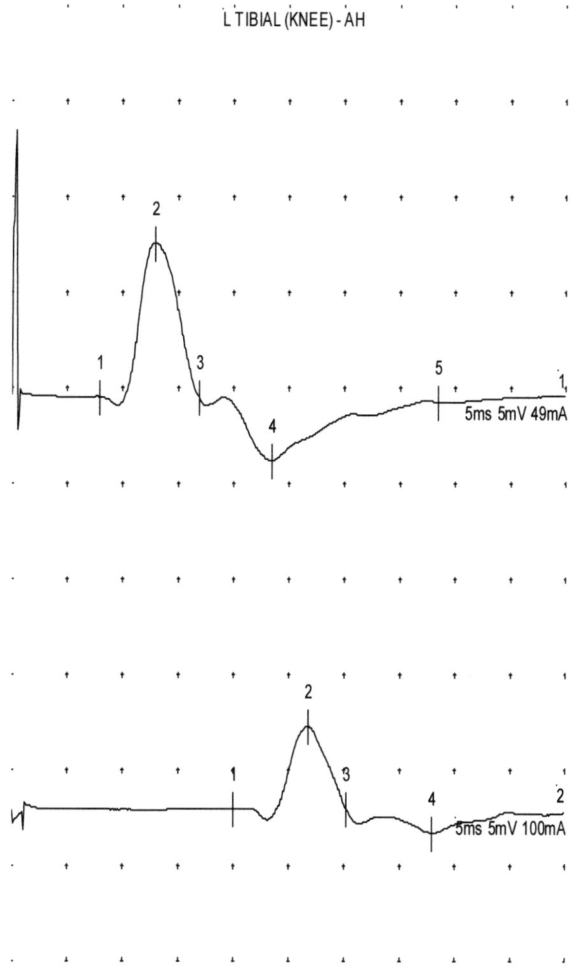

Fig. 5.

Most pediatric patients who have the peripheral neuropathy associated with diabetes mellitus are not detectable clinically. Both vibratory and tactile perception thresholds are not reliable. Most patients with diabetes are asymptomatic. Approximately 40% can be detected with a careful clinical examination. A larger percentage, approximately 60% can be detected with neurophysiological tests. It is important to identify which patients have diabetic neuropathy because they are at higher risk for retinopathy and nephropathy (Nelson, 2006). Presentations of diabetic neuropathy in clinidren to childern include Carpal Tunnel Syndrome (CTS) (seen in 1/5 of type I diabetics and 1/3 of type 2 diabetics), 3rd nerve with sparing of the pupil, intercostals neuropathy (severe abdominal and chest pain that can mimic cardiac disease), chronic inflammatory demyelinating polyradiculopathy, small fiber neuropathy, autonomic neuropathy (seen in 16% of type I diabetics and 22% of type

II diabetics), and in the case of our patient, amyotrophy. Diabetic amyotrophy is a consequence of uncontrolled diabetes mellitus. It usually presents as progressive proximal greater than distal lower extremity weakness, muscle wasting, and significant weight loss. It is a rare complication of pediatric patients and often occurs with significant peripheral neuropathy (Trotta, 2004).

Symptoms of autonomic neuropathy can be seen in 15-20% of adolescent patients with long-standing diabetes. Autonomic neuropathy impairs the epinephrine response to hypoglycemia and thus places patients at risk for severe complications. Multiple systems can be involved with diabetic autonomic Neuropathy including the cardiovascular and gastrointestinal systems (Trotta, 2004). Please refer to the excellent review written by Trotta et al, 2004 for a discussion of the symptoms of autonomic neuropathy associated with Diabetes Mellitus in children.

Although some degree of neuropathy cannot be avoided in even the best controlled patients, controlling sugars is the best way to slow down progression and complications.

8. Case #7

History: A 2 year old girl is referred to the neurophysiology laboratory for absent reflexes. Per her mother, she had been developmentally normal for the first 8 months of her life. At this point, her development became stagnant. She developed increased tone, never attained the abilities to crawl, stand, or walk. She was able to sit but lost this ability several months before the test. Her mother stated that she had an abnormal MRI. Review of the report indicates that she has a leukodystrophy.

Physical examination highlights: The patient was awake with eyes open. She did not track consistently. Despite increased tone in her trunk and extremities, she had absent reflexes. During her appointment in the neurophysiology laboratory for nerve conduction studies, the patient had several 10-15 second seizures with a semiology of head and eye deviation to the right and lip smacking.

Studies: NCV demonstrates a generalized demyelinating neuropathy. Further bloodwork revealed a very low level of arylsulfatase.

Diagnosis: Metachromatic Leukodystrophy (MLD).

Inborn errors of metabolism are rare but important causes of neuropathy in childhood. Causes of inborn errors of metabolism that are associated with peripheral neuropathy include metachromatic leukodystrophy. Metachromatic leukodystrophy has multiple forms based on the mutation as well as the age of onset. Our patient has the most severe form (infantile) which is generally fatal in one to two decades. MLD can also present in childhood, adolescence, and young adulthood. These forms are less progressive and the neuropathic component can be more prominent. No cure exists for this disease but bone marrow transplant can be helpful. In some studies, it was able to significantly slow down the progression or halt the disease for short period of time from a cognitive standpoint. However, the peripheral neuropathy component continued. Patients with the later onset forms of metachromatic leukodystrophy have presented with peripheral neuropathy without clinical evidence of CNS involvement (de Silva, 1993). Very rarely, a patient can have peripheral nervous system involvement without apparent central nervous system involvement (Coulter-Mackie, 2001).

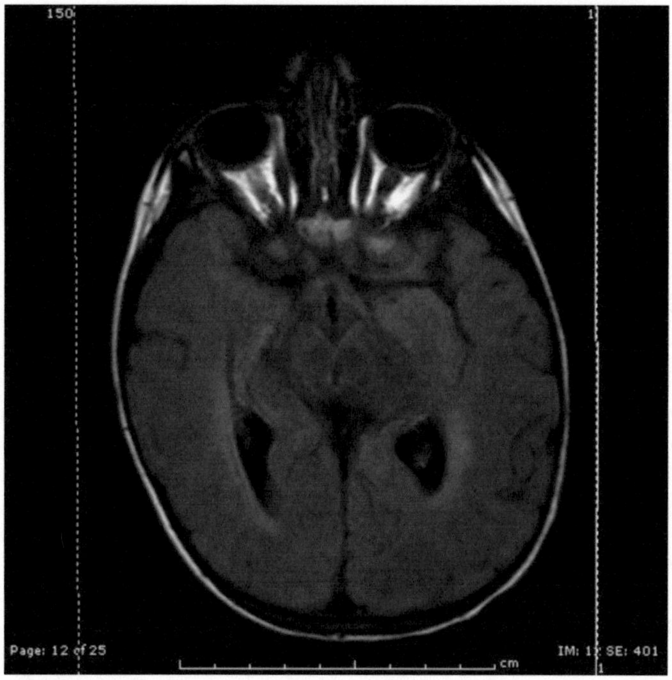

Fig. 7. T1 FLAIR image of patient with MLD

Krabbe's disease is an autosomal recessive disorder of galactocerebrosidase metabolism abnormality resulting in galactocerbrosidase beta galactosidase deficiency. Neurophysiological features include a demyelinating motor neuropathy on NCV and denervation on EMG. Like Metachromatic Leukodystrophy, there are different forms of the disease characterized by the time of their onset. The early infantile form can result in death after quick progression, sometimes by the second birthday. Other forms include the late infantile form (presents between 1.5 and 3 years), juvenile form (presents from 3-10 years) and the late onset form (presents later than 10 years of age) that makes up 10-15% of the patients. Late onset Krabbe's disease has been reported to present initially only as a peripheral neuropathy before the clinical onset of CNS manifestations. However, typically, the peripheral neuropathy associated with Late Onset Krabbe's disease is one of many other symptoms including limb weakness, termor, ataxia, nystagmus, blindness, psychomotor regression, and bulbar symptoms (Marks, 1997).

Other disorders associated with neuropathy include, Refsum, Mucopolysaccharidoses (which can present with bilateral Carpal tunnel syndrome) (Gschwind, 1992), Lowe's, and mitochondrial disorders (Wierzbicki, 2002; Charnas, 1998; Moosa, 1970). Other leukoencephalopathies associated with peripheral neuropathy include Fabry's Disease, Adrenoleukodystrophy/Adrenomyeloleukodystrophy, hypomyelination with congenital cataract, and Cockayne Syndrome (Kohlschutter, 2010).

POLG-1 mutations have been described in patients who present with a CMT- like appearance but tested negative for PMP-22 and related abnormalities. Profound sensory ataxia is seen in this phenotype. SANDO (sensory ataxic neuropathy with dysphagia and ophthalmoplegia) is another mitochondrial cytopathy that is associated with peripheral neuropathy (Harrowe, 2008).

9. Conclusion

Pediatric neuropathy presentations are quite varied. Evaluation of these disorders can be challenging in this population. Careful history and review of the available diagnostic work-up is essential. EMG/NCV studies continue to be an important tool in the evaluation of a child with neuropathy. Genetic classification and testing has been improving our diagnostic abilities. It is important to decipher as quickly as possible which ones warrant prompt treatment.

10. References

Agrawal, S., et al. (2007). Management of Children with Guillain Barre Syndrome. *Archives of Disease In Childhood* 92: ep161-ep168.

Andrews, I. and Sanders, D. (2003). Chapter 34: Juvenile Myasthenia Gravis. In *Neuromuscular Disorders of Infancy, Children, and Adolescence, A Clinician's Approach,* H.R. Jones, D.C. DeVivo, and B. T. Darras pp 575-597.

Antonellis, A., et al (2003). Glycyl tRNA Synthetase Mutations in Charcot-Marie Tooth Disease Type 2D and Distal Spinal Muscular Atrophy Type V. *American Journal of Human Genetics,* 72,1293-1299

Asbury, A. and Cornblath, D. (1990). Assessment of Current Diagnostic Criteria for Guillain Barre Syndrome. *Annals of Neurology,* 27, S21-24.

Boerkoel, C. et al (2001). Periaxin Mutations Cause Recessive Dejerine Sottas Neuropathy. *American Journal of Human Genetics,* 325-333

Charnas, L., et al. (1988). MRI findings and Peripheral Neuropathy in Lowe's Syndrome. *Neuropediatrics* 1988 19: 7-9.

Cosi, V. and Versino, M. (2006). Guillain-Barre Syndrome. *Neurological Sciences,* 27:S47-51.

Coulter-Mackie, M., et al. (2002). Isolated peripheral neuropathy in atypical Metachromatic Leukodystrophy: A Recurrent Mutation. Canadian Journal of Science 2002 29: 159-163.

De Silva, K., and J. Pearce (1973). Neuropathy of Metachromatic Leukodystrophy. *Journal of Neurology, Neurosurgery, and Psychiatry,* 36: 30-33.

Dubourg, O., et al (2001). Clinical, electrophysiological and molecular genetic characteristics of 93 patients with X-linked Charcot –Marie-Tooth Disease. *Brain,* 124, 1958-1967.

Evgrafov, O., et al (2004). Mutant small heat shock protein 27 causes axonal Charcot-Marie-Tooth disease and distal hereditary motor neuropathy. *Nature Genetics,* 36,602-606

Felice, K. and Jones, R. (1996). Pediatric Ulnar Mononeuropathy: Report of 21 Electromyography-Documented Cases and Review of the Literature. *Journal of Child Neurology* 11: 116-120.

Figueroa, A., et al. (1980). The Role of Folate Deficiency in the Development of a Peripheral Neuropathy Caused By Anticonvulsants. *Journal of the Neurological Sciences,* 48: 315-323.

Fraser, J. and Olney, R. (1992). The Relative Diagnostic Sensitivity of Different F-wave Parameters in Various Polyneuropathies. *Muscle and Nerve,* 15: 912-918.

Gorson, Kenneth, et al (1996). Prospective evaluation of MRI Lumbosacral nerve root enhancement in acute Guillain-Barre Syndrome. *Neurology,*47,813-817

Graf, W., et al (1996). Severe Vincristine Neuropathy in Charcot-Marie-Tooth Disease Type 1A. *Cancer* 77:1356-62.

Gschwind, C. and Tonkin, M. (1992). Carpal Tunnel Syndrome in Children with Mucopolysacharidosis and Related Disorders. *Journal of Hand Surgery* 17A:44-7.

Gutman, L. and Gutman, L. (1999). Critical Illness Neuropathy and Myopathy. *Archives of Neurology,* 56: 527-528.

Harel, L., et al (2002). Peripheral Neuropathy in Pediatric Systemic Lupus Erythromatosus. *Pediatric Neurology,* 27, 53-56.

Harrower, T., et al (2008) POLG1 Mutation Manifesting as Autosomal Recessive Axonal Charcot-Marie-Tooth Disease. *Archives of Neurology,* 65, 133-136

Hayakasa, K, et al (1993). De novo mutation of the myelin P0 gene in Dejerine -Sotts Disease (hereditary motor and sensory neuropathy type III), *Nature Genetics,* 5, 266-268.

Ho, T., et al. (1997). Patterns of Recovery in the Guillain Barre Syndromes. *Neurology,* 48: 695-700.

Hughes, R. et al (2003). Practice Parameter: Immunotherapy for Guillain Barre Syndrome: Report of the Quality Standards Subcommittee of the American Academy of Neurology, *Neurology,* 61,736-740.

Jones, R. (1986). Compressive Neuropathy in Childhood: A Report of 14 Cases. *Muscle and Nerve* 9: 720-723.

Kautio, A., et al. (2008). Amitriptyline in the treatment of Chemotherapy Induced Neuropathic Symptoms. *Journal of Pain and Symptom Management* 35: 31-39.

Kellens, T., et al (1993). Deletion of the serine 34 codon from the major peripheral myelin protein P0 gene in Charcot-Marie-Tooth disease type 1b. *Nature Genetics,* 5,35-38

Kuwabara, S., et al. (2004). Sensory Nerve Conduction in Demyelinating and Axonal Guillain Barre Syndromes. *European Neurology,* 51: 196-198.

Kohlschutter, A., et al. (2010). Leukodystrophies and Other Genetic Metabolic Leukoencephalopathies In Children and Adults. *Brain and Development,* 32: 82-89.

Levin, K, et al (1991). Childhood Peroneal Neuropathy From Bone Tumors. *Pediatric Neurology,* 7: 308-309.

Lopate,G., et al. (2005). Treatment of Chronic Inflammatory Demyelinating Polyneuropathy with High-Dose Intermittent Intravenous Methylprednisolone. *Archives of Neurology* 62: 249-252.

Markowitz, J., et al. (2008). Child Neurlogy: Chronic Inflammatory Demyelinating Polyradiculoneuropathy in Children. *The Journal of Neurology,* 71:e74-78.

Marks, H., et al. Krabbe's Disease Presenting as A Peripheral Neuropathy (1997). *Muscle and Nerve,* 20: 1024-1028.

McLeod, J. and Penny, R. (1969). Vincristine neuropathy: an electrophysiological and histological study. *Journal of Neurology, Neurosurgery, and Psychiatry,* 32, 297-304.

McGee, K. (2002). The role of a child life specialist in a pediatric radiology department. *Pediatric Radiology* 33: 467-474.

Moosa, A. and Dubowitz, V. (1970). Peripheral Neuropathy in Cockayne's Syndrome. *Archives of Disease in Childhood* 45: 674-677.

Mori, M., et al. (2001). Clinical Features of Miller Fischer Syndrome. *Neurology,* 56: 1104-1106.

Nelson, D., et al (2006) Comparison of Conventional and Non-Invasive techniques for the early identification of diabetic neuropathy in children and adolescents with type I diabetes. *Pediatric Diabetes, 7, 305-310.*

NINDS fact sheet on Charcot-Marie-Tooth Disease. (2011) http://www.ninds.nih.gov/disorders/charcot_marie_tooth/detail_charot_marie_tooth.htm.

Oh, S. et al. Changes in Permeability Caused by Connexin 32 Mutations Underlie X-Linked Charcot-Marie-Tooth Disease. *Neuron,*19, 927-938

Packer, R., et al (1994). Outcome for children with medulloblastoma treated with radiation and cisplatin, CCNU, and vincristine chemotherapy. *Journal of Neurosurgery,* 81, 690-698.

Petersen, B., et al (1999). Critical Illness Neuropathy in Pediatric Intensive Care patients. *Pediatric Neurology,* 21, 749-753

Preston, D. and Shapiro, B. (1998). Polyneuropathy, In *Electromyography and Neuromuscular Disorders Clinical and Electrophysiologic Correlations,* D. Prestion and B. Shapiro, pp. *389-420.*

Priolo, T., et al. (2008). Childhood Thalidomide Neuropathy: A Clinical and Neurophysiological Study. *Pediatric Neurology,* 38: 196-199.

Quasthoff, S. and H. Hartung (2002). Chemotherapy-Induced Peripheral Neuropathy. Journal of Neurology 249: 9-17.

Reddy, A. and Witek, K. (2003). Neurological Complications of Chemotherapy for Children with Cancer. *Current Neurology and Neuroscience Reports,* 3: 137-142.

Rees, J., et al (1995). Campylobacter Jejuni Infection and Guillain-Barre Syndrome. *The New England Journal of Medicine,* 333, 1374-1379

Roa, B., et al (1993). Dejerine-Sottas Syndrome Assicuated with Point Mutation in the peripheral myelin protein 22 (PMP22) gene. *Nature Genetics,* 5, 269-273.

Rotta, F., et al (2000). The spectrum of chronic inflammatory demyelinating polyneuropathy. *Journal of the Neurological Sciences,* 173, 129-139.

Servais, L., et al. (2001). Anterior Spinal Artery Syndrome After Aortic Surgery in a Child. *Pediatric Neurology,* 24: 310-312.

Shanbag, P. ,et al. (2003). Intravenous Immunoglobulins in Severe Guillain-Barre Syndrome in Childhood. *Indian Journal of Pediatrics,* 70: 541-543.

Shahar, E., et al. (2003). Outcome of Severe Guillain Barre Syndromes in Children: Comparison Between Untreated Cases Versus Gamma-Globulin Therapy. *Clinical Neuropharmacology,* 26: 84-87.

Simmons, Z., et al. Chronic Inflammatory Demyelinating Polyradiculoneuropathy in Children: I. Presentation, electrodiagnostic syudies, and initial clinical course, with comparison to adults. *Muscle and Nerve,* 20, 1008-1015.

Simmons, Z., et al (1997). Chronic Inflammatory Demyelinating Polyradiculoneuropathy in Children: II. Long-Term Follow-Up, with Comparison to Adults. *Muscle and Nerve,*20, 1569-1575.

Simmons, Z. (2010). Treatment and Management of Autoimmune Neuropathies, In *Neuromuscular Disorders Treatment and Management,* T. Bertorini, pp. 215-229.

Strauss, R. and K. Das (2000). Thalidomide Induced Sensory Neuropathy. *Journal of Pediatric Gstroenterology,* 32: 322-324.

Thompson, S. et al. (1984). Cisplatin Neuropathy Clinical, Electrophysiological, Morphological, and Toxologic Studies. *Cancer,* 54:1269-1275.

Trotta, D., et al (2004). Diabetic Neuropathy in Children and Adolescents. *Pediatric Diabetes,*4, 47-55.

Van der Berg, L., et al (1991). Anti GM1 antibodies in patients with Guillain Barre Syndrome. *Journal of Neurology, Neurosurgery, and Psychiatry,* 55, 8-11.

Verhamme, C., et al (2009). Oral high dose ascorbic acid treatment for one yeat in young CMT1a patients: a randomized, double-blind, placebo-controlled phase II trial. *British Medical Journal.*

Wolf, S., et al. (2008). Chemotherapy Induced PIN: Prevention and Treatment Strategies. *European Journal of Cancer* 44: 1507-1515.

Wierzbicki, A., et al (2002). Refsum's disease: a peroxisomal disorder affecting phytanic acid alpha oxidation. *Journal of Neurochemistry* 80: 727-735.

8

Neuropathies Associated with Cosmetic Surgeries

Alexander Cárdenas-Mejía, Xitlali Baron, Colin Coulter, Javier Lopez-Mendoza and Claudia Gutiérrez
Postgraduate Course in Plastic and Reconstructive Surgery, Universidad Nacional Autonoma de México, General Hospital "Dr. Manuel Gea González", México City Mexico

1. Introduction

Plastic, aesthetic and reconstructive surgery encompasses a wide range of surgical procedures for various parts of the body such as the face, neck, breast, body contouring and surgery on the upper and lower limbs.

In the last two decades the number of aesthetic procedures across the world has increased significantly. Although aesthetic surgery is not new its current popularity has rapidly increased due to the improved outcomes of techniques using autologous tissue as well as minimally invasive techniques which cause less scarring following surgical procedures[1].

However with this increase in the number of procedures, the number of postoperative complications has also risen although in the majority of cases these are minor[1].

Major complications are rare and frequently related to factors unique to the patient (such as anatomical variants) rather than with the technical aspects of the surgical procedure [1].

Nerve injury is a rare complication in patients who undergo aesthetic surgery; nonetheless, whatever the cause of the injury, it can lead to moderate disability in some patients.

Iatrogenic nerve lesions caused during aesthetic surgery can present in two ways. One is with a sensory change such as dysesthesia, anesthesia or chronic untreatable pain. The other is a change in motor function manifesting either as partial or complete loss of function or synkinesis. Both outcomes can lead to physical and emotional disability.

Plastic, aesthetic and reconstructive surgeons should have in mind all of the possible nerve injuries during the procedures. A thorough understanding of anatomy as well as changes with age is very important for the surgeons.

There are some nerve injuries which are unavoidable and form an inherent part of the surgical procedure with the full knowledge of the surgeon and the patient. These include procedures such as mammoplasty (augmentation, reduction or mastopexy) and dermolipectomies. In these procedures sectioning and injury to the nerve is unavoidable and sensory changes usually recover after a period of time.

2. Incidence

Across the international medical literature, it is clear that the incidence of nerve injuries differs according to the surgical area and the type of nerve.

Sensory nerves are at greater risk but injuries to them are not widely reported. However weakness of the temporal branch of the facial nerve has been reported in around 0.7% of patients[4,6,29].

Forehead lifting; 50% of procedures result in some degree of decreased sensation to the forehead[30]. Body contouring procedures carry a high risk of injury to the sensory nerves. Breast reduction; Schlenz[7] reports sensory changes in up to 47.8% of patients. Breast augmentation; Ducic[21] reports the presence of chronic pain in 7% of patients. Abdominoplasty; Bufoni[31] reports sensory changes to the hypogastric area in up to 75% of patients. Calf augmentation; several papers report no nerve complications following surgery[24,25,26] but the nerves at risk are the medial sural nerve and the saphenous nerve which innervate the posterior part of the leg. Upper limb; Knoetgen[9] reports two cases (an incidence of 5%) of nerve-related complications during brachioplasties with injury to the medial antebrachial cutaneous nerve (MACN) in the arm.

The majority of the literature relating to iatrogenic nerve injuries caused by surgery concentrates on orthopaedic patients. However there are some documented reports of such injuries following aesthetic surgery procedures as well [2].

These reports should be interpreted with caution. The majority of data comes from referral hospitals which see a high volume of patients. In these cases, the reported rates are very low probably owing to the vast experience of plastic surgeons that treat a high number of patients in these circumstances.

A detailed neurological examination is required to identify the deficits. Motor weakness may be obvious or the patient will bring it to the attention of the surgeon. On the other hand the sensory deficits at first may be mildly uncomfortable to the patient, but are usually well tolerated and may not be a major source of complaint for the patient.

Facial surgeries; Rhytidectomies carry the highest incidence of nerve injuries predominantly causing sensory changes. Damage to the great auricular nerve is reported in 1-7% of cases. Nerve injuries affecting the forehead typically show motor deficits in 0.5-3% of cases. These can result from damage to any of the branches of the facial nerve: marginal mandibular 3%, temporal 1.5%, cervical 1.75%, zygomatic and buccal 0.2%. The incidence increases if the procedure is performed endoscopically and when it is combined with ultrasound-assisted liposuction. The next most common procedures resulting in nerve injuries are blepharoplasties, rhinoplasties and genioplasties with some reported cases of isolated nerve injury [3,4,5,6].

Breast surgeries; reduction mammoplasty utilizing the superior pedicle technique shows the highest incidence of sensory changes to the nipple-areola complex as high as 47.8%[7].

Body contouring procedures; ultrasound-assisted liposuction causes the greatest incidence of sensory nerve lesions with reports of hyperesthesia in up to 79% of patients. This is followed by gluteal implantation which causes paresthesia in 4-20% of patients and paresis in 1.5% while only 1% of patients receiving gluteal lipoinjections suffer from paresthesia[8].

The limbs; brachioplasties represent the highest rate of nerve injuries of up to 5% with injuries to the medial antebrachial cutaneous nerve. In the lower limbs the incidence is much lower with reports of damage to the medial sural cutaneous nerve and the medial saphenous nerve during the placement of calf implants[9, 10,11].

3. Mechanism of injury

The mechanism of injury varies between cases. It can be due to direct nerve traction caused by the use of retractors, direct mechanical injury, thermal or ultrasound injury, nerve laceration from instrument usage or damage by physical manipulation of the nerve.

Nerve entrapment or compression may also result due to sutures or the formation of scar tissue, haematomas or even poor positioning of the patient[7]. Other concomitant therapies such as radiation or chemotherapy can cause neuritis or neuropathy with or without compression. The position of the patient during the surgical procedure such as having the patient in the prone position can increase the risk of nerve injuries such as plexopathy[2, 12].

4. Diagnosis

It should be emphasised that early diagnosis with appropriate treatment is necessary to ensure that optimum nerve function is restored. The deficits can get worse if patients have to wait longer for evaluation.

In the case of a late diagnosis nerve reconstruction is more difficult resulting in sub optimal nerve function. As Sunderland described, once atrophy of the motor end plate begins after 3 to 6 months, only partial reconstruction can be achieved[2].

The diagnosis of nerve damage requires a complete neurological examination evaluating any sensory or motor impairment by validated scales i.e. British Medical Council Scale for Muscle Strength (BMRC) while sensory changes can be evaluated either by using the same scale or applying the Seddon classification.

Electrophysiological studies are an integral part of the evaluation to elucidate the site and possibly extent of the injury. The information gained ideally in the first 2-4 months will indicate which therapeutic options are most appropriate.

Measuring the quality of life using the standardised scale SF-36[2] can be worthwhile.

The above recommendations do not apply in the case of injuries to the facial nerve. The standardised scale recommended for use in these patients is the House-Brackmann scale. However some authors consider the Sunnybrook Facial Grading System to provide a better evaluation since it does not only group the patients into one of five possible categories (as the HB scale does) but also provides a more precise measurement scale assigning a score of between 0 and 100 to the patient. It also incorporates an evaluation of synkinesis by the fourth outpatient clinic. However for this group of patients the SF-36 scale is not useful. Frijters et al. (2008) reported no statistically significant relationship between injuries to branches of the facial nerve and SF-36 scores.[13]

Electrophysiological studies including nerve conduction studies of sensory and motor nerves and electromyography should be performed at the time of the diagnosis and during follow-up monitoring.

Somatosensory Evoked Potentials tests, electroneurography and electromyography are very helpful in diagnosing nerve injury [14].

<table>
<tr><th>STANDARDIZED QUESTIONNAIRES</th><th colspan="3">EVALUATION</th><th>TOTAL SCORE</th><th>WHO EVALUATES</th><th>SUBJECT OF EVALUATION</th></tr>
<tr><td rowspan="6">HOUSE BRACKMANN</td><td colspan="3">NORMAL SYMMETRICAL FUNCTION IN ALL AREAS</td><td>1</td><td rowspan="6">INTERRATER</td><td rowspan="6">FACIAL PARALYSIS</td></tr>
<tr><td colspan="3">SLIGHT WEAKNESS NOTICEABLE ONLY ON CLOSE INSPECTION. COMPLETE EYE CLOSURE WITH MINIMAL EFFORT. SLIGHT ASYMMETRY OF SMILE WITH MAXIMAL EFFORT. SYNKINESIS BARELY NOTICEABLE, CONTRACTURE OR SPASM ABSENT.</td><td>2</td></tr>
<tr><td colspan="3">OBVIOUS WEAKNESS, BUT NOT DISFIGURING. MAY NOT BE ABLE TO LIFT EYEBROW COMPLETE EYE CLOSURE AND STRONG BUT ASYMMETRICAL MOUTH MOVEMENT WITH MAXIMAL EFFORT. OBVIOUS, BUT NOT DISFIGURING SYNKINESIS, MASS MOVEMENT OR SPASM.</td><td>3</td></tr>
<tr><td colspan="3">OBVIOUS DISFIGURING WEAKNESS. INABILITY TO LIFT BROW. INCOMPLETE EYE CLOSURE AND ASYMMETRY OF MOUTH WITH MAXIMAL EFFORT. SEVERE SYNKINESIS, MASS MOVEMENT, SPASM</td><td>4</td></tr>
<tr><td colspan="3">MOTION BARELY PERCEPTIBLE. INCOMPLETE EYE CLOSURE, SLIGHT MOVEMENT CORNER MOUTH SYNKINESIS, CONTRACTURE, AND SPASM USUALLY ABSENT</td><td>5</td></tr>
<tr><td colspan="3">NO MOVEMENT, LOSS OF TONE, NO SYNKINESIS, CONTRACTURE, OR SPASM</td><td>6</td></tr>
<tr><td rowspan="9">SUNNYBROOK FACIAL GRADING SYSTEM</td><td rowspan="3">RESTING SYMMETRY</td><td>PALPEBRAL FISSURE</td><td>NORMAL
NARROW
WIDE</td><td rowspan="9">0 - 100
0: COMPLETE FACIAL PARALYSIS
100: NORMAL FACIAL FUNCTION</td><td rowspan="9">INTER AND INTRARATER</td><td rowspan="9">FACIAL PARALYSIS</td></tr>
<tr><td>NASOLABIAL FOLD</td><td>NORMAL
ABSENT
LESS
OR MORE PRONOUNCED</td></tr>
<tr><td>CORNER OF THE MOUTH (TO THE NORMAL SIDE)</td><td>NORMAL
DROOPED
PULLED UP/OUT</td></tr>
<tr><td rowspan="5">SYMMETRY OF VOLUNTARY MOVEMENT</td><td>FOREHEAD WRINKLE</td><td rowspan="5">1 (NO MOVEMENT)

5 (MOVEMENT COMPLETE)</td></tr>
<tr><td>GENTLE EYE CLOSURE</td></tr>
<tr><td>OPEN MOUTH SMILE</td></tr>
<tr><td>SNARL</td></tr>
<tr><td>LIP PUCKER</td></tr>
<tr><td>SYNKINESIS</td><td>DEGREE OF</td><td>0 (NO SYNKINESIS)
3 (SEVERE SYNKINESIS)</td></tr>
</table>

SHORT FORM-36 HEALTH SURVEY	PHYSICAL FUNCTIONING	0 – 100 100: HIGHER LEVELS OF WELL FUNCTIONING OR WELL BEING	SELF REPORT QUESTIONNARIE	LIFE QUALITY
	ROLE LIMITATIONS DUE TO PHYSICAL HEALTH PROBLEMS			
	BODILY PAIN			
	GENERAL HEALTH PERCEPTIONS			
	VITALITY			
	SOCIAL FUNCTIONING			
	ROLE LIMITIATIONS DUE TO EMOTIONAL PROBLEMS			
	GENERAL MENTAL HEALTH			

Table 1. Scales to evaluate facial paralysis and sequelae

Electromyography has proven to be the most useful test in the study of these types of injuries. It evaluates and registers the electrical activity produced by skeletal muscles measuring the electrical potential generated by the muscle cells.

Electromyography is performed 14 to 21 days after the injury when Wallerian degeneration of the axons has occurred. However in the acute phase, it is not possible to distinguish the extent of the axonal degeneration until the 3rd to 14th day[14]. In acute injuries increased spontaneous activity including positive waves and fibrillation potentials are noted. When the motor end plates are reinnervated electromyography shows polyphasic action potentials[15].

In circumstances where electrophysiological studies do not detect a loss of axonal continuity or Wallerian degeneration it is advisable to have a period of "watchful waiting" with regular nerve conduction studies to confirm that nerve transmission is not deteriorating[15, 16].

In any of the cases described above, patients presenting with a nerve injury should always be referred to a specialist in order to start the most appropriate treatment as early as possible.

5. Facial surgery

In facial surgery nerve injuries have been reported following procedures such as blepharoplasties, rhinoplasties, genioplasties and most commonly in rhytidectomies[16].

There have been some distressing reports of blindness following blepharoplasties. Data collected regarding rhinoplasties has reported cases of sensory loss of the nose-tip and injuries resulting from genioplasties have caused anesthesia or dysesthesia affecting the lips, chin and in some cases, paresthesia or paralysis of the lower lip.

However rhytidectomies are the commonest cause of facial nerve injuries. Patients can present with paresis with loss of function of the facial nerve- an event which can have a significant psychological impact for the patient[14].

The majority of nerve injuries following rhytidectomies show sensory loss with the great auricular nerve being the most commonly affected. This is followed by injuries resulting in loss of motor function affecting in decreasing order the following divisions of the facial nerve: temporal, marginal mandibular, buccal and zygomatic.

There are some reports that rhytidectomies performed endoscopically on the upper third and upper half of the face can lead to complications such as transitory paresis of the temporal and zygomatic branches of the facial nerve showing recovery within six months after the procedure. When the procedure is carried out using ultrasound-assisted liposuction the incidence of motor nerve injuries is 7.6% (affecting the marginal mandibular branch)[17].

Although an uncommon outcome from aesthetic surgery of the neck, injury to the spinal accessory nerve has been documented following cervicofacial lift and is most likely due to scar formation developing around the nerve.[32]

About 20% of injuries affecting the motor function of the facial nerve following rhytidectomies fail to show any spontaneous recovery of function.

The facial nerve and its branches travel along the anteromedial aspect of the parotid gland, running in a deep plane towards the superficial muscular and aponeurotic system (SMAS). The facial muscles are therefore innervated by the facial nerve from a deep position with the exception of the muscles elevating the corner of the mouth: buccinator and mentalis. With this in mind it is therefore necessary to perform a superficial dissection of the SMAS in order to avoid nerve-related complications[2, 14, 16].

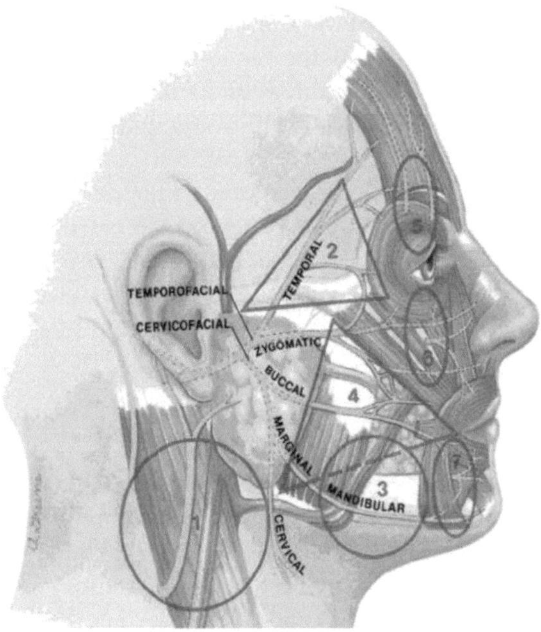

Fig. 1. Zeckel´s nerve risk zones during face lift; major to minor risk; 1= great auricular nerve, 2= frontal branch of facial nerve, 3= marginal branch of facial nerve, 4= buccal branch of facial nerve, 5= supraorbital nerve, 6= infrorbital nerve, 7= mental nerve

Furthermore dissections of the posterior aspect of the sternocleidomastoid muscle ought to be undertaken with caution from beneath the mastoid process where the great auricular nerve runs more superficially thus increasing the risk of injury. Care must therefore be taken when using electrocautery while dissecting the superficial nerves.

Permanent damage to the nerve results in hypoesthesia or, in patients with a neuroma, painful dysesthesia in the lower two thirds of the ear and the skin of the neck and cheek.
The temporal branch of the facial nerve poses the greatest risk of motor damage followed by the marginal mandibular and buccal branches. In terms of anatomical regions, the temporo-frontal region, the angle of the mandible and the pre-parotid region are the riskiest areas in terms of nerve injury[4, 8].
The temporal branch of the facial nerve is the thickest and is located anterior and caudal to the frontal branch of the superficial temporal artery in 91% of cases. Seckel locates the temporal branch in an area he describes as *Facial Zone 2*, where the nerve branch originates below the parotid gland at the level of the zygomatic arch before innervating the frontal muscle. Injury to the nerve results in paralysis of this muscle but orbicular function remains intact owing to the dual innervation it receives from the inferior zygomatic branches. This presents clinically as paralysis on the affected side of the forehead with ptosis of the eyebrow and a loss of symmetry during animation on that side[4, 18].
In the middle third of the face the branches of the facial nerve can be damaged when carrying out deep dissection in front of the anterior border of the parotid gland. In the inferior third of the face the marginal branch can be damaged when carrying out deep dissection from beneath the inferior border of the mandible.
In subperiosteal rhytidectomies and other procedures where the tissue is elevated above the zygomatic arch, the superficial layer of the deep temporal fascia can be damaged when penetrating the superficial temporal fat pad.
Injury to the nerve results in asymmetry of the lower lip especially when opening the mouth and when smiling. If the triangular muscle of the lips is denervated, the corner of the mouth cannot be moved and the lower lip cannot be lowered making it impossible to show the inferior teeth on the affected side. At rest, the zygomatic muscles, which are normally innervated, are not opposed because the triangular muscle of the lips has no tone and the commissure of the mouth is held in such a way that the lower lip lies above the teeth when at rest.
One way of damaging the marginal mandibular nerve is by electrocautery while trying to control bleeding from the facial vein or less frequently from the facial artery. Both are found medially and deep to the marginal mandibular branch. The electric current can be passed to the nerve causing damage.

6. Breast surgery

The surgical procedures performed on the breast which can cause nerve injuries and chronic neurogenic pain include breast reconstruction, breast reduction, mastoplexy and breast lifting[21].
The symptoms can be due to neuromas-in-continuity with the intercostal nerve branches caused either by direct compression or by scar formation resulting from nerve traction or dissection.
Ducic describes the different zones of the breast which are susceptible to nerve injury as the superior, inferior, medial, lateral, central or the nipple-areola complex (NAC)[21].
In surgery of the mammary gland, preserving the innervation of the nipple-areola complex has become a fundamental matter of importance. Nerve injuries affecting the NAC are most commonly expected during breast reduction surgery[7].

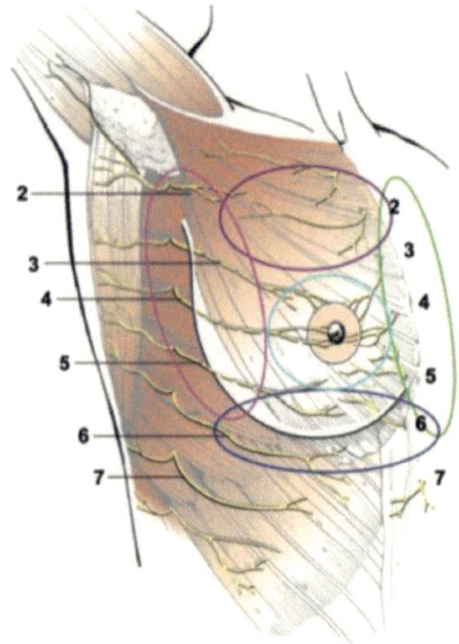

Fig. 2. Ducic´s danger zones for nerve injuries, resulting in chronic posoperative breast pain

The mammary gland is innervated by the medial branches of the first to sixth intercostal nerves and the lateral branches of the second to seventh intercostal nerves[21].

Innervation of the NAC is supplied by the anterior and lateral branches of the third, fourth and fifth intercostal nerves. The nipple is innervated by the anterior and lateral branches of the fourth intercostal nerve with additional innervations supplied by the lateral branches of the third to fifth nerves and the anterior branches of the second to fifth[7, 22].

The anterior branches run superficially through the subcutaneous tissue emerging superficially in the medial border of the areola. These branches can be damaged when the areola size is reduced. The lateral branches pass deeply through the pectoral fascia ending in the superficial posterior border of the complex in 93% of cases. These branches are damaged when the tissue is resected occurring most frequently during the breast reduction technique using the superior pedicle (Lejour, Lassus)[7, 22].

In breast augmentation, transareolar access can damage the third and fourth intercostal branches, inframmamary incisions can injure the fifth and sixth intercostal nerves, transaxillar access may injure the second intercostal nerve and incisions made in the infraumbilical region (not currently used) can damage the tenth. In breast reconstruction the third to seventh intercostal nerves may be damaged, including the lateral, inferior and medial zones. During mastopexy the third and fourth intercostal nerves are damaged with the central zone of the breast being predominantly affected. The most common nerve injury presenting in cases of breast reduction is caused by a simultaneous injury affecting the central, inferior and lateral zones. In light of this, the majority of authors (Giorgiade, McKissock and Wuringuer) agree that techniques using the inferior pedicle are the only ones where innervation of the NAC is preserved [7, 21].

Some authors do not recognize the importance of nerve injuries to the NAC, making reference to reports of reinnervation with free-nipple-grafts through the dermal plexus using the supraclavicular and third intercostal nerve[22].

7. Body contouring

The neuropathies reported in body contouring procedures can be due to direct nerve injury, compression or traction.

The position of the patient, appropriate cushioning and knowledge of the anatomy are crucial to avoid nerve injury[16].

Temporary paresthesia is frequently reported around the site of surgery owing to direct laceration of the cutaneous nerves. Tight clothing can also elicit this effect where temporary inflammation causes paresthesia fading after 48 hours or once the external compression has been removed[16].

Direct nerve injuries which have been reported include those to the lateral femoral cutaneous nerve, the iliohypogastric nerve and the ilioinguinal nerve during abdominoplasty procedures.

The lateral femoral cutaneous nerve is the longest branch of the lumbar plexus emerging from the dorsal branch of the second, third and fourth lumbar nerves[23].

The lateral femoral cutaneous nerve can be located 2cm medial to the anterior superior iliac spine. It passes through psoas major emerging from its lateral inferior border advancing through the inguinal ligament towards the thigh[16, 23].

In the thigh, the anterior division of the femoral nerve gives off cutaneous branches which supply sensation to the anterior surface of the thigh and muscular branches to the pectineus and sartorius muscle[23].

The posterior division of the femoral nerve originates from the saphenous nerve which supplies sensation to the anterior and medial part of the leg. Its muscular branches innervate the quadriceps femoris. A weak patellar tendon reflex is the clearest objective sign of femoral neuropathy. This causes instability of the knee joint by weakness of the quadriceps.

Abdominoplasty is the most frequent cause of damage to this nerve, especially when retractors are used. Transverse incisions of the abdomen and a thin body habitus are also additional risk factors[23].

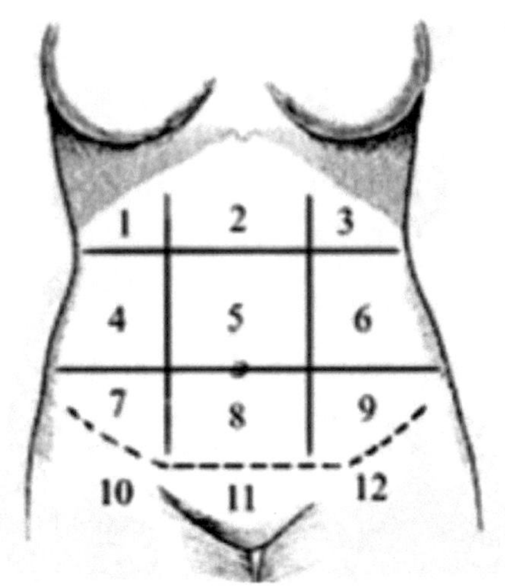

Fig. 3. Bufoni´s zones to evaluate sensibility of the abdomen after abdominoplasty. Zone 4 is the area that takes longer time for recovery and sometimes will never recover.

Gluteal lipoinjections are another one of the aesthetic surgical procedures where complications of this type are described. These include damage to the sciatic nerve which can occur in three different ways: direct injury by the cannula, extrinsic compression by injected adipose tissue or intrinsic compression by accidental injection of fat into the nerve sheath. The majority of minor injuries present as transient paresthesia or hyperesthesia and self-limiting muscle weakness but serious injuries such as axonotmesis of the nerve can also present in this way.[1]

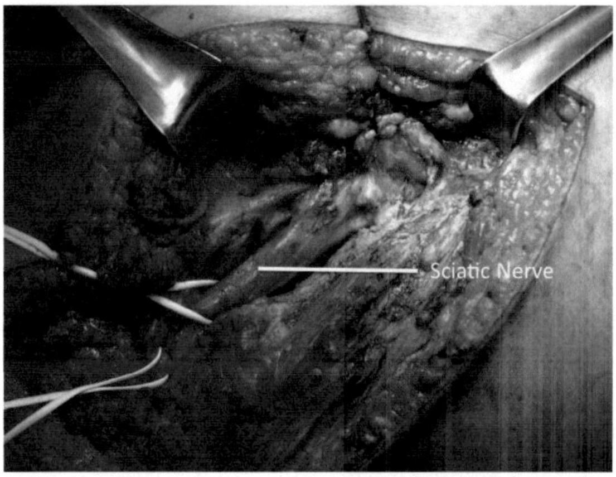

Fig. 4. Sciatic nerve lipoinjected during a gluteal lipoinjection. We reported good recovery after neurolysis.

In procedures on the gluteal region, Meieta reports a rate of 20% of transient paresthesia in the intramuscular region following gluteal implantation which returns to normal after three weeks of treatment with gabapentin[8].

Bruner et al. report transient sciatic paresthesia in 4% of patients for two to three weeks in 261 patients and a transient loss of sciatic motor function in two patients (1.5%) with restoration of motor function in one to two weeks and an improvement in the paresthesia in one to two months.

Mendieta describes a frequency of transient paresthesia in less than 1% of gluteal lipoinjections and Restrepo & Ahmed also report this outcome without quantifying the amount[8].

With this in mind it is important to have as thorough an understanding of the gluteal region as it is for the rest of the body's anatomy.

8. Aesthetic surgery on the limbs

The medial antebrachial cutaneous nerve can be damaged during brachioplasty. An incidence of 6% has been reported with the presence of paresthesia that resolves over the course of 13 months up to the most severe injury being complex regional pain syndrome type II[9].

The medial antebrachial cutaneous nerve and the medial brachial nerve originate from the medial cord in 78% of cases and from the inferior trunk in 22%. It emerges from the axilla travelling medially to the brachial artery. It runs adjacent to the basilic vein or posterior to it. Although not all authors agree that the nerve runs continuously alongside the basilic vein its location in relation to the cubital nerve is medial and posterior[9,16].

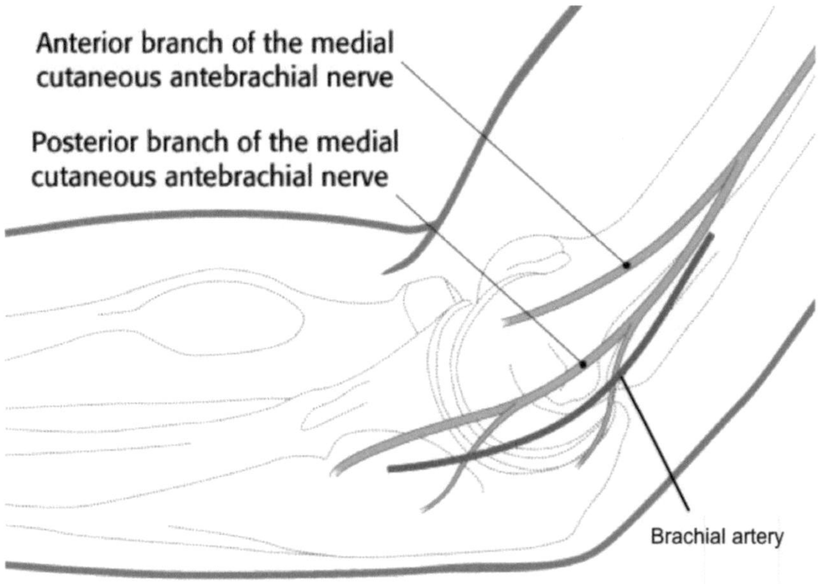

Fig. 5. Medial cutaneous branch and his terminal branches, anatomy landmarks.

The medial antebrachial cutaneous nerve and the medial brachial nerve are two constant structures which run below the deep facia on the edge of the intermuscular septum in the arm, perforating the fascia as it moves superficially to approximately 14cm to the medial condyle (from 8 to 21cm) dividing itself into two branches, anterior and posterior. The posterior branch innervates the region peripheral to the medial epicondyle while the anterior branch moves towards the proximal end of the forearm to innervate it. From the site where it becomes superficial, the nerve perforates the deep fascia , this is what causes the risk of damage during brachioplasty. This risk is greatest when the surgical site is located in the intermuscular septum, a location preferred by many authors, since it is where scarring can easily be hidden.

To avoid injury during brachioplasty it is advisable to leave a margin of 1cm of adipose tissue around the deep fascia during the surgical procedure[9].

In the lower limb, damage to the medial sural cutaneous nerve and the medial saphenous nerve can occur during calf implantation. This can be avoided by preserving the fascial connection across the medial aspect of the leg[24, 25, 26].

9. Medical treatment

Early identification of nerve injury is important to initiate therapeutic intervention[16].

Once the injury has been diagnosed and the extent of it has been determined, one can offer conservative management for those who present with first or second degree paralysis; the re-myelinization and regeneration of the nerve should lead to a complete recovery. In these cases physical therapy will also help with the restoration of function[27].

10. Drugs

There are drugs which are indicated for use in the conservative management of the patient's injury, as adjuvant therapy to the surgical procedure whose primary or secondary function is to help with nerve regeneration[28].

Although there are not enough studies, the use of steroids in nerve injuries is safe and probably effective when administering a dose of 1 mg/kg/day for 7-10days or with steroid injections if there are no contraindications to their use[28].

Other drugs used in the regeneration of nerve fibres include Etioxine, Zofenopril, Nimodipine and Tacrolimus.

Other drugs can be used but their function is to control neuropathic pain and include Gabapentin, B Complex and Pregabalina.

11. Surgical treatment

The estimated extent of axonal loss is the best indicator of expected recovery. The injuries which show less than 50% of sensory/motor loss will show recovery, in some cases over the course of a year. However if after four months of treatment the patient still does not show signs of nerve repair and the EMG does not show signs of nerve regeneration one ought to consider surgical intervention[2].

In the case of nerve injuries with axonotmesis demonstrated by electrical conduction studies, one ought to carry out end-to-end (primary) neurorrhaphy as soon as possible.

When it is possible, this procedure offers better results compared with injuries that are repaired using interposition nerve grafts or by nerve transfers. Nerve transfers can sometimes cause synkinesis in the face[13].

Nerve repair can be epinerual and perineural or one can use surgical adheshives for the appostion of nerves without needing to perform neurorrhaphy[14].

One ought to follow the basic principles of nerve suturing which are to alleviate the tension and to avoid excessive scarring and fibrosis at the site of anastomosis[14].

Other alternatives are nerve conduits which are currently used for the interposition of nerve grafts and cross-face neurotizations. In some cases though it may not be possible to sacrifice a healthy nerve[14].

And finally, in other procedures one may also consider the use of muscle replacement and aesthetic treatments.

Nowadays the use of stem cell injections and growth factors is being added to all surgical techniques[14].

12. Prevention

In each surgical procedure it is recommended that the neuronal structure be preserved as well as taking caution when using different surgical positions to avoid nerve injuries especially when the patient is in the prone position since this has been known to cause vascular events and nerve injuries such as plexopathy[12].

Nerve injuries during surgery are not always avoidable and sometimes lead to permanent motor and/or sensory loss.

During the surgical procedure one ought to use blunt instruments for the dissection, avoid the use of manoeuvring or blocking and also avoid excessive use of electrocautery.

Being conscious of the possible appearance of nerve injuries one can take appropriate measures to avoid them and early detection of the injury will help the recovery of the patient.

13. References

[1] Cárdenas A, Rodriguez J, Leon D, Taylor J, Gutierrez C. Bilateral Sciatic Nerve Axonotmesis After Gluteal Lipoaugmentation. Ann Plast Surg. 63: 4, 2009.
[2] Ko¨mu¨rcu¨ F, Zwolak P, Benditte-Klepetko H, Deutinger M. Management Strategies for Peripheral Iatrogenic Nerve Lesions. Annals of Plastic Surgery. Volume 54, Number 2, 2005.
[3] Grotting J, Beckenstein M. Cervicofacial Rejuvenation using ultrasound- assisted lipectomy. Vol 107. No. 3. 2001
[4] Zani R, Fadul R, Dias Da Rocha M, Santos R, Chaves m, Masako L. Facial nerve in rhytidoplasty: anatomic study of its trajectory in the overlying skin and the most common sites of injury. Annals of Plastic Surg Volume 51, number 3. 2003.
[5] Cordier B, De la Torre J, Al Hakeem M, Rosenberg L. Rejuvenation of the midface by elevating the malar fat pad: review of technique, cases and complications. Plast. Reconstr. Surg. 110: 1526, 2002.
[6] Chang S, Pusic A, Rohrich R. A systematic reviem of comparison of efficacy and complication rates among face lift techniques. Plast. Reconstr. Surg. 127: 423, 2011.
[7] Schlenz I, Rigeñ S, Schemper M, Kuzbari R. Alteration of Nipple and Areola Sensitivity by Reduction Mammaplasty: A Prospective Comparison of Five Techniques. Plast Recontr. Surg. 115: 743, 2005
[8] Bruner T, Roberts T, Nguyen K. Complications of buttocks augmentation: Diagnosis, management and prevention. Clin in Plastic Surg. 33 (2006) 449. Clin Plastic Surg 33 (2006) 449–466
[9] Knoetgen J, Moran S. Long-term outcomes and complications associated with brachioplasty: a retrospective review and cadaveric study. Plast. Reconstr. Surg. 117: 7. 2219. 2006.
[10] Niechajev I. Calf Augmentation and Restoration. Sweden Plast. Reconstr. Surg. 116: 295, 2005
[11] Aiache A. Calf Implantation. Plast. Reconstr. Surg. 83 : 1989.
[12] Shermak M, Shoo B, Deune G. Prone positioning precautions in plastic surgery. Plast. Reconstr. Surg. 117: 5. 1584. 2006.
[13] Frijters E, Hofer S, Mureau M. Long-term subjective and objective outcome after repair of traumatic facial nerve injuries. Ann Plast Surg 2008: 61: 181-187.
[14] Greywoode J, Hao H, Artz G, Heffelfinger R. Management of traumatic facial nerve injuries. Facial Plastic Surgery Vo. 26.No. 6.2010
[15] Hadlock T, Kowaleski J, Lo D, Mackinnon S, Heaton J. Rodent facial nerve recovery after selected lesions and repair techniques. Plast. Reconstr. Surg. 125: 99, 2010.
[16] Michaels J, Coon D, Rubin P. Complications in postbariatric body contouring: postoperative management and treatment. Plast. Reconstr. Surg. 127: 1693, 2011
[17] Grotting J, Beckenstein M. Cervicofacial Rejuvenation using ultrasound- assisted lipectomy. Vol 107. No. 3. 2001
[18] Rodriguez-Bruno K,Papel D. Rhytidectomy: principles and practice emphasizing safety. Facial Plastic Surgery Vo. 27.No. 1. 2011

[19] Rovak J, Tung T, Mackinnon S. The surgical management of facial nerve injury. Seminars in plastic surgery . Vol. 18 No. 1. 2004.
[20] Saylam C, Ucerler H, Orhan M, Uckan A, Cuneyt O. Localization of the mandibular branch of the facial nerve. The Journal of Crnaiof Surg. Vol 18, Number 1. 2007.
[21] Ducic I, Seibith L, Iorio M. Chronic postoperative breast pain: danger zones for nerve injuries. Plast. Reconstr. Surg. 127: 41, 2011
[22] Greuse M, Hamdi M, DeMey A. Breast sensitivity after vertical mamaplasty. Plast Reconstr Surg. Vol. 107, No. 4. 2001
[23] Pechter E, Smith P. Transient Femoral Neuropathy after abdominoplasty. Ann Plast Surg 2008;61: 492–493
[24] Gustein R. Augmentation of the Lower Leg: A New Combined Calf-Tibial Implant. Plast. Reconstr. Surg. 117: 817, 2006.
[25] Niechajev I. Calf Augmentation and Restoration. Sweden Plast. Reconstr. Surg. 116: 295, 2005.
[26] Aiache A. Calf Implantation. Plast. Reconstr. Surg. 83 : 1989.
[27] Novak C. Rehabilitation strategies for facial nerve injuries. Seminars in plastic surgery. Vol. 18 No. 1. 2004.
[28] Lindsay R, Heaton J, Edwards C. Smitson C, Hadlock T. Nimodipine and Acceleration of Functional Recovery of the Facial Nerve After Crush Injury. Arch Facial Plast Surg. 2010;12(1):49-52
[29] Matarasso A, Elkwood A, Rankin M, Elkowitz M. National Plastic Surgery Survey: Face Lift Techniques and complications. Plast Reconstr Surg 2000;106:1185-1195
[30] Behmand R, Guyuron B. Endoscopic Forehead Rejuvenation, long term results. Plast Reconstr Surg 2006; 117(4):1137-1143
[31] Bufoni FA, Xerfan N, Masako FL, Sensibility of the abdomen after abdominoplasty. Plastic Reconstr Surg. 2004;114:577-582
[32] Seror P. Accesory nerve lesion after cervicofacial lift: clinical and electrodiagnosis evaluations of two cases. Muscle Nerve 2009;39(3):400-405

Part 4

Advances in Therapy of Peripheral Neuropathies

9

Multimodal Analgesia for Neuropathic Pain

Jorge Guajardo Rosas, Faride Chejne Gomez
and Ricardo Plancarte Sanchez
*Pain Clinic Department, Instituto Nacional de Cancerologia Mexico City,
Centro Medico American British Cowdray,
Mexico*

1. Introduction

Neuropathic pain can be caused by a number of different diseases such as diabetes mellitus (DM), herpes zoster, Human Inmunodeficiency virus (HIV), cancer or secondary to treatment i.e. radiotherapy, chemotherapy or surgery. Alterations in the nerve pathways such as trigeminal or nerve roots can lead to pain.
Another study from Mayo Clinic reported neuropathic pain in 66% of insulin-dependent diabetic patients and 59% in non-insulin dependent diabetic patients (Davies 2006). Epidemiological study in Minnesota reported an annual incidence of postherpetic neuralgia to be 11.6 per 100,000 people per year, similar to seen in UK with a lifetime incidence of 70/100, 000. (Dyck 1993)
Traditionally, neuropathic pain has been classified into peripheral and central, taking into account the anatomical location of the lesion or anatomical dysfunction. The current definition of neuropathic pain indicates that it is "pain that arises as a direct result of an injury or illness affecting the somatosensory system" (Treede 2008). Several recent studies have shown that neuropathic pain may adversely affect the overall quality of life including physical and emotional health (Oster 2005), which are associated with significant social costs (O ' Connor 2009).
Neuropathic pain is associated with suffering, disability, decreased quality of life and increased costs. The exact prevalence is unknown. German Studies state that 37% of patients with chronic low back pain have predominantly neuropathic pain, in terms of painful diabetic neuropathy occurs in 16% in patients with diabetes in the UK, one third of these patients had never received Treatment for this type of pain. In the United States two-thirds of patients with painful diabetic neuropathy workers reported absence from work or decreased productivity due to pain and only one fifth of these employees were satisfied with their treatment prescribed analgesic (Bouhassira 2008).
Of the various etiologies of neuropathic pain DM needs the most attention due to the increasing number of patients expected by 2025. It is estimated that the present number of 246 million people worldwide will increase to 380 million especialy in developing countries. Though estimated 80% of these patients live in developing or under developed countries only 20% increased will be in the budget to treat this condition (Walters1992/Davies 2006).
These epidemiological data support that neuropathic pain has severe impact on the economic, social and emotional aspects of patient population.

Neuropathic pain is considered a diagnostic and therapeutic challenge because it can often be the result of a diverse group of diseases, which differ in etiology, and symptomatology. In some disorders the clinical picture may or may not be related to the anatomical distribution.

Although a primary goal of pain management is to relieve pain using a single agent, the reality is that monotherapy rarely provides adequate relief from chronic neuropathic pain. In these complex and refractory situations, combination therapy using two or more agents with synergistic mechanisms of action (eg, gabapentin + tramadol) is frequently necessary. In clinical practice, some patients begin to respond to a particular monotherapy, but often are restricted by dose-related side effects. In such cases, combination therapy with two or more agents with different modes of action at suboptimal doses may provide the additive effects or even synergistic effects necessary for optimal pain relief without compromising the side-effect profile of each agent. (NEJ 2005)

2. Clinical efficacy

Under the umbrella of the IASP (International Association for Study of Pain) a chapter or group with special interest in neuropathic pain (NeuPSIG) held a consensus to develop evidence-based guidelines for the pharmacological treatment of neuropathic pain that took into account the clinical efficacy, adverse effects, the impact on quality of life related to health, and costs. (Connor 2009)

Three classes of drugs were recommended as first line of treatment for neuropathic pain: antidepressants, which inhibit both norepinephrine and serotonin reuptake (tricyclic antidepressants and selective inhibitors and inhibitors of norepinephrine reuptake [SNRIs]), the ligand calcium channel blockers, gabapentin and pregabalin, and topical lidocaine (lidocaine patch 5%).

Opioids and tramadol are recommended as second-line treatment in generalexcept in certain specific clinical situations in which they can be considered for first-line use.

Other medications are considered third-line therapy. The guidelines recognize that an effective drug combination for neuropathic pain may provide greater analgesia than the use of single drugs (monotherapy) (NEJ 2005), although this therapy can often be associated with more side effects or risk of drug interactions. However, the combination therapy was incorporated into a management strategy for patients with partial response to treatment with first-line drugs.

Four steps should be performed that may require treatment, dose adjustment or additional monitoring of therapy

Step 1.

- Establishing the diagnosis of neuropathic pain.
- Assess pain
- Establish and treat the cause of neuropathic pain.
- Identify relevant comorbidities (eg, heart, kidney or liver disease, depression) that may require treatment or dose adjustment or additional monitoring of therapy
- Explain the diagnosis and treatment plan for the patient and set realistic expectations

Step 2.

- Initiate therapy for the disease causing neuropathic pain.
- Start the treatment of symptoms with one or more of the following:

A ligand calcium channel alpha 2-delta (gabapentin)

- For patients with peripheral neuropathic pain localized topical lidocaine used alone or in combination with one of the other first-line therapies

- For patients with acute neuropathic pain, Neuropathic pain due to cancer, exacerbations or episodes of severe pain and / or when the system of pain relief during the assessment of a first-line drug to an effective dose is required, opioid analgesics or tramadol may be used alone or in combination with one of the first-line therapies
- Assess the patient for non-pharmacological treatments and to initiate, if necessary

Step 3.

- Reassess the pain and often assess the quality of life related to health.
- If pain relief is adequate (for example, the average pain reduced to ≤ 3 / 10) and tolerable side effects, continue the treatment.
- If there is partial relief of pain (for example, the average is still ≥ 4 / 10) after appropriate treatment, add one of the other four first-line drugs.
- If no or inadequate pain relief (eg, reduction of <30%) after appropriate treatment should be changed to an alternative first-line drug

Step 4.

- If the tests of first-line drugs alone and in combination fail, consider the second-and third-line and / or referral to a pain specialist (2009)

Importantly, the doses used (start, qualifications and maximum) and the duration of clinical trials are appended in the table below.

The duration of the trials with the use of gabapentin was 3-10 weeks with 4 weeks use of tramadol.

3. Treatment of neuropathic pain and pharmacological classes

3.1 Antidepressants

TCAs are often listed as first-line drugs for neuropathic pain. Typically, this class of agents is separated into two categories based on their chemical structure: tertiary and secondary amines. TCAs appear to affect pain transmission via multiple mechanisms including reuptake inhibition of both serotonin and norepinephrine at spinal cord receptor sites, including projections to the brain stem and dorsal horn nuclei. It has been postulated that the tertiary agents maintain a more balanced chemical profile, providing inhibition of both serotonin and norepinephrine. In contrast, the secondary amines appear to provide more reuptake inhibition of norepinephrine. The analgesic properties of TCAs appear to be independent of their antidepressant properties. Other possible mechanisms of action include: alpha-adrenergic blockade; anticholinergic effects; antihistaminic effects; reuptake inhibition of dopamine; effects on gamma-aminobutyric acid (GABA)-B and adenosine; potassium, calcium and, most importantly, sodium channel blockade; N-methyl-D-aspartic acid (NMDA)-receptor antagonism.

The secondary amines (eg, desipramine and nortriptyline) appear to be as effective as the tertiary agents (eg, imipramine and amitriptyline) as analgesics in neuropathic pain and produce markedly fewer side effects This favorable side-effect profile makes secondary amine TCAs more clinically appropriate for many patients.

3.2 Anticonvulsants

As with epilepsy, the hallmark characteristic of neuropathic pain is thought to be neuronal hyperexcitability. Some of the known mechanisms of action of anticonvulsants include blockade of the membrane sodium currents, effects on calcium conductance, activation of the gamma-aminobutyric acid (GABA) inhibitory system by direct or indirect means, and reduction of the activity of the excitatory neurotransmitter glutamate. The net result is the depression of synaptic transmission and the elevation of the threshold for repetitive firing of nociceptive neurons, as well as a reduction in discharges of the dorsal root ganglion cells.

To date, only five agents have been evaluated in randomized double-blind clinical trials. These are carbamazepine, gabapentin, lamotrigine, phenytoin, and pregabalin. Of these, carbamazepine and phenytoin require intensive monitoring of serum levels and maintain a fairly extensive adverse effect profile. Lamotrigine use is limited by a risk of Stevens–Johnson syndrome and other serious dermatological adverse events. Gabapentin produces markedly fewer adverse effects than many other anticonvulsants, and does not require blood tests.

Gabapentin has recently been shown to be an effective treatment option for both DPN and PHN in two large multicenter, randomized, double-blind, placebo-controlled, parallel group trials. Gabapentin was also compared to amitriptyline in a small-scale prospective, randomized, double-blind, double-dummy, crossover study in DPN. Although both drugs provided analgesia, no significant difference was shown between gabapentin and amitriptyline with respect to pain scores or global pain assessment. The authors concluded that gabapentin is an effective alternative to amitriptyline for treatment of DPN pain, but could not be recommended over amitriptyline due to cost.

The most common side effects of gabapentin are drowsiness, somnolence, and generalized fatigue. These side effects are usually transient, lasting an average of 2 to 3 weeks. Treatment should be initiated at 300 mg at bedtime, with a test dose of 100 mg at bedtime for elderly patients. The dose is then increased by 300 mg every 3 to 5 days, until the patient has adequate pain relief. The median effective daily dose ranges between 900 and 1800 mg, although some patients respond to daily doses as low as 100 mg and others require 3600 mg. Gorson and colleagues reported that doses less than 900 mg per day (300 mg TID) are either ineffective or only minimally effective for the treatment of painful diabetic neuropathy. The average age of the patients evaluated in this report was 62 years. Because of its short half-life, gabapentin should be administered on a TID schedule. The drug is excreted unchanged by the kidneys, with clearance directly proportional to creatinine clearance. Therefore, dosage reduction may be needed in patients with renal impairment. As a result of the lack of drug–drug interactions, gabapentin may be an attractive agent for patients receiving multiple medications.

Stacey (2005) identified several randomized, double-blind clinical trials (level 2 evidence) demonstrating that gabapentin had significantly greater efficacy than placebo in PHN (at 1800 to 3600 mg/day) and DPN (900 to 3600 mg). In DPN, gabapentin showed comparable efficacy to amitriptyline. Controlled clinical trials suggest that carbamazepine (100 to 4000 g/day) is effective in TGN and DPN, but not PHN or central pain (all level 2 evidence). Compared to the first-generation anticonvulsants, gabapentin has a more favorable safety and tolerability profile. Pregabalin (300 or 600 mg/day) also appears to be effective in some types of neuropathic pain, with level 2 evidence indicating that 50% of patients with PHN achieved a decrease in pain of 50% or more. Sodium valproate has demonstrated efficacy in painful DPN (level 2 evidence), but the evidence for other anticonvulsants (levetiracetam, oxcarbazepine, topiramate, zonisamide) in the treatment of neuropathic pain was not as good. These results were in accordance with those from earlier studies. Anticonvulsants are thought to hold significant promise in the treatment of CRPS. Carbamazepine has a traditional and perhaps clinically important place in this indication, and gabapentin holds significant promise (level 4 evidence).

3.3 Opioids and tramadol

Opioid agonists work by mimicking the activity of enkephalins and endorphins in the central descending pathways of the pain-processing loop. By binding to mu-opioid receptors in the central nervous system, opioid agonists dampen neuronal excitability and elicit pain relief. Despite concerns regarding the efficacy of opioids in neuropathic pain, several double-blind RCTs (level 2 evidence) have demonstrated that oxycodone, morphine, and methadone can be modestly effective in PHN, DPN, phantom limb pain, and other types of neuropathic pain. A recent review demonstrated that opioids had significant efficacy over placebo for neuropathic pain in intermediate-term studies. Although reported adverse events with opioids were common, they were not life-threatening. When compared to treatment with TCAs, opioids were as effective but resulted in a greater number of dropouts. Nevertheless, patients who finished the study preferred treatment with opioids over TCA.

Tramadol is a centrally acting agent with a weak affinity for mu-opioid receptors and weak reuptake inhibition of the neurotransmitters norepinephrine and serotonin. It has shown utility in a variety of pain syndromes, most notably neuropathic pain. Treatment should generally be initiated at a dose of 50 mg daily and increased by 50 mg increments every 3 to 5 days. Adverse events increase with more rapid dose titration. Effective daily doses range between 100 and 400 mg, administered in divided doses four times daily. The most common adverse effects of tramadol are dizziness, vertigo, nausea, constipation, headache, and somnolence. In addition, patients with a history or potential for seizure activity should avoid use of this agent.

3.4 Topical agents

Topical agents work locally, directly at the site of application, with minimal systemic effects. Lidocaine, like other local anesthetics, seems to act through inhibition of voltage-gated sodium channels. Capsaicin is thought to elevate the pain threshold in which it is applied through depletion of the nociceptive neurotransmitter, substance P, from the terminals of unmyelinated C fibers. It also causes degeneration of substance P-positive epidermal nerve fibers. Ketamine works through antagonism of the NMDA receptors and clonidine is thought to act at the presynaptic alpha-2 adrenergic receptors, subsequently inhibiting release of norepinephrine.

The evidence supporting the 5% lidocaine patch for the treatment of neuropathic pain is strong. The lidocaine patch is effective in PHN (level 2 evidence), with minimal risk of drug interactions or systemic adverse effects. However, the current approved dose of 12-hour on/12-hour off was found to be insufficient for some patients. The lidocaine patch also has shown efficacy in DPN (level 2 evidence), with the number needed to treat in some studies comparing favorably to those of other treatments for neuropathic pain. Complete or some pain relief has been noted in patients with myofascial pain (two-thirds of whom had lower back pain) and in those with lower back pain. Both types of pain may result, in part, from neuropathic mechanisms. The lidocaine patch also may be useful in the treatment of CRPS.

Capsaicin cream (0.075%) was evaluated in several clinical studies for DPN and PHN (both level 2 evidence). Although results were inconsistent, clinical experience suggests it may occasionally be effective in individual circumstances. Capsaicin also has partial efficacy in CRPS (level 3 evidence). Level 3 evidence was noted for the efficacy of ketamine gel in the treatment of neuropathic pain.

3.5 Anesthetics for systemic use

Abnormal electrical activity in injured nerves and neuromas is partly generated by abnormal accumulation of sodium channels. Therefore, a sodium channel-blocking agent may help to relieve neuropathic pain. Such medications include intravenous lidocaine (which also depresses C-fiber polysynaptic evoked activity and thus suppresses dorsal horn neurons to the C-fiber input), oral mexiletine (which has a similar mode of action to lidocaine), and oral tocainamide. The GABAergic system in the spinal cord also plays a pivotal role in modulating pain control and as a result, baclofen (a GABA-B-receptor agonist) has been shown to be effective for neuropathic pain.

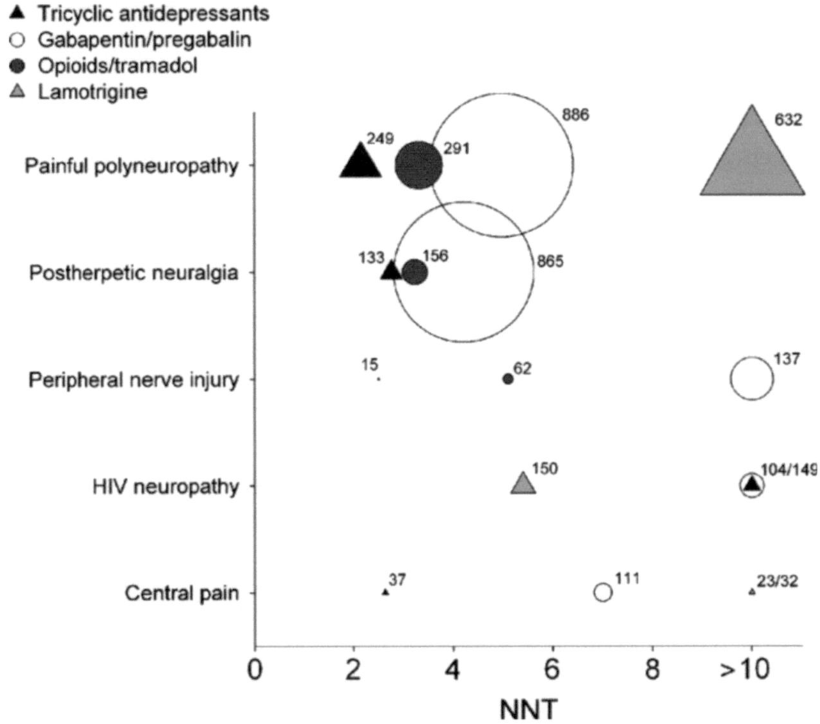

Fig. 1. Combined number-needed-to-treat (NNT) values for various drug classes in all central and peripheral neuropathic pain conditions (not including trigeminal neuralgia, cancer-related neuropathic pain, or radiculopathies).The circle sizes indicate the relative number (given in parentheses) of patients who received active treatment drugs in trials for which dichotomous data were available. It is important to note that because studies on tricyclic antidepressants (TCAs), selective serotonin reuptake inhibitors (SSRIs), and opioids are mainlycrossover trials and studies on SNRIs and gabapentin or pregabalin are mainly parallel-group design studies, a direct comparison of NNT values across drug classes cannot be made. Adapted from Finnerup et al. The evidence for pharmacological treatment of neuropathic pain. Pain 2010;150:573–81.
Abbreviations: BTX-A = botulinum toxin A; ns = absolute risk difference not signifi cant; SNRIs = mixed serotoninnorepinephrine reuptake inhibitors.

Mexilitene, an orally available lidocaine congener antiarrhythmic, has been evaluated in several double-blind clinical trials for treatment of painful diabetic neuropathy. Only one of these trials demonstrated significant pain relief with mexilitene, and even then only limited nighttime pain relief with high doses (675 mg per day). Mexilitene is not a benign drug, and as such has a less than favorable adverse effect profile. Common adverse effects include chest pain, dizziness, gastrointestinal disturbances, palpitations, and tremor. As with other antiarrhythmics, mexilitene may worsen existing arrhythmia. The daily effective dose

ranges between 450 and 675 mg, usually administered on a thrice daily schedule. As a function of its questionable efficacy and its toxicity, mexilitene should be considered an option only when other measures have failed.
In clinical practice, a combination of two or more drugs is often needed to achieve satisfactory pain relief, although there have been few trials done to support this clinical observation. However, combination therapy with gabapentin and extended-release morphine in patients with postherpetic neuralgia or painful diabetic neuropathy and extended-release morphine and pregabalin in different neuropathic pain síndromes (neuropathic back pain, postherpetic neuralgia, radiculopathy, painful diabetic neuropathy) had higher pain relief with lower doses compared with administration of one drug alone. These results have also been confirmed for the combination of nortriptyline and gabapentin, as well as for pregabalin and topical lidocaine, in patients with painful diabetic neuropathy and postherpetic neuralgia. Taken together, these results substantiate the usefulness of combination therapy in patients with neuropathic pain.

4. Conclusions

Although a primary goal of pain management is to relieve pain using a single agent, the reality is that monotherapy rarely provides adequate relief from chronic neuropathic pain. In these complex and refractory situations, combination therapy using two or more agents with synergistic mechanisms of action (eg, gabapentin + lamotrigine or tramadol + gabapentin) is frequently necessary. In clinical practice, some patients begin to respond to a particular monotherapy, but often are restricted by dose-related side effects. In such cases, combination therapy with two or more agents with different modes of action at suboptimal doses may provide the additive effects or even synergistic effects necessary for optimal pain relief without compromising the side-effect profile of each agent. However, it is essential that a careful patient history is taken before initiating a polypharmacy regimen.

5. References

[1] Treede RD, Jensen TS, Campbell JN, et al. Neuropathic pain: redefinition and a grading system for clinical research purposes. *Neurology*. 2008; 70(18):1630-1635.
[2] Oster G, Harding G, Dukes E, Edelsberg J, Cleary PD. Pain, medication use, and health-related quality of life in older persons with postherpetic neuralgia: results from a population-based survey. *J Pain*. 2005;6(6):356-363.
[3] O'Connor AB. Neuropathic pain: a review of the quality of life impact, costs, and cost-effectiveness of therapy. *Pharmacoeconomics*. 2009;27(2):95-112.
[4] Bouhassira D, Lanteri-Minet M, Attal N, Laurent B, Touboul C. Prevalence of chronic pain with neuropathic characteristics in the general population. Pain 2008;136:380–7.
[5] Freynhagen R, Baron R, Gockel U, Tolle TR. painDETECT: a new screening questionnaire to identify neuropathic components in patients with back pain. Curr Med Res Opin 2006;22:1911–20.
[6] Davies M, Brophy S, Williams R, Taylor A. The prevalence, severity, and impact of painful diabetic peripheral neuropathy in type 2 diabetes. Diabetes Care 2006; 29:1518–22.
[7] Dyck PJ, Kratz KM, Karnes JL, et al. The prevalence by staged severity of various types of diabetic neuropathy, retinopathy, and nephropathy in a population-based cohort: the Rochester Diabetic Neuropathy Study.*Neurology*. 1993;43:817–824.
[8] Walters DP, Gatline W, Mullee MA, Hill RD. The prevalence of diabetic distal sensory neuropathy in an English community. *Diabet Med*. 1992;9:349–353.

[9] Ziegler D, Gries FA, Spuler M, Lessmann F. The epidemiology of diabetic neuropathy. *J* Diabetes Complications. 1992;6:49–57

[10] Finnerup N, Sindrup S. The evidence for pharmacological treatment of neuropathic pain. PAIN. 2010; 573–581.

[11] O'Connor A, Dworkin R. Treatment of Neuropathic Pain: An Overview of Recent Guidelines. The American Journal of Medicine (2009) 122, S22–S32

[12] Gilron I, Bailey J.Morphine, Gabapentin, or Their Combination for Neuropathic Pain. N Engl J Med 2005;352:1324-34

[13] Leon-Casasola O. Multimodal, Multiclass, Multidisciplinary Therapy, The Key to Better Analgesia in the 21st Century?. Clin J Pain 2010;26:S1–S2

[14] Dworkin R, O'Connor A. Recommendations for the Pharmacological Management of Neuropathic Pain: An Overview and Literature Update Mayo Clin Proc. 2010; 85(3)(suppl):S3-S14

[15] Pharmacological Management of Neuropathic Pain. PAIN CLINICAL UPDATE, nov 2010.

[16] Baron R, Binder A.Neuropathic pain: diagnosis, pathophysiological mechanisms, and treatment. Lancet Neurol 2010; 9: 807–19

[17] Codd E, Martinez R Tramadol and several anticonvulsants synergize in attenuating nerve injury-induced allodynia. Pain 134 (2008) 254–262

[18] Zepeda T, Hernández Santos J, Manejo del dolor neuropático en el paciente diabético con Tramadol vía oral comparado con la administración del mismo asociado a la Amitriptilina o Gabapentina. Revista Mexicana de Anestesiología, Publicación Oficial de la Sociedad Mexicana de Anestesiología, A.C.VOLUMEN 1, No. 2. Abril - Junio 2001

[19] Mendoza H, García M. Gabapentina/tramadol para el tratamiento del dolor neuropático intratable crónico: un estudio de eficacia y seguridad. Revista Médica Latina. ISSN, 1692-5122. Año 7, No. 2, Febrero 2009

[20] Keskinbora K, Pekel A. Gabapentin and an Opioid Combination Versus Opioid Alone for the Management of Neuropathic Cancer Pain: A Randomized Open Trial. J Pain Symptom Manage 2007;34:183e189

[21] Granados-Soto V, Argüelles C. Synergic Antinociceptive Interaction between Tramadol and Gabapentin after Local, Spinal and Systemic Administration. Pharmacology 2005;74:200–208

[22] Dai X. Brunson C. Gender differences in the antinociceptive effect of tramadol, alone or in combination with gabapentin, in mice. J. Biomed Sci. March 2008.

[23] Morello CM, Leckband SG, Stoner CP, Moorhouse DF, Sahagian GA. Randomized double-blind study comparing the efficacy of gabapentin with amitriptyline on diabetic peripheral neuropathy pain. *Arch Intern Med.* 1999;159:1931–1937.

[24] Backonja M-M, Serra J. Pharmacologic management part 1: better-studied neuropathic pain diseases. *Pain Med.* 2004;5(suppl 1):S28–S47.

[25] Backonja M-M, Serra J. Pharmacologic management part 2: lesser-studied neuropathic pain diseases. *Pain Med.* 2004;5(suppl 1):S48–S59.

[26] Stacey BR. Management of peripheral neuropathic pain. *Am J Phys Med Rehabil.* 2005;84: S4–S16.

[27] Harden RN. Pharmacotherapy of complex regional pain syndrome. *Am J Phys Med Rehabil.* 2005;84: S17–S28.

[28] Wright JM, Oki JC, Graves L III. Mexiletine in the symptomatic treatment of diabetic peripheral neuropathy. *Ann Pharmacother.* 1997;31:29–34

10

Cell Therapy for Diabetic Neuropathy

Julie J. Kim and Young-Sup Yoon
Emory University
USA

1. Introduction

A debilitating consequence of diabetes mellitus (DM) is neuropathy which globally affects between 20 -30% of diabetic patients and up to 50% [1, 2]. The lifetime incidence of diabetic neuropathy (DN) is estimated to be up to 45% for type 2 diabetic patients and 59% for type 1 diabetic patients in USA. The risk of DN rises with age, duration of DM, and vascular disease. Characterized by damages in the arms and legs, peripheral neuropathy is the most common complication of DM.

The pathophysiology of DN is promoted by several risk factors: microvascular disease, neural hypoxia, and hyperglycemia-induced effects. At the molecular level, the primary cause of diabetic complications is known to be hyperglycemia, which disrupts cellular metabolism by the formation of reactive oxygen species (ROS). In the aspect of nerve functions, ROS formation increases neuron's susceptibility to damage. In addition, hyperglycemia impedes production of angiogenic and neurotrophic growth factors, which are necessary for normal function of neurons and glial cells and maintenance of vascular structure.

The most common presentation of nerve damage due to the effects of hyperglycemia is neuropathic pain. Peripheral neuropathy may cause foot deformities such as hammertoes and unnoticed sores and infections in the numb areas of the foot. Improperly treated infection frequently extends to the bone and requires an amputation of the foot.

There have not been any definitive disease-modifying treatments to reverse DN. The current treatment focuses on tight glycemic control which can reduce potential risk factors for further nerve damage and DN-associated pain management. In many studies, deficiency of neurotrophic factors and lack of vascular support have been regarded as key factors in the development DN. Therefore, cell therapy has recently emerged as an attractive therapeutic strategy to meet the needs of both neurotrophic and vascular deficiencies of DN.

2. Symptoms, signs and diagnostic tests

DN most often starts with hypesthesia (diminished sensation) of the lower extremities, which extends to a stocking-glove distribution. The most feared complications are foot pain, ulcerations and amputation, which increase morbidity and mortality thereby reduce the patient's quality of life [3]. Proper diagnosis of the etiology of DN depends on the pattern of sensory loss, reflex test, electrodiagnostic studies, and imaging. In electrodiagnostic studies, nerve conduction velocity and magnitude are measured by electrically stimulating nerves.

Peripheral nerve imaging such as ultrasound and magnetic resonance imaging (MRI) are used for evaluating the extent of peripheral nerve pathology. They give insight to which type of nerve fiber is affected.

3. Pathophysiology

DN, nerve damage caused mainly by glycemic dysregulation, is the most common complication of DM. Prolonged hyperglycemic episodes result in a complex series of metabolic and vascular damages which contribute to the multi-factorial etiology of DN [4, 5]. The major pathogenetic factors are hyperglycemia-induced metabolic derangements which cause excess oxidative stress and loss of neurovascular support.

In general, immediate pathologic effects of hyperglycemic episodes are metabolic in nature. However, electrophysiologic and morphologic alterations seem to be late occurrences. There are various pathologic changes that occur in DN. Pathologic changes in peripheral nerve are endoneurial microangiopathy, nerve demyelination, loss of nerve fibers, axonal degeneration, axonal dystrophy and Schwann cell abnormalities[6, 7-9].

3.1 Oxidative stress to cellular damage

Hyperglycemia-induced oxidative stress has been proposed as a single unifying mechanism of neurodegeration in DM by Brownlee et al. [10]. Hyperglycemia cause metabolic abnormalities which result in mitochondrial superoxide overproduction in peripheral nerves [11] and supporting vasculatures [10, 12].

Hyperglycemic environment induces activation of 5 pathways involved in the pathogenesis of diabetic microvascular complications [13]. These include: the polyol pathway[14]; nonenzymatic glycation of proteins which increases advanced glycation end-products (AGEs) [15, 16]; hexosamine pathway flux [17]; protein kinase C (PKC) pathway [18] which triggers stress responses; and the poly ADP-ribose polymerase (PARP) pathway [19, 20]. Increased activity of the 5 pathways deplete antioxidants which are necessary for antioxidant defense system against free radicals. The hyperglycemia-mediated superoxide overproduction perturbs the five pathways, and thereby causes metabolic and vascular imbalance and initiates the progression of neurovascular dysfunction [21-23].

In polyol pathway of glucose metabolism, aldose reductase catalyzes the NADPH-dependent conversion of glucose to sorbitol [14]. Aldose reductase also competes with glutathione reductase in NADPH-dependent production of Glutathione (GSH), a major antioxidant in cells. A high level of glucose overactivates the polyol pathway thereby depleting NADPH necessary for GSH antioxidant production. Consequently, insufficient GSH level contributes to accumulation of ROS.

In hexosamine pathway of glucose metabolism, its overactivation diminishes antioxidant production. This also increases posttranslational modification of specific amino acid residues on cytoplasmic and nuclear proteins, and thereby changes their functions [17].

In DM, high levels of AGEs is found in extracellular matrix. Thus, plasma proteins enhanced with advanced glycation bind to Receptor for AGEs (RAGE) on cells such as macrophages and vascular endothelial cells. This activates pleiotropic transcription factors such as nuclear factor kappa-light-chain-enhancer of activated B cells (NF-kB) which results in multiple pathological changes in gene expression. The interaction between RAGE and AGEs is shown to cause pro-inflammatory gene activation [24]. Myelin is considered a major target for such non-enzymatic modification by glucose. Reactive and degenerative Schwann cell changes lead to demyelination which is the dominant lesion of peripheral neuropathy. The decrease in the density of myelins affects both large and small nerve fibers. Hyperglycemic condition causes consistent demyelination and axonal degeneration and presents aberrations in nerve regeneration.

Activation of PKC pathway leads to inhibition of Na+/K+ ATPase which in turn leads to decreased endothelial nitric oxide synthase (eNOS). Consequently, eNOS reduction results in blood-flow abnormalities and vascular occlusion caused by increased transforming growth factor beta (TGF-B) and plasminogen activator inhibitor-1 (PAI-1). PKC pathway activation also increase NF-kB expression which results in proinflammatory response and dysfunction in sending electrical signals in neurons. As a result, the nerve conduction level diminishes, and thereby obstructs nerve regeneration.

In healthy cells, ROS production is tightly controlled. The antioxidant defense system of a cell responds to the environmental changes [25]. However, in diabetic environment, cells end up with accumulated ROS which alter proteins and their functions. Superoxide accumulation can have direct, toxic damages to Schwann cells. This leads to decreased neuron insulation causing ineffective signaling, weakened immunologic perineurial blood-nerve-barrier, and reduced nerve regeneration. Studies showed that oxidative stress impairs vasodilation of epineural blood vessels, resulting in ischemia to the neural tissue [26-28].

3.2 Loss of neurotrophic and vascular support

Oxidative stress majorly contributes to the development of DM complications, both microvascular and macrovascular [13]. The confluence of metabolic and vascular disturbances in nerve causes impairment of neural function. There are clear evidences that insufficient vascular support and neurotrophic factors play a major pathophysiologic role in DN. Studies show decreases in nerve and angiogenic growth factors in nerves from animals with experimental DN [29, 30]. The emphasis placed on the fact that animals with DN show a deficiency in growth factors with both angiogenic and neurotrophic function. This seems to play significant role in pathogenesis of DN.

3.2.1 Growth factor deficiency

There are specific growth factors that guide blood vessels and nerves to their tissue targets, and their deficiency plays a significant role in the pathogenesis of DN. Many representative growth factors display pleiotropic effects which are both neurotrophic and angiogenic [31]. To underline their duality, the growth factors that have both angiogenic and neurotrophic effects are referred to as, "angioneurin" [32]. For example, vascular endothelial growth factor (VEGF) was originally discovered as growth factors specific for endothelial cells [33]. While VEGF was originally known to play a key role in promoting angiogenesis, studies showed that it directly affects the neural growth, neural survival and protection (neurotrophic), and axonal outgrowth (neurotropic) [31]. Thus, VEGF which was once regarded as a specific angiogenic factor is now implicated in neuroprotection.

Similarly, nerve growth factor (NGF), known to promote neurotrophic and neurotropic effects in neuronal cells [34-36], also have angiogenic effect on endothelial cells. Since nerve growth factors (NGF) promote maintenance, survival and regeneration of nerves, a decrease in NGF synthesis causes functional deficit of nerve fibers [37].

VEGF and NGF are not the only examples of angioneurin. Another representative angioneurin involved in pathogensis of DN is insulin-like growth factor (IGF) [38-40]. IGFs are know to promote growth and differentiation of neurons. In addition, IGFs is also found to exert favorable effects on angiogenesis [41]. Insulin deficiency in diabetic state causes reduction in IGFs level in circulation. This abnormal metabolism of angioneurins adds to pathogenesis of DN. Several studies have shown that diabetic animals showing decreased level of angioneurins highly correlates with reduced neural and vascular function [42, 43].

3.2.2 Vascular deficiency

Initially, the focus has been on the hyperglycemia-induced metabolic changes and their direct neuronal effects. However, studies in animal models showed that they also have vascular targets linked to neuropathy [44].

The vascular alterations observed in human and animal models of DN include: thickening of basement membrane of vasa nervorsa[6, 36, 45-48] strongly related to severity of DN [45, 49, 50], decrease in nerve conduction velocity (NCV) in rats with impaired vasodilation in epineurial arterioles [26-28]., changes in luminal areas of endoneurial capillaries, and changes in endoneurial capillary density. Studies on measures of luminal areas of endoneurial capillaries showed different findings. Rodent and feline models of DN showed increase in luminal areas of endoneurial capillaries[51-54].

Conversely, studies on human showed various results. They showed that luminal areas increased [45, 46, 55], unaltered [36, 48, 56], or decreased [6, 47, 49, 57, 58]. Similar to measures of luminal areas, the measured density of endoneurial capillaries also showed mixed results. Studies on animal models showed that the density was increased [53, 59], unaltered [60], or decreased [42, 43, 61]. As well as in human, the results were mixed. A study showed that the density of endoneurial capillaries was increased in patients of early stage DM than healthy subjects [56], while the density of those with established neuropathy and late stage DM was similar to that of normal people [36, 45, 49].

The complex series of oxidative stress-related metabolic changes result in reduced nerve perfusion and ischemia [23, 62]. Impaired blood supply to nerve and ganglion and endoneurial hypoxia play a significant role in causing DN. Specifically, impairment of blood supply to neural tissues through vasa nervorum, blood vessels of peripheral nerves prompt pathogenic mechanisms of DN [62].

Thrainsdottir et al. [56] reported vascular structural alterations caused by early diabetic condition. Blood vessel number in diabetic nerves increased in response to ischemia in early DM. However, the blood vessel number decreased due to impaired neovascularization under prolonged diabetic condition [6].

One of the major pathogenic factors in the development of DN is reduced nerve blood flow (NBF). Various clinical and experimental studies give evidence that amelioration of NBF improved nerve functions. Studies on diabetic patients reported decrease in endoneurial blood flow and presence of hypoxia compared to healthy subjects. Direct measures of nerve perfusion revealed that DN strongly correlated with decreased sural nerve blood flow [63, 64]. A study by Tesfaye et al. [63] also showed that patients suffering from DN had impoverished endoneurial microenvironment.

Overall, the results of various studies indicate that vascular deficiency is highly represented in established DN. As observed, there was an increased number of capillaries in response to ischemia in early stage DM. Eventually, the number of capillaries decreased. It is plausible that chronic diabetic condition disturbed neovascularization and regeneration [51, 65, 66].

Therefore, debilitating microvascular dysfunction and pathogenic mechanisms altering the the surrounding vascularity damage the peripheral nerve.

3.3 Multifactorial etiology of DN

DN is caused by damages in vessels, neurons, and Schwann cells. Hyperglycemia induces metabolic abnormalities cause overproduction of reactive oxygen species (ROS), activation of inappropriate inflammation pathways, and decreased level of antioxidants such as glutathione. These abnormalities render endothelial and neural cells more susceptible to angioneurin deficiency which finally causes deterioration of neurovascular support in nerves. Ischemia (a restriction in blood supply) and damaged perfusion further stimulates hyperactivity of pathogenic cycles in endothelial cells, neurons, and Schwann cells - resulting in nerve degeneration.

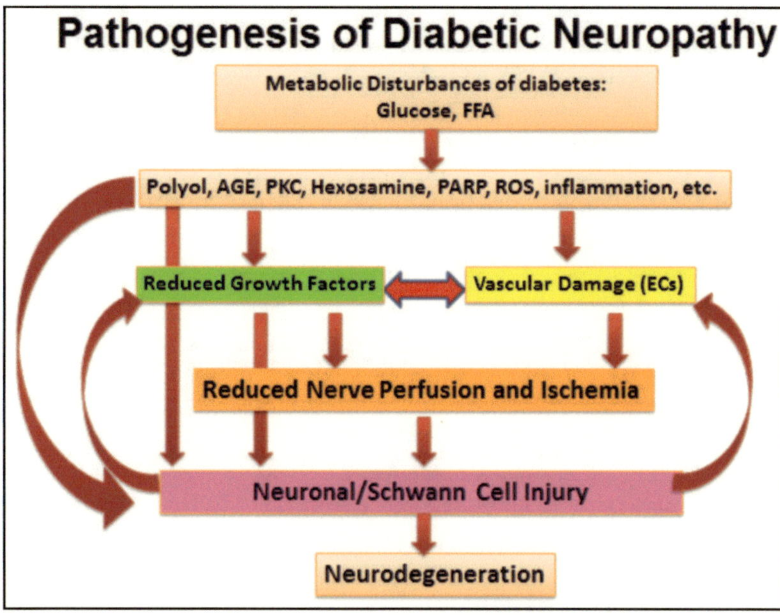

Fig. 1. The proposed pathways that lead to the pathogenesis of DN and interactions at the level of each proposed mechanism. Polyol = Polyol pathway; ECs = endothelial cells.

4. Treatment options and cell therapy

Current treatment strategies focus on preventing neuropathy, slowing its progression, and reducing symptoms and pain. Symptomatic treatment options which are only partially effective include lifestyle interventions, physical therapies, drug-therapies and complementary therapies. Several potential therapies exist for the treatment of DN based on neurovascular pathogenesis. They include: gene, protein, and cell therapies.

Emerging evidence is that angiogenic factors such as VEGF-A, VEGF-C, SHh, and statin can restore microcirculation of the affected nerves and induced functional improvement in DN [61, 62, 67]. On the other hand, lack of neurotrophic factors has emerged as an important pathogenic mechanism of DN [29, 30]. Administration of neurotrophic factors such as NGF

[68], IGF1 and IGF2 [38, 39], ciliary neurotrophic factor (CNTF) [69], or glial cell line-derived neurotrophic factor (GDNF) [70] was shown to ameliorate DN in animal models.

These findings suggest that a therapy targeting both angiogenic and neurotrophic processes may be more advantageous for the treatment of DN. As stem or progenitor cells have such pleiotrophic effects, cell therapy can be more effective than single gene or protein therapy. Cell therapy can provide multiple angiogenic and neurotrophic factors as well as specific type of cells required for vascular or neuronal regeneration (Fig 1). Currently, various bone marrow (BM) cells were shown to have favorable effects for treating DN.

4.1 Therapeutic potential of bone marrow mononuclear cells

Bone marrow (BM) is a source mononuclear cells (MNCs). Bone marrow-derived mononuclear cells (BM-MNCs) are heterogeneous group of cells which include at least: endothelial progenitor cells (EPCs) and the mesenchymal stem cells (MSCs). MSCs are speculated to differentiate into the cellular components of vascular structures [71]. An advantage of using circulating or BM-derived cells is that they can be harvested from a patient's own peripheral blood or bone marrow, and re-introduced back to the patient [72, 73].

Studies have shown the beneficial effects of using BM-MNCs. They improved neovascularisation by increasing levels of angiogenic factors such as VEGF, FGF-2, and angiopoietin-1 [102, 103]. In patients with ischemia, BM-MNCs transplantation has also been reported to be beneficial [104]. Because bone marrow derived MSC transplantation has been shown to be an option in treating ischemic diseases [74], there was an in interest of using similar strategy in treating DN.

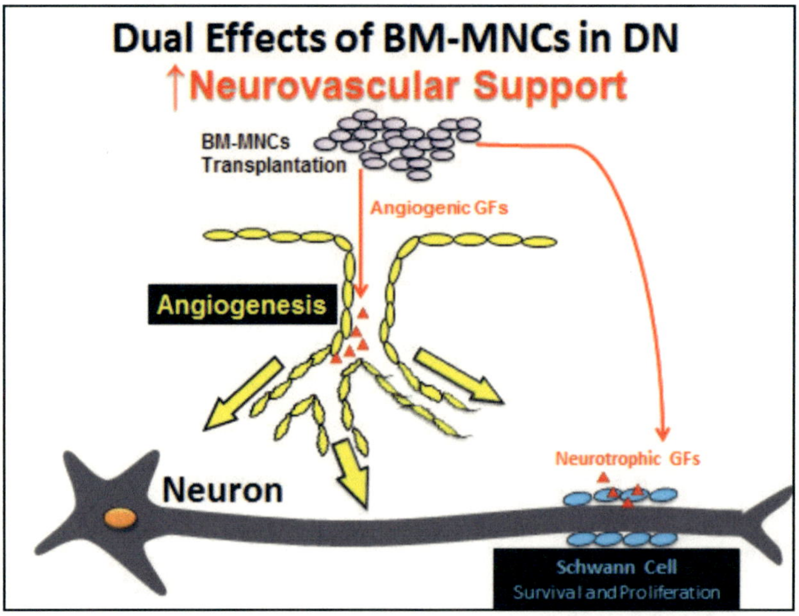

Fig. 2. BM-MNCs induce paracrine effects by releasing angiogenic and neurotrophic growth factors (GFs) thereby increasing neurovascular support in the nerves.

An advantage of using BM-MNCs as source of cell therapy is that they are rather easy to acquire. They can be isolated from bone marrow by centrifugation and do not require ex

vivo culture system. Other advantages of using the BM-derived cells that MSCs and EPCs have proved their therapeutic effects in various clinical and experimental studies of DN.
For example, a study by Hasegawa showed that peripheral blood mononuclear cells (PB-MNCs) or BM-MNCs implantation in rats with DN partially recovered blood flow and improved the NCV of the sciatic nerve [60].
A study by Kim et al. [43] reported that intramuscular transplantation of BM-MNCs preferentially homed in vasa nervorum and increased expression of various angiogenic and neurotrophic factors in the nerves [43]. The study also showed improvement of nerve vascularity and normalization of NCV suggesting that BM-MNC-induced neovascularization is a consequence of angiogenesis (Fig 2). Overall, the emphasis must be placed on the idea that BM-MNCs induce neovascularization and improve manifestations of DN by their ability to promote angiogenesis. Also the safety of autologous BM-derived cells was reported by clinical trials [75].

4.2 Endothelial progenitor cells and vasculogenesis

There are two processes involved in blood vessel formation: vasculogenesis and angiogenesis. Vasculogenesis is the process of formation of blood vessels from *de novo* productions of endothelial cells which may have differentiated from angioblasts or endothelial progenitor cells [76]. Conversely, angiogenesis is the pre-existing vessel growth by vessel formation blood vessels through proliferation and migration of endothelial cells [77]. Thus, endothelial cells are of great interest because of their ability to form blood vessels thereby potential to regenerate vascular dysfunction in DN.
Endothelial progenitor cells (EPCs) are a heterogeneous subset of BM-MNCs. EPCs are capable for differentiation within endothelial cell lineage and are identified according to expression of hematopoietic stem cell and endothelial cell surface markers. EPCs were initially identified by their expression of surface markers VEGF receptor-2 and CD34 [78-80] However, later studies also used CD133 expression to identify EPCs [4, 81] . The precise defintion and characterization of EPCs are still controversial due to the fact that they don't have a unique marker that solely identifies the EPCs. Various types of EPCs have been known as different culture methods give rise to EPCs with distinct characteristics [82]. Derived from mononuclear cells or monocytes, "Early EPCs", have a short proliferation period which is up to a few weeks [83-85]. Conversely, "Late EPCs" have rapid and longer proliferation period and shaped like cobblestones [83, 86]. The early and late EPCs also express different set of cell surface markers. In addition, therapeutic potential of early EPCs has been reported but that of late EPCs is still questioned [83, 86].
The question of whether the differentiation of EPCs plays a vital role in the recovery of damaged tissue function is still controversial.. Some studies showed that differentiation of EPCs into endothelial lineage cells and they were incorporated into blood vessel formation [87, 88]. However, more recent studies have argued against the fact that EPCs did not differentiate into ECs [89, 90]. Although the major therapeutic effects are not through endothelial differentiation but angiogenesis, overall evidence clearly suggests that BM-derived EPCs partake blood vessel formation through vasculogenesis.
Despite such discrepancies, studies on EPC transplantation in DN animal models appear to reach the consensus that EPCs' therapeutic effects and promotion of neovascularization are primarily caused by paracrine or humoral action, not endothelial differentiation [84, 91]. One study showed that cord-blood derived EPCs was effective for treating DN [92]. This

study claimed that mechanistically, the therapeutic effects are due to the increased differentiation of EPCs into endothelial cells in hind limb muscles, which then led to an increase in sciatic nerve blood flow. However, this study did not demonstrate the fate of the EPCs in tissues, nor did it address the mechanisms by which transplanted EPCs increase neovascularization in muscles or nerve. Given that most recent studies have argued against the endothelial differentiation of EPCs as a major mechanism for neovascularization, endothelial differentiation does not appear to underlie such magnitude of therapeutic effects toward DN [84, 91].

A study by Jeong et al. [42] reported direct augmentation of neural neovascularization in sciatic nerves of mice with DN after local intramuscular injection of BM-derived EPCs. The injected EPCs preferentially homed to peripheral nerves but much less to the muscles. This showed that muscular neovascularization is not the mechanism at work. Also, the study showed EPCs have durable engraftment into diabetic nerve. The engraftment lasted up to 12 weeks, which is a unique behavior of EPCs in peripheral nerves because EPCs normally disappear within a couple of weeks in other tissue types. Another novel finding was that engrafted EPCs were localized close to the vasa nervorum which is the blood supply to the peripheral nerves. These findings clearly indicated that BM-derived EPCs exerted therapeutic effects by directly tartgeting the nerves. At the molecular level, the study showed significantly increased levels of angiogenic and neurotrophic factors in the EPC-injected nerves. They include: VEGF-A[62, 93], FGF-2[94], BDNF[95], SHh[61, 96], and stromal cell derived factor (SDF)-1α [97, 98]. These factors are known to have effects on both angiogenesis and neuro-protection [62, 99, 100], suggesting dual angioneurotrophic effects of EPCs. More direct evidence of such dual effects of EPCs were demonstrated by proliferation of endothelial cells and schwann cells and decreased apoptosis of Schwann cells at the histology level. This study showed previously unexpected and distinct properties of BM-derived EPCs such as peripheral neurotropism, sustained engraftment, vascular localization of EPCs, dual angioneurotrophic effects and reversal of various functional and pathologic features of DN [42, 43, 60, 92].

4.3 Mesenchymal stem cells

Mesenchymal stem cells (MSCs) are multipotent cells which are found in nearly all postnatal organs and tissues [101]. The adherent nature of MSCs makes them easy to expand in culture and an attractive candidate to use in cell therapy. Also, MSCs are particularly attractive therapeutic agents because of their ability to self-renew, differentiate into multilineage cell types [102, 103], and locally secrete angiogenic cytokines, including basic fibroblast growth factor (bFGF) and VEGF [74, 104-106]. These factors were reported to prompt neovascularization [107] and have support for neural regeneration [99, 108]

MSC transplantation was reported to be a therapeutic agent in the treatment of cardiovascular disease. Similarly, it was plausible that MSCs may also be an effective therapeutic agent for the DN treatment [74, 109] through the paracrine effects of bFGF and VEGF [110] and their potential to differentiate into neural cells such as astrocytes [111], oligodendrocytes [112], and Schwann cells [113, 114].

A study by Shibata et al. [109] suggested that the MSC transplantation on thigh muscles of STZ-induced rats with DN achieved therapeutic effects. Diabetic rats showed hypoalgesia, decreased nerve conduction velocity (NCV), decreased sciatic nerve blood flow (SNBF), decreased capillary number-to-muscle fiber ratio in muscles. These variables were improved by intramuscular MSC injection. MSC injection in diabetic rats seems to produce bFGF and VEGF which eventually showed increased muscular and neural blood flow leading to functional improvement [109]. Although MSCs seem to have some ameliorating , paracrinal effects on diabetic nerve fibers [109] they did not seem to differentiate into neural cells.

Despite the beneficial effects of MSC transplant in experimental DN shown previously, there appears to be major limitation in using MSCs for DN therapy. Study by Jeong et al. [115] showed that BM-derived MSCs may undergo chromosomal abnormalities and formed malignant tumors after injection into mice with DN. This study alerts careful monitoring of chromosomal status for transplantation of MSCs from in vitro expansion.

5. Conclusion

Intensive symptomatic treatment and tight glycemic control benefits and amerliorates nerve dysfunction and pain in some patients with DN. However, favorable outcomes of cell therapy using BM-MNCs, EPCs and MSCs emphasize the importance of targeting multiple pathophysiology for effective therapy and the need for future clinical trial. Particularly, EPCs' synergistic action of neurotrophic, angiogenic and vasculogenic properties show great potential as a therapeutic agent.

Cell therapy may not be a standard treatment option for all stages of DN because different stages of DN are marked by different structural or functional changes. At present, cell therapy may be applied to those patients who suffer from intractable symptoms, acute exacerbation, or combined diseases such as diabetic foot ulcers or critical limb ischemia. However, there are a few remaining concerns in cell therapy strategy. The effectiveness of the patient's own cells needs to be evaluated considering the possibility that BM cells derived from diabetic subjects may be impaired in therapeutic potential. Experiments using the autologous cells derived from diabetic subjects are necessary to address these concerns. Also, the long-term effects of cell therapy need to be tested.

6. Acknowledgment

This work was supported in part by NIH grants RO1HL084471, RC1GM092035, AMDCC pilot and feasibility grant, and HHSN268201000043C (Program of Excellence in Nanotechnology Award); NSF EBICS grant; and Stem Cell Research Center of the 21st Century Frontier Research Program grant SC4300, funded by the Ministry of Science and Technology, Republic of Korea. The authors declare no competing financial interests.

7. References

[1] Rathur, H.M. and A.J. Boulton, *Recent advances in the diagnosis and management of diabetic neuropathy.* The Journal of bone and joint surgery. British volume, 2005. 87(12): p. 1605-10.

[2] Wild, S., et al., *Global prevalence of diabetes: estimates for the year 2000 and projections for 2030.* Diabetes care, 2004. 27(5): p. 1047-53.

[3] Dalla Paola, L. and E. Faglia, *Treatment of diabetic foot ulcer: an overview strategies for clinical approach.* Current diabetes reviews, 2006. 2(4): p. 431-47.

[4] Feldman, E.L., et al., *New insights into the pathogenesis of diabetic neuropathy.* Curr Opin Neurol, 1999. 12(5): p. 553-63.
[5] Verrotti, A., et al., *New trends in the etiopathogenesis of diabetic peripheral neuropathy.* J Child Neurol, 2001. 16(6): p. 389-94.
[6] Malik, R.A., et al., *Sural nerve pathology in diabetic patients with minimal but progressive neuropathy.* Diabetologia, 2005. 48(3): p. 578-85.
[7] Yagihashi, S., S. Yamagishi, and R. Wada, *Pathology and pathogenetic mechanisms of diabetic neuropathy: correlation with clinical signs and symptoms.* Diabetes Res Clin Pract, 2007. 77 Suppl 1: p. S184-9.
[8] Fernyhough, P., S.K. Roy Chowdhury, and R.E. Schmidt, *Mitochondrial stress and the pathogenesis of diabetic neuropathy.* Expert Rev Endocrinol Metab, 2010. 5(1): p. 39-49.
[9] Lauria, G., et al., *Axonal swellings predict the degeneration of epidermal nerve fibers in painful neuropathies.* Neurology, 2003. 61(5): p. 631-6.
[10] Brownlee, M., *The pathobiology of diabetic complications - A unifying mechanism.* Diabetes, 2005. 54(6): p. 1615-1625.
[11] Obrosova, I.G., *How does glucose generate oxidative stress in peripheral nerve?* Neurobiology of Diabetic Neuropathy, 2002. 50: p. 3-35.
[12] Yu, T., J.L. Robotham, and Y. Yoon, *Increased production of reactive oxygen species in hyperglycemic conditions requires dynamic change of mitochondrial morphology.* Proceedings of the National Academy of Sciences of the United States of America, 2006. 103(8): p. 2653-8.
[13] Giacco, F. and M. Brownlee, *Oxidative stress and diabetic complications.* Circulation research, 2010. 107(9): p. 1058-70.
[14] Oates, P.J., *Polyol pathway and diabetic peripheral neuropathy.* Int Rev Neurobiol, 2002. 50: p. 325-92.
[15] Sugimoto, K., M. Yasujima, and S. Yagihashi, *Role of advanced glycation end products in diabetic neuropathy.* Curr Pharm Des, 2008. 14(10): p. 953-61.
[16] Obrosova, I.G., et al., *An aldose reductase inhibitor reverses early diabetes-induced changes in peripheral nerve function, metabolism, and antioxidative defense.* FASEB J, 2002. 16(1): p. 123-5.
[17] Goldberg, H.J., C.I. Whiteside, and I.G. Fantus, *The hexosamine pathway regulates the plasminogen activator inhibitor-1 gene promoter and Sp1 transcriptional activation through protein kinase C-beta I and -delta.* J Biol Chem, 2002. 277(37): p. 33833-41.
[18] Koya, D. and G.L. King, *Protein kinase C activation and the development of diabetic complications.* Diabetes, 1998. 47(6): p. 859-66.
[19] Garcia Soriano, F., et al., *Diabetic endothelial dysfunction: the role of poly(ADP-ribose) polymerase activation.* Nat Med, 2001. 7(1): p. 108-13.
[20] Ilnytska, O., et al., *Poly(ADP-ribose) polymerase inhibition alleviates experimental diabetic sensory neuropathy.* Diabetes, 2006. 55(6): p. 1686-94.
[21] Cameron, N.E. and M.A. Cotter, *Effects of protein kinase Cbeta inhibition on neurovascular dysfunction in diabetic rats: interaction with oxidative stress and essential fatty acid dysmetabolism.* Diabetes Metab Res Rev, 2002. 18(4): p. 315-23.
[22] Cameron, N.E., et al., *Inhibitors of advanced glycation end product formation and neurovascular dysfunction in experimental diabetes.* Ann N Y Acad Sci, 2005. 1043: p. 784-92.

[23] Cameron, N.E., et al., *Vascular factors and metabolic interactions in the pathogenesis of diabetic neuropathy.* Diabetologia, 2001. 44(11): p. 1973-88.

[24] Bierhaus, A., et al., *Diabetes-associated sustained activation of the transcription factor nuclear factor-kappaB.* Diabetes, 2001. 50(12): p. 2792-808.

[25] Vincent, A.M., et al., *Oxidative stress in the pathogenesis of diabetic neuropathy.* Endocrine reviews, 2004. 25(4): p. 612-28.

[26] Coppey, L.J., et al., *Preventing superoxide formation in epineurial arterioles of the sciatic nerve from diabetic rats restores endothelium-dependent vasodilation.* Free Radic Res, 2003. 37(1): p. 33-40.

[27] Coppey, L.J., et al., *Slowing of motor nerve conduction velocity in streptozotocin-induced diabetic rats is preceded by impaired vasodilation in arterioles that overlie the sciatic nerve.* Int J Exp Diabetes Res, 2000. 1(2): p. 131-43.

[28] Coppey, L.J., et al., *Effect of antioxidant treatment of streptozotocin-induced diabetic rats on endoneurial blood flow, motor nerve conduction velocity, and vascular reactivity of epineurial arterioles of the sciatic nerve.* Diabetes, 2001. 50(8): p. 1927-37.

[29] Leinninger, G.M., A.M. Vincent, and E.L. Feldman, *The role of growth factors in diabetic peripheral neuropathy.* J Peripher Nerv Syst, 2004. 9(1): p. 26-53.

[30] Anand, P., *Neurotrophic factors and their receptors in human sensory neuropathies.* Prog Brain Res, 2004. 146: p. 477-92.

[31] Lazarovici, P., C. Marcinkiewicz, and P.I. Lelkes, *Cross talk between the cardiovascular and nervous systems: neurotrophic effects of vascular endothelial growth factor (VEGF) and angiogenic effects of nerve growth factor (NGF)-implications in drug development.* Curr Pharm Des, 2006. 12(21): p. 2609-22.

[32] Zacchigna, S., D. Lambrechts, and P. Carmeliet, *Neurovascular signalling defects in neurodegeneration.* Nat Rev Neurosci, 2008. 9(3): p. 169-81.

[33] Simovic, D., et al., *Improvement in chronic ischemic neuropathy after intramuscular phVEGF165 gene transfer in patients with critical limb ischemia.* Arch Neurol, 2001. 58(5): p. 761-8.

[34] Salis, M.B., et al., *Nerve growth factor supplementation reverses the impairment, induced by Type 1 diabetes, of hindlimb post-ischaemic recovery in mice.* Diabetologia, 2004. 47(6): p. 1055-63.

[35] Emanueli, C., et al., *Nerve growth factor promotes angiogenesis and arteriogenesis in ischemic hindlimbs.* Circulation, 2002. 106(17): p. 2257-62.

[36] Giannini, C. and P.J. Dyck, *Ultrastructural morphometric abnormalities of sural nerve endoneurial microvessels in diabetes mellitus.* Ann Neurol, 1994. 36(3): p. 408-15.

[37] Vinik, A.I., *Diabetic neuropathy: pathogenesis and therapy.* Am J Med, 1999. 107(2B): p. 17S-26S.

[38] Schmidt, R.E., et al., *Insulin-like growth factor I reverses experimental diabetic autonomic neuropathy.* Am J Pathol, 1999. 155(5): p. 1651-60.

[39] Zhuang, H.X., et al., *Insulin-like growth factors reverse or arrest diabetic neuropathy: effects on hyperalgesia and impaired nerve regeneration in rats.* Exp Neurol, 1996. 140(2): p. 198-205.

[40] Lopez-Lopez, C., D. LeRoith, and I. Torres-Aleman, *Insulin-like growth factor I is required for vessel remodeling in the adult brain.* Proceedings of the National Academy of Sciences of the United States of America, 2004. 101(26): p. 9833-8.

[41] Granata, R., et al., *Insulin-like growth factor binding protein-3 induces angiogenesis through IGF-I- and SphK1-dependent mechanisms.* J Thromb Haemost, 2007. 5(4): p. 835-45.
[42] Jeong, J.O., et al., *Dual angiogenic and neurotrophic effects of bone marrow-derived endothelial progenitor cells on diabetic neuropathy.* Circulation, 2009. 119(5): p. 699-708.
[43] Kim, H., et al., *Bone marrow mononuclear cells have neurovascular tropism and improve diabetic neuropathy.* Stem Cells, 2009. 27(7): p. 1686-96.
[44] Cameron, N.E. and M.A. Cotter, *The relationship of vascular changes to metabolic factors in diabetes mellitus and their role in the development of peripheral nerve complications.* Diabetes/metabolism reviews, 1994. 10(3): p. 189-224.
[45] Britland, S.T., et al., *Relationship of endoneurial capillary abnormalities to type and severity of diabetic polyneuropathy.* Diabetes, 1990. 39(8): p. 909-13.
[46] Malik, R.A., et al., *Microangiopathy in human diabetic neuropathy: relationship between capillary abnormalities and the severity of neuropathy.* Diabetologia, 1989. 32(2): p. 92-102.
[47] Malik, R.A., et al., *Endoneurial localisation of microvascular damage in human diabetic neuropathy.* Diabetologia, 1993. 36(5): p. 454-9.
[48] Sima, A.A., et al., *Endoneurial microvessels in human diabetic neuropathy. Endothelial cell dysjunction and lack of treatment effect by aldose reductase inhibitor.* Diabetes, 1991. 40(9): p. 1090-9.
[49] Bradley, J., et al., *Morphometry of endoneurial capillaries in diabetic sensory and autonomic neuropathy.* Diabetologia, 1990. 33(10): p. 611-8.
[50] Khawaja, K.I., et al., *Clinico-pathological features of postural hypotension in diabetic autonomic neuropathy.* Diabet Med, 2000. 17(2): p. 163-6.
[51] Sugimoto, K. and S. Yagihashi, *Effects of aminoguanidine on structural alterations of microvessels in peripheral nerve of streptozotocin diabetic rats.* Microvasc Res, 1997. 53(2): p. 105-12.
[52] Yasuda, H., et al., *Effect of prostaglandin E1 analogue TFC 612 on diabetic neuropathy in streptozocin-induced diabetic rats. Comparison with aldose reductase inhibitor ONO 2235.* Diabetes, 1989. 38(7): p. 832-8.
[53] Uehara, K., et al., *Effects of cilostazol on the peripheral nerve function and structure in STZ-induced diabetic rats.* J Diabetes Complications, 1997. 11(3): p. 194-202.
[54] Estrella, J.S., et al., *Endoneurial microvascular pathology in feline diabetic neuropathy.* Microvasc Res, 2008. 75(3): p. 403-10.
[55] Yasuda, H. and P.J. Dyck, *Abnormalities of endoneurial microvessels and sural nerve pathology in diabetic neuropathy.* Neurology, 1987. 37(1): p. 20-8.
[56] Thrainsdottir, S., et al., *Endoneurial capillary abnormalities presage deterioration of glucose tolerance and accompany peripheral neuropathy in man.* Diabetes, 2003. 52(10): p. 2615-22.
[57] Dyck, P.J., et al., *Capillary number and percentage closed in human diabetic sural nerve.* Proceedings of the National Academy of Sciences of the United States of America, 1985. 82(8): p. 2513-7.
[58] Malik, R.A., et al., *Transperineurial capillary abnormalities in the sural nerve of patients with diabetic neuropathy.* Microvasc Res, 1994. 48(2): p. 236-45.

[59] Artico, M., et al., *Morphological changes in the sciatic nerve of diabetic rats treated with low molecular weight heparin OP 2123/parnaparin.* Anat Histol Embryol, 2002. 31(4): p. 193-7.

[60] Hasegawa, T., et al., *Amelioration of diabetic peripheral neuropathy by implantation of hematopoietic mononuclear cells in streptozotocin-induced diabetic rats.* Exp Neurol, 2006. 199(2): p. 274-80.

[61] Kusano, K.F., et al., *Sonic hedgehog induces arteriogenesis in diabetic vasa nervorum and restores function in diabetic neuropathy.* Arterioscler Thromb Vasc Biol, 2004. 24(11): p. 2102-7.

[62] Schratzberger, P., et al., *Reversal of experimental diabetic neuropathy by VEGF gene transfer.* J Clin Invest, 2001. 107(9): p. 1083-92.

[63] Tesfaye, S., et al., *Impaired blood flow and arterio-venous shunting in human diabetic neuropathy: a novel technique of nerve photography and fluorescein angiography.* Diabetologia, 1993. 36(12): p. 1266-74.

[64] Newrick, P.G., et al., *Sural nerve oxygen tension in diabetes.* British medical journal, 1986. 293(6554): p. 1053-4.

[65] Zochodne, D.W. and C. Nguyen, *Increased peripheral nerve microvessels in early experimental diabetic neuropathy: quantitative studies of nerve and dorsal root ganglia.* J Neurol Sci, 1999. 166(1): p. 40-6.

[66] Kennedy, J.M. and D.W. Zochodne, *Influence of experimental diabetes on the microcirculation of injured peripheral nerve: functional and morphological aspects.* Diabetes, 2002. 51(7): p. 2233-40.

[67] Ii, M., et al., *Neuronal nitric oxide synthase mediates statin-induced restoration of vasa nervorum and reversal of diabetic neuropathy.* Circulation, 2005. 112(1): p. 93-102.

[68] Apfel, S.C., *Neurotrophic factors in the therapy of diabetic neuropathy.* Am J Med, 1999. 107(2B): p. 34S-42S.

[69] Mizisin, A.P., et al., *Ciliary neurotrophic factor improves nerve conduction and ameliorates regeneration deficits in diabetic rats.* Diabetes, 2004. 53(7): p. 1807-12.

[70] Anitha, M., et al., *GDNF rescues hyperglycemia-induced diabetic enteric neuropathy through activation of the PI3K/Akt pathway.* J Clin Invest, 2006. 116(2): p. 344-56.

[71] Silva, G.V., et al., *Mesenchymal stem cells differentiate into an endothelial phenotype, enhance vascular density, and improve heart function in a canine chronic ischemia model.* Circulation, 2005. 111(2): p. 150-6.

[72] Tacken, P.J., et al., *Dendritic-cell immunotherapy: from ex vivo loading to in vivo targeting.* Nat Rev Immunol, 2007. 7(10): p. 790-802.

[73] Prochazka, V., et al., *Autologous bone marrow stem cell transplantation in patients with end-stage chronical critical limb ischemia and diabetic foot.* Vnitr Lek, 2009. 55(3): p. 173-8.

[74] Kinnaird, T., et al., *Local delivery of marrow-derived stromal cells augments collateral perfusion through paracrine mechanisms.* Circulation, 2004. 109(12): p. 1543-9.

[75] Abdel-Latif, A., et al., *Adult bone marrow-derived cells for cardiac repair: a systematic review and meta-analysis.* Arch Intern Med, 2007. 167(10): p. 989-97.

[76] Risau, W., *Mechanisms of angiogenesis.* Nature, 1997. 386(6626): p. 671-4.

[77] Carmeliet, P. and R.K. Jain, *Angiogenesis in cancer and other diseases.* Nature, 2000. 407(6801): p. 249-57.

[78] Gehling, U.M., et al., *In vitro differentiation of endothelial cells from AC133-positive progenitor cells.* Blood, 2000. 95(10): p. 3106-12.

[79] Peichev, M., et al., *Expression of VEGFR-2 and AC133 by circulating human CD34(+) cells identifies a population of functional endothelial precursors.* Blood, 2000. 95(3): p. 952-8.

[80] Shi, Q., et al., *Evidence for circulating bone marrow-derived endothelial cells.* Blood, 1998. 92(2): p. 362-7.

[81] Simmons, Z. and E.L. Feldman, *Update on diabetic neuropathy.* Curr Opin Neurol, 2002. 15(5): p. 595-603.

[82] Lin, Y., et al., *Origins of circulating endothelial cells and endothelial outgrowth from blood.* J Clin Invest, 2000. 105(1): p. 71-7.

[83] Hur, J., et al., *Characterization of two types of endothelial progenitor cells and their different contributions to neovasculogenesis.* Arterioscler Thromb Vasc Biol, 2004. 24(2): p. 288-93.

[84] Rehman, J., et al., *Peripheral blood "endothelial progenitor cells" are derived from monocyte/macrophages and secrete angiogenic growth factors.* Circulation, 2003. 107(8): p. 1164-9.

[85] Kalka, C., et al., *Transplantation of ex vivo expanded endothelial progenitor cells for therapeutic neovascularization.* Proceedings of the National Academy of Sciences of the United States of America, 2000. 97(7): p. 3422-7.

[86] Yoon, C.H., et al., *Synergistic neovascularization by mixed transplantation of early endothelial progenitor cells and late outgrowth endothelial cells: the role of angiogenic cytokines and matrix metalloproteinases.* Circulation, 2005. 112(11): p. 1618-27.

[87] Peters, B.A., et al., *Contribution of bone marrow-derived endothelial cells to human tumor vasculature.* Nat Med, 2005. 11(3): p. 261-2.

[88] Yeh, E.T., et al., *Transdifferentiation of human peripheral blood CD34+-enriched cell population into cardiomyocytes, endothelial cells, and smooth muscle cells in vivo.* Circulation, 2003. 108(17): p. 2070-3.

[89] O'Neill, T.J.t., et al., *Mobilization of bone marrow-derived cells enhances the angiogenic response to hypoxia without transdifferentiation into endothelial cells.* Circulation research, 2005. 97(10): p. 1027-35.

[90] Ziegelhoeffer, T., et al., *Bone marrow-derived cells do not incorporate into the adult growing vasculature.* Circulation research, 2004. 94(2): p. 230-8.

[91] Cho, H.J., et al., *Role of host tissues for sustained humoral effects after endothelial progenitor cell transplantation into the ischemic heart.* J Exp Med, 2007. 204(13): p. 3257-69.

[92] Naruse, K., et al., *Therapeutic neovascularization using cord blood-derived endothelial progenitor cells for diabetic neuropathy.* Diabetes, 2005. 54(6): p. 1823-8.

[93] Schratzberger, P., et al., *Favorable effect of VEGF gene transfer on ischemic peripheral neuropathy.* Nat Med, 2000. 6(4): p. 405-13.

[94] Abe, K. and H. Saito, *Neurotrophic effect of basic fibroblast growth factor is mediated by the p42/p44 mitogen-activated protein kinase cascade in cultured rat cortical neurons.* Brain Res Dev Brain Res, 2000. 122(1): p. 81-5.

[95] Kermani, P., et al., *Neurotrophins promote revascularization by local recruitment of TrkB+ endothelial cells and systemic mobilization of hematopoietic progenitors.* J Clin Invest, 2005. 115(3): p. 653-63.

[96] Calcutt, N.A., et al., *Therapeutic efficacy of sonic hedgehog protein in experimental diabetic neuropathy.* J Clin Invest, 2003. 111(4): p. 507-14.

[97] Chalasani, S.H., et al., *The chemokine stromal cell-derived factor-1 promotes the survival of embryonic retinal ganglion cells.* J Neurosci, 2003. 23(11): p. 4601-12.

[98] Mirshahi, F., et al., *SDF-1 activity on microvascular endothelial cells: consequences on angiogenesis in in vitro and in vivo models.* Thromb Res, 2000. 99(6): p. 587-94.

[99] Nakae, M., et al., *Effects of basic fibroblast growth factor on experimental diabetic neuropathy in rats.* Diabetes, 2006. 55(5): p. 1470-7.

[100] Masaki, I., et al., *Angiogenic gene therapy for experimental critical limb ischemia: acceleration of limb loss by overexpression of vascular endothelial growth factor 165 but not of fibroblast growth factor-2.* Circ Res, 2002. 90(9): p. 966-73.

[101] Porada, C.D., E.D. Zanjani, and G. Almeida-Porad, *Adult mesenchymal stem cells: a pluripotent population with multiple applications.* Current stem cell research & therapy, 2006. 1(3): p. 365-9.

[102] Pittenger, M.F., et al., *Multilineage potential of adult human mesenchymal stem cells.* Science, 1999. 284(5411): p. 143-7.

[103] Jackson, L., et al., *Adult mesenchymal stem cells: differentiation potential and therapeutic applications.* Journal of postgraduate medicine, 2007. 53(2): p. 121-7.

[104] Kinnaird, T., et al., *Bone-marrow-derived cells for enhancing collateral development: mechanisms, animal data, and initial clinical experiences.* Circulation research, 2004. 95(4): p. 354-63.

[105] Iwase, T., et al., *Comparison of angiogenic potency between mesenchymal stem cells and mononuclear cells in a rat model of hindlimb ischemia.* Cardiovascular research, 2005. 66(3): p. 543-51.

[106] Al-Khaldi, A., et al., *Postnatal bone marrow stromal cells elicit a potent VEGF-dependent neoangiogenic response in vivo.* Gene therapy, 2003. 10(8): p. 621-9.

[107] Masaki, I., et al., *Angiogenic gene therapy for experimental critical limb ischemia: acceleration of limb loss by overexpression of vascular endothelial growth factor 165 but not of fibroblast growth factor-2.* Circulation research, 2002. 90(9): p. 966-73.

[108] Schratzberger, P., et al., *Reversal of experimental diabetic neuropathy by VEGF gene transfer.* The Journal of clinical investigation, 2001. 107(9): p. 1083-92.

[109] Shibata, T., et al., *Transplantation of bone marrow-derived mesenchymal stem cells improves diabetic polyneuropathy in rats.* Diabetes, 2008. 57(11): p. 3099-107.

[110] Wang, X., et al., *Hsp20-engineered mesenchymal stem cells are resistant to oxidative stress via enhanced activation of Akt and increased secretion of growth factors.* Stem Cells, 2009. 27(12): p. 3021-31.

[111] Wislet-Gendebien, S., et al., *Astrocytic and neuronal fate of mesenchymal stem cells expressing nestin.* Brain research bulletin, 2005. 68(1-2): p. 95-102.

[112] Hermann, A., et al., *Efficient generation of neural stem cell-like cells from adult human bone marrow stromal cells.* Journal of cell science, 2004. 117(Pt 19): p. 4411-22.

[113] Keilhoff, G., et al., *Transdifferentiated mesenchymal stem cells as alternative therapy in supporting nerve regeneration and myelination.* Cellular and molecular neurobiology, 2006. 26(7-8): p. 1235-52.

[114] Dezawa, M., et al., *Sciatic nerve regeneration in rats induced by transplantation of in vitro differentiated bone-marrow stromal cells.* The European journal of neuroscience, 2001. 14(11): p. 1771-6.

[115] Jeong, J.O., et al., *Malignant tumor formation after transplantation of short-term cultured bone marrow mesenchymal stem cells in experimental myocardial infarction and diabetic neuropathy.* Circulation research, 2011. 108(11): p. 1340-7.

11

Cell Therapy for Ischemic Peripheral Neuropathy

Yousuke Katsuda, Ken Arima, Hisashi Kai and Tsutomu Imaizumi
Division of Cardio-Vascular Medicine, Department of Medicine
Kurume University School of Medicine
Japan

1. Introduction

Critical limb ischemia due to chronic peripheral arterial occlusive disease, such as arteriosclerosis obliterans and Buerger's disease (thromboangiitis obliterans), damages peripheral nerves and results in an ischemic neuropathy. Clinical and electro-physiologic features of ischemic neuropathy are sensorimotor polyneuropathy with axonal features as previously reported. In particular, symptoms of ischemic neuropathy include painful burning, sensory impairment, and reflex loss. Although ischemic peripheral neuropathy is a major complication of critical limb ischemia resulting in impaired quality of life, effective treatment for ischemic neuropathy is not available at present.

Recently, it has been reported that therapeutic angiogenesis using vascular endothelial growth factor (VEGF) gene transfer for critical limb ischemia improves ischemic neuropathy in animals or humans. Furthermore, Cuevus et al. reported that transplantation of bone marrow stromal cells improved peripheral nerve function in rats.

We reported that therapeutic angiogenesis using autologous transplantation of bone marrow mononuclear cells (BM-MNCs) for peripheral artery disease increased limb perfusion and improved clinical conditions, such as ischemic pain, claudication and ischemic ulcer. BM-MNCs contain various kinds of cell lineages, such as $CD34^{+}$ cells or bone marrow stromal cells, in addition to various growth factors, such as VEGF. Thus, such cells or growth factors can work beneficially for ischemic peripheral neuropathy.

Therefore, in this chapter, we tried to clarify whether cell therapy with autologous transplantation of BM-MNCs improves ischemic neuropathy with critical ischemic limb in humans.

2. Patients and methods

2.1 Study subjects

We prospectively examined 39 patients having chronic bilateral critical limb ischemia, defined as angiographic documentation of severe large artery stenosis or occlusion associated with limb pain at rest and/or non-healing ischemic ulcers. All the patients fulfilled the inclusion criteria and did not have any exclusion criteria for therapeutic angiogenesis using BM-MNCs as described previously. Briefly, they were not candidates for non-surgical or surgical revascularization. We excluded patients with poorly controlled diabetes mellitus (HbA1C>6.5% and proliferative retinopathy) or with evidence of malignant disorder for the past 5 years. Furthermore, patients in whom neurological scales could not be evaluated due to huge ulcer or limb amputation were excluded. Finally, 14 patients undergoing autologous transplantation of BM-MNCs were enrolled in this study. Age and sex matched 23 healthy volunteers were served as controls to examine neurophysiologic scales (Healthy group). The protocol was approved by the Institutional Ethic Committee of the Kurume University. Written informed consent was obtained from all subjects.

2.2 Collection and transplantation of BM-MNCs

Bone marrow cells were collected from the iliac crest under general anesthesia. We sorted mononuclear cells on CS-3000 blood-cell separator (Baxter, Deerfield, USA) by a density gradient centrifugation method and concentrated them to a final volume of about 30ml immediately after aspiration. We injected the cells with 26-gauge needle into the gastro-cunemius muscle of the more ischemic limb (treated limb), and injected saline into the opposite limb (control limb). We injected about 0.5ml of BM-MNCs or saline into each injection site (50 sites, 1-1.5cm deep).

2.3 Clinical features

The severity of rest pain was described and scored by patient from 0 (none) to 10 (maximum) points using visual analogue scale (VAS). Pain free walking distance was separately measured twice as ischemic status before and 4 weeks after transplantation of BM-MNCs. Also, the detailed nature of pain was recorded to exclude symptoms that could be attributable to tissue ischemia rather than neuropathy. To distinguish neuropathic symptoms from ischemic ones, numbness, painful burning, and paresthesia in the toes of foot were defined neuropathic in origin. We excluded symptoms when they exclusively appeared during walk or by use (i.e. foot elevations). Two examiners evaluated the neurological scales. The examiners were blinded to the findings of patients' clinical profile, treatment and to each other's results. The existence of neuropathic symptom was described and scored by the patient from 0 to 1 point (0=without neuropathic symptom, 1=with neuropathic symptom) as neurologic sensory score (NSS). We tested untreated limb to assess the natural course of the disease as control limb. Each patient was evaluated 1 week before and 4 weeks after treatment.

2.4 Neurophysiologic scales

Two examiners evaluated the neurological scales. The examiners were blinded to the findings of patients' clinical profile, treatment and to each other's assessment. Conduction studies were performed using techniques described elsewhere (Neuropack MEB-2200, Nihon Kohden Co. ltd, Japan). Briefly, motor nerve conduction velocities (MNCV) of the tibial nerve were measured. Tibial compound muscle action potentials (CMAP) were also recorded with surface disk electrodes from the abductor hallucis. Sensory nerve conduction velocities (SNCV) or sensory nerve action potentials (SNAP) of the sural nerve were measured. All determinations were made with the patient supine and at the surface temperature between 29-32°C. The same examiner using the identical anatomical landmarks and distances performed repeated studies after treatment. Quantitative vibration threshold time (QVT) was measured using standard techniques by a tuning fork to determine the thresholds of vibration in the legs. We performed these neurophysiologic testing before and 4 weeks after treatment. We also measured MNCV, SNCV, CMAP and SNAP of the healthy group at baseline.

2.5 Assessment of blood flow

We measured ankle brachial pressure index (ABPI) 1 week before and 4 weeks after implantation, the ratio of simultaneously measured systolic pressure of brachial and posterior tibial arteries (ABI-form, Colin, Japan). Digital subtraction angiography (DSA) was performed with the strictly fixed amount of contrast agent, force of contrast injection, and position of the catheter tip at 1 week before and 4 weeks after transplantation. Two radiologists who were blinded to treatment evaluated collateral vessels independently. Angiograms were assessed when contrast flow in the main conducting arteries was most clearly visible. Angiographic evaluation was presented as changes in DSA score: 3+ (rich collateral development), 2+ (moderate), 1+ (slight), 0 (no changes), and 1- (decreased).

2.6 Statistical analysis

Data were expressed as mean ± SD. Differences between the two groups were analyzed by paired or unpaired Student's *t* test when appropriate. Univariate correlations were analyzed by a Pearson's correlation. Differences with a $p < 0.05$ were considered statistically significant.

3. Results

3.1 Patient's characteristics

Patient's characteristics are shown in Table 1. Nine patients were Buerger's disease and 5 ASO. They all had undergone optimal medical or surgical treatment prior to this study. The average numbers of transplanted mononuclear cells of CD34 positive cells were $4.89 \pm 5.21 \times 10^9$ and $5.46 \pm 4.25 \times 10^7$, respectively (Table 1). During follow up period, no one had major adverse event, such as any cause of death and cardiovascular event.

Patient	Age (y.o.)	sex	Diagnosis	No. of MNCs ($\times 10^9$)	No. of $CD34^+$ cells ($\times 10^7$)
1	67	M	TAO	2.58	2.63
2	29	M	TAO	2.9	8.48
3	72	F	TAO	1.07	0.92
4	69	M	ASO	1.83	6.82
5	43	M	TAO	4.14	7.18
6	63	M	ASO	1.39	1.17
7	75	M	ASO	1.70	5.03
8	40	M	TAO	5.12	17.05
9	61	M	TAO	13.5	3.3
10	50	M	TAO	16.90	6.5
11	62	M	TAO	11.9	8.3
12	78	M	ASO	1.80	2.9
13	55	F	TAO	2.38	5.1
14	65	F	ASO	1.20	1.1
mean±SD	59.2±14.2			4.89±5.21	5.46±4.25

Abbreviations y.o.: years old, M: male, F: female, MNCs: mononuclear cells, TAO: thromboangiitis obliterans, ASO: arteriosclerosis obliterans

Table 1. Patients characteristics and number of implanted cells.

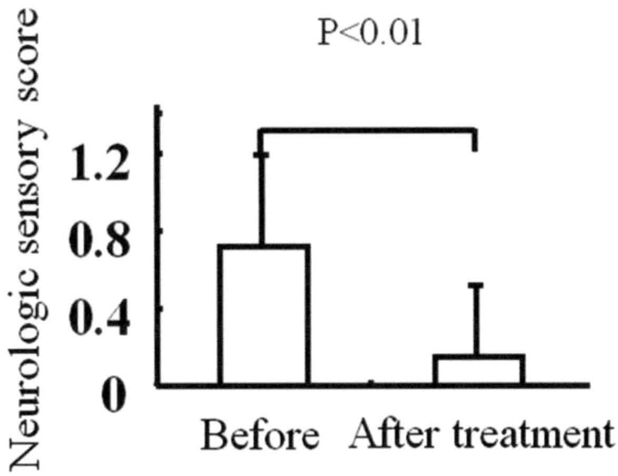

Fig. 1. Neurologic sensory score.

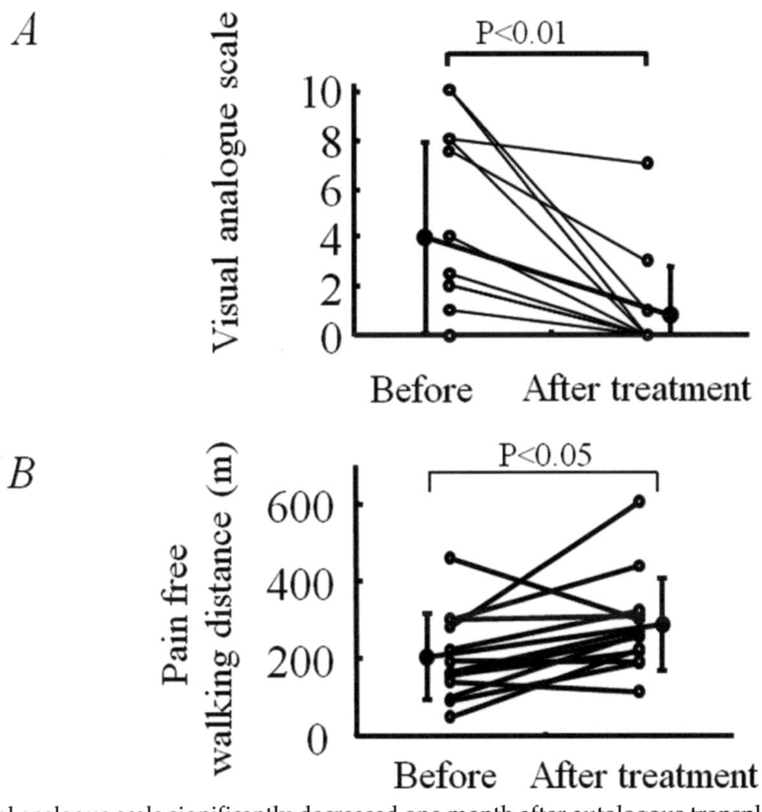

Panel A: Visual analogue scale significantly decreased one month after autologous transplantation of BM-MNCs.

Panel B: Pain free walking time significantly increased one month after autologous transplantation of BM-MNCs.

Open circles indicate individual value. Closed circle indicate average value.

Fig. 2. Improvement of ischemic symptoms.

3.2 Subjective symptoms

Before treatment, 10 of 14 patients (71.4%) had neuropathic symptoms with average NSS of 0.71±0.47 (Figure 1). Four weeks after treatment, only 2 patients had neuropathic symptoms, and averaged NSS was decreased to 0.14±0.36 ($p<0.01$ vs. before treatment, Figure 1). VAS significantly improved (3.93±3.92 to 0.79±1.79, $p<0.01$, Figure 2A) after treatment. Pain free walking distance significantly increased (201±110 to 317±197, $P<0.05$, Figure 2B) after treatment

3.3 Nerve functions

MNCV and CMAP could be measured in the treated limb of all patients, and in the control limb of 12 patients. SNCV and SNAP could be measured 11 of 14 patients in the treated limb, and 10 of 14 patients in the control limb. Figure 3 shows the representative waveform of MNCV and CMAP before and one month after treatment. Before treatment, both MNCV and CMAP were significantly smaller in the treated limb than those in the healthy group (Table 2). Treatment significantly increased both MNCV and CMAP only in the treated limb (Table 2) but not in the control limb. MNCV was recovered to the level of healthy group but CMAP was still depressed after transplantation of BM-MNCs (Table 2). SNCV and SNAP of the patients did not differ to those of the healthy group. SNCV and SNAP were not improved by treatment (Table 2). QVT was significantly improved only in the treated limb, but not in the control limb after treatment (Table 2).

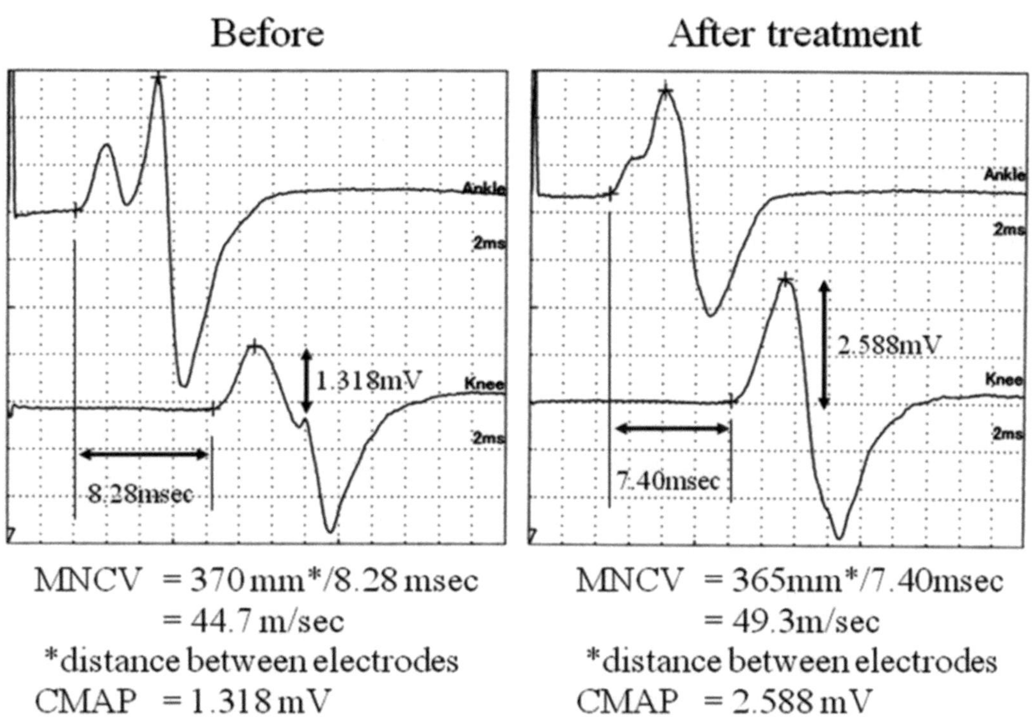

Fig. 3. Representative waveforms of MNCV and CMAP. MNCV and CMAP increased one month after autologous transplantation of BM-MNCs.

Nerve function	Healthy group N=23	Patients N=14			
		before	after	before	after
		Control limb		Treated limb	
MNCV (m/sec)	50.4±6.94	47.3±3.0	44.8±3.0	41.1±6.5**	43.9±6.2
CMAP (mV)	5.3±2.8	4.9±4.3	5.2±5.2	2.3±2.7*	3.6±3.5¶*
SNCV (m/sec)	50.0±10.7	49.5±3.7	48.3±4.5	46.8±4.3	46.5±4.9
SNAP (μV)	10.2±8.9	8.4±2.1	8.6±3.1	7.6±3.8	8.7±4.4
QVT (sec)	NM	10.5±3.2	11.1±4.0	9.2±2.7	11.5±3.5

Values are expressed as mean±SD. Differences between the two groups were analyzed by paired or unpaired Student's t test. Univariate correlations were analyzed by a Pearson's correlation. Abbreviations VAS: visual analogue scale, MNCV: motor nerve conduction velocity, CMAP: compound muscle action potential, SNCV: sensory nerve conduction velocity, SNAP: sensory nerve action potential, QVT: quantitative vibration threshold time. N/A: not available, NM: not measured, SD: standard deviation
*: p<0.05 vs. healthy group, **: p<0.01 vs. healthy group, ¶: p<0.05 vs. before treatment, :p<0.01 vs. before treatment.

Table 2. Effects of nerve functions. (Based on data originally presented by Arima, K. et al.).

3.4 Assessment of blood flow

Before treatment, ABPI was significantly decreased in the treated and control limbs. After treatment, ABPI was significantly increased only in the treated limb (0.59±0.24 to 0.70±0.20, P=0.035), but not in the control limb (0.89±0.20 to 0.89±0.20, N.S.). DSA score in the treated limb was significantly increased after treatment (0.0±0.0 to 0.86±0.77, p<0.05, Figure 4).

4. Discussion

The major findings of this study are the following two. First, autologous transplantation of BM-MNCs significantly improved subjective ischemic and neuropathic symptoms in patients with critical limb ischemia. Second, autologous transplantation of BM-MNCs improved not only peripheral blood perfusion but also peripheral nerve function.

4.1 Neuropathy in patients with critical limb ischemia

Several studies have reported neuropathy at the frequency of 5-31% in patients with chronic and critical limb ischemia. The mechanisms of neuropathy in patients with limb ischemia are multifocal because they have frequently have associated disease like diabetes mellitus. Weinberg et al reported that the degree of ischemia, as estimated with ABPI, correlated with clinical neuropathy. Thus it is suggested that limb ischemia is the major factor of peripheral neuropathy in patients with critical limb ischemia.

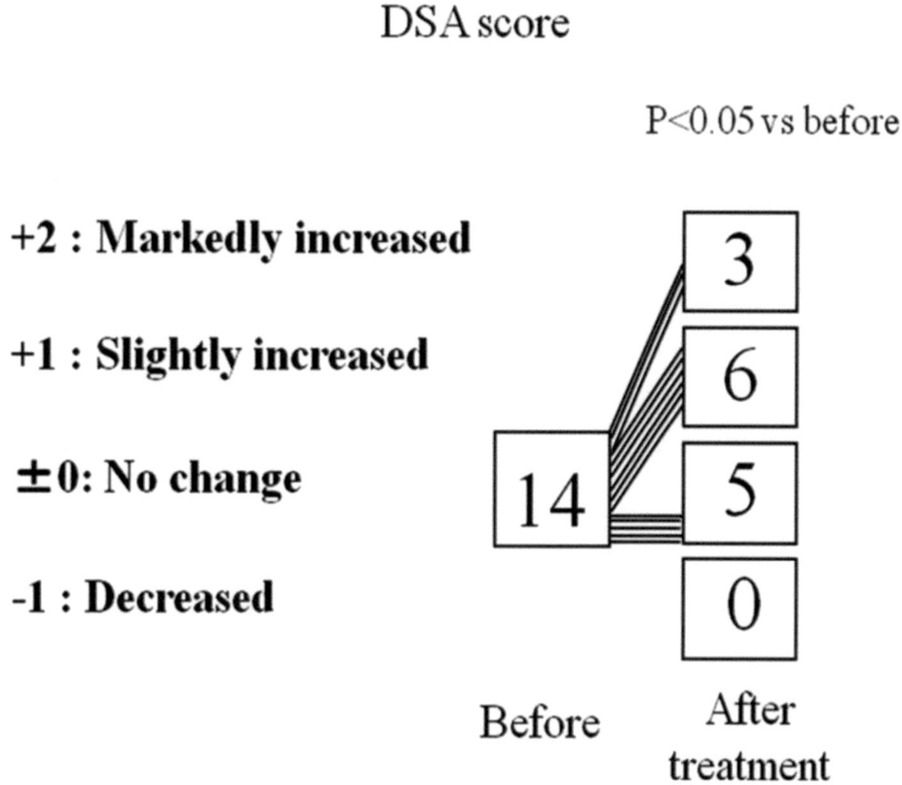

Fig. 4. Time course of DSA score after autologous transplantation of BM-MNCs in the treated limb. In the treated limb, DSA score significantly improved one month after autologous transplantation of BM-MNCs (P<0.05). DSA indicates digital subtraction angiography.

In this study, our patients had not only ischemic symptoms (rest pain and claudication) but also neuropathic symptoms. Because ABPI was significantly decreased and because we excluded patients with diabetes mellitus, we think the nature of neuropathic symptoms is related to limb ischemia. Furthermore, nerve function in the patients was severely impaired compared with the healthy group. Thus, the etiology of peripheral neuropathy in our patients was probably ischemic in its origin. Although our patients had bilateral limb ischemia, the nerve function at baseline was impaired only in the treated limb. The reason is not clear at present but the difference in the severity of limb ischemia may explain it.

Apart from MNCV or CMAP, SNCV and SNAP of ischemic limb before treatment were similar to those of healthy subject. The reason of such different effect of limb ischemia on motor and sensory nerves is unknown, but may be due to the size of nerve fibers. The size of motor nerve (5-15 micrometer) is larger than sensory nerve (0.5-13 micrometer). Previous pathologic studies reported that decrease in the population of large myelinated fibers was observed in ischemic peripheral neuropathy. The damage of nerve fiber may be smaller for the sensory nerve than the large motor nerve in the presence of ischemia, which may account for the preserved SNCV and SNAP.

4.2 Autologous transplantation of BM-MNCs improved neuropathy

Recently, we reported that autologous transplantation of BM-MNCs increased limb perfusion and improved symptoms and ulcers in human ischemic limb. In this study, we confirmed our previous findings that autologous transplantation of BM-MNCs significantly improved ABPI and DSA score in treated limbs. This treatment significantly improved not only ischemic pain (VAS, pain free walking time) but also neuropathic symptoms. Furthermore, transplantation of BM-MNCs significantly improved objective peripheral nerve functions (MNCV, CMAP and QVT) in the treated limb, but saline injection did not affect the nerve functions. These results indicated that the effects of the treatment were not related to natural course or non-specific effects. Thus, it is concluded that autologous transplantation of BM-MNCs improved not only peripheral blood perfusion but also ischemic peripheral neuropathy.

4.3 Mechanisms of improvement of peripheral neuropathy

The several mechanisms may contribute to the improvement of peripheral nerve function. First, the improvement may be caused by better blood perfusion after autologous transplantation of BM-MNCs. On this issue several conflicting results were reported.

There were several therapeutic strategies for improving blood perfusion, such as surgical revascularization or therapeutic angiogenesis induced by VEGF gene transfer. Hunter et al. examined electrophysiological changes of nerves after surgical revascularization. They reported no improvement of multiple electrophysiological outcome measures after surgical revascularization, suggesting that ischemic neuropathy may be an irreversible condition. On the other hand, Simovic et al. reported that VEGF gene transfer improved the neuropathic symptoms, CMAP and QVT, but not nerve conduction velocity. They speculated that the differences of efficiency between surgical revascularization and VEGF gene transfer were related to the size of restored vessels after treatments. In fact, surgical revascularization mainly restores blood flow of large vessels, and neovascularization from angiogenic cytokines, such as VEGF, principally involves small vessels including the vasa-nervorum (<180 micrometer), the nutrient arteries of peripheral nerves. Furthermore, it is reported that VEGF gene transfer improves peripheral nerve perfusion and function through regeneration of vasa-nervorum in rats with streptozotocin-induced diabetes. In this study, electrophysiological study showed improvement of nerve functions in addition to neuropathic symptoms. It is reported that variety of cytokines, such as VEGF, are contained in transplanted bone-marrow fluid or secreted by transplanted BM-MNCs. Thus, such various angiogenic cytokines might have improved nerve perfusion and function in this study.

Second, nerve regeneration might have occurred after transplantation of BM-MNCs. It is reported that VEGF also has regenerative and protective function for peripheral nerve. Furthermore, Cuevas et al. reported that implantation of bone-marrow stromal cells improved peripheral nerve function via nerve regeneration in animals. They reported that implanted cells participated in nerve regeneration through their differentiation in Schwann-like cells and also in the production of trophic factors. Because transplanted BM-MNCs used in this study presumably contain various kinds of cells such as bone-marrow stromal cells as previously reported, it may be speculated that transplantation of BM-MNCs might have regenerated the damaged peripheral motor nerve. Of course, we have no evidence.

Limitations of this study need to be addressed. First, this study was an observational open-label study with no placebo control group. Next, the number of patients enrolled in this study was small. Further large sized controlled clinical study is needed to confirm our findings. Finally, we treated patients with critical limb ischemia who had undergone optimal medical and surgical treatment. Thus, it is not known whether autologous transplantation of BM-MNCs is effective for the earlier stage of patients.

5. Conclusions

In conclusion, these results suggested that cell therapy with autologous transplantation of BM-MNCs improves ischemic neuropathy with critical ischemic limb in humans.

6. Acknowledgement

This study was supported in part by Kimura Memorial Heart Foundation Research Grant: by grants for Cardiovascular Disease (16C-6) from the Ministry of Health, Labor, Welfare: by a Grant for Science Frontier Promotion Program and Grants-In-Aid from the Ministry of Education, Culture, Sports, Science, and Technology of Japan. We thank Kimiko Kimura for technical assistance.

7. References

Arima, K. & Katsuda, Y. & Takeshita, Y. & Saito, Y. & Toyama, Y. & Katsuki, Y. & Ootsuka, M. & Koiwaya, H. & Sasaki, K. & Kai, H. & Imaizumi, T. (2010). Autologous transplantation of bone marrow mononuclear cells improved ischemic peripheral neuropathy in humans, *J. Am. Coll. Cardiol*, Vol. 56, No. 3, (July 2010), pp. 238-239, ISSN 0735-1097

Cahill, BE. & Kerstein MD. (1987). Ischemic neuropathy. *Sug Gynecol Obstet* Vol.165, No. 5, (November 1987), pp. 469-74, ISSN 0039-6087

Cuevas, P. & Carceller, F. & Dujovny, M. & Garcia-Gomez, I. & Cuevas, B. & Gonzalez-Corrochano, R. & Diaz-Gonzalez, D. & Reimers, D. (2002) Peripheral nerve regeneration by bone marrow stromal cells. *Neurol Res.* Vol. 24, No. 7, (October, 2002), pp. 634-8, ISSN 0161-6412

Cuevas, P. & Carceller, F. & Garcia-Gomez, I. & Yan, M. & Dujovny, M. (2004). Bone marrow stromal cell implantation for peripheral nerve repair. *Neurol Res.* Vol. 26, No. 2, (April, 2004), pp. 230-2, ISSN 0161-6412

Farinon, AM. & Marbini, A. & Gemignani, F. & Govoni, E. & Bragaglia, MM. & Sianesi, M. & Tedeschi, F. (1984) Skeletal muscle and peripheral nerve changes caused by chronic arterial insufficiency - Significance and clinical correlations - Histological, histochemical and ultrastructural study. *Clin Neuropathol.* Vol. 3, No. 6, (November 1984), pp. 240-52, ISSN 0722-5091

Hunter, GC. & Song, GW. & Nayak, NN. & Zapotoxski, D. & Guernsey, JM. (1988) Peripheral nerve conduction abnormalities in lower extremity ischemia: the effects of revascularization. *J Surg Res.* Vol. 45, No. 1, (July 1988), pp. 96-103, ISSN 0022-4804

Isner, JM. & Pieczek, A. & Schainfeld, R. & Blair, R. & Haley, L. & Asahara, T. & Rosenfield, K. & Razvi, S. & Walsh, K. & Symes, JF. (1996). Clinical evidence of angiogenesis after arterial gene transfer of ph VEGF165 in patient with ischaemic limb. *Lancet.* Vol. 348, No. 9034, (Aug 10), pp. 370-374, ISSN 0140-6736

Kamihata, H. & Matsubara, H. & Nishiue, T. & Fujiyama, S. & Tsutsumi, Y. & Ozono, R. & Masaki, H. & Mori, Y. & Iba, O. & Tateishi, E. & Kosaki, A. & Shintani, S. & Murohara, T. & Imaizumi, T. & Iwasaka, T. (2001). Implantation of bone marrow mononuclear cells into ischemic myocardium enhances collateral perfusion and regional function via side supply of anigioblasts, angiogenic ligands, and cytokines. *Circulation.* Vol. 104, No. 9, (August 2001), pp. 1046-52, ISSN 1524-4539

Mufson, I. (1952) Diagnosis and treatment of neural complications of peripheral arterial obliterative disease. *Angiology,* Vol. 3, No. 5, (October 1952), pp 392-3, ISSN 0003-3197

Saito, Y. & Sasaki, K. & Katsuda, Y. & Murohara, T. & Takeshita, Y. & Okazaki, T. & Arima, K. & Katsuki, Y. & Shintani, S. & Shimada, T. & Akashi, H. & Ikeda, H. & Imaizumi, T. (2007) Effect of autologous bone-marrow cell transplantation on ischemic ulcer in patients with Buerger's disease. *Circ J.* Vol. 71, No. 8, (July 2007), pp. 1187-92, ISSN 1346-9843

Schratzberger, P. & Schratzberg, G. & Silver, M. & Curry, C. & Kearney, M. & Magner, M. & Alroy, J. & Adelman, LS. & Veinberg, DH. & Ropper, AH. & Isner, JM. (2000). Favorable effect of VEGF gene transfer on ischemic peripheral neuropathy. *Nat Med.* Vol. 6, No. 6, (March 2000), pp. 405-13, ISSN 1078-8956

Schratzberger, P. & Walter, DH. & Rittig, K. & Bahlmann, FH. & Pola, R. & Curry, C. & Silver, M. & Krainin, JG. & Weinberg, DH. & Ropper, AH. & Isner, JM. (2001) Reversal of experimental diabetic neuropathy by VEGF gene transfer. *J Clin Invest.* Vol. 107, No. 9, (May 2001), pp. 1083-92, ISSN 0021-9738

Simovic, D. & Isner, JM. & Rooper, AH. & Pieczedk, A. & Weinverg, DH. (2001). Improvement in chronic ischemic neuropathy after intramuscular phVEGF165 gene transfer in patients with critical limb ischemia. *Arch Neurol,* Vol. 58, No. 5, (May 2001), pp. 761-8, ISSN 0003-9942

Strokebaum, E. & Lambrechts, D. & Carmeliet P. (2004). VEGF: once regarded as a specific angionenic factor, now implicated in neuroprotection. Bioessays. Vol. 26, No. 9, (September 2004), pp. 943-954, ISSN 0265-9247

Tateishi-Yuyama, E. & Matsubara, H. & Murohara, T. & Ikeda, U. & Shintani, S. & Masaki, H. & Amano, K. & Kishimoto, Y. & Yoshimoto, K. & Akashi, H. & Shimada, K. & Iwasaka, T. & Imaizumi, T. (2002). Therapeutic angiogenesis for patients with limb ischaemia by autologous transplantation of bone-marrow cells: a pilot study and a randomized controlled trial. *Lancet.* Vol. 360, No. 9331, (August 2002), pp. 427-35, ISSN 0140-6736

Weinberg, DH. & Simovic, D. & Isner, J. & Ropper, AH. (2001). Chronic ischemic monomelic neuropathy from critical limb ischemia. *Neurology,* Vol. 57, No 6, (September 2001), pp. 1008-12, ISSN 00283878

12

Gene and Cell Therapy for Peripheral Neuropathy

Deirdre M. O'Connor, Thais Federici and Nicholas M. Boulis
Department of Neurosurgery, Emory University, Atlanta, GA, USA

1. Introduction

Peripheral neuropathy describes a range of degenerative processes that affect the peripheral nervous system and are largely untreatable. These neuropathies affect both sensory and motor fibers and include diabetic neuropathy, chemical neuropathy, post-herpetic neuralgia and peripheral nerve injury. Other causes of neuropathy include alcoholism, nutritional deficits, Guillian-Barre syndrome, AIDS related neuropathy and neuropathy caused by toxins such as heavy metals. Current treatments focus on pain management and on microsurgical intervention such as nerve grafting (Federici and Boulis 2009). Therapies that focus on promoting axon growth and regeneration subsequent to peripheral nerve degeneration or injury are suboptimal.

1.1 Peripheral nerve injury

Damage to peripheral nerves results in demyelination and axonal degeneration. Axonal degeneration can happen in several ways. Wallerian degeneration happens when the continuity of the nerve fibre is interrupted through traumatic, toxic, ischemic or metabolic events (Dubovy 2011). In neurodegenerative processes, there is progressive degeneration of the axons towards the cell body which remains intact over a longer period of time. This degenerative process is referred to as distal axonopathy or dying back axonal degeneration (Hoke 2006). Research on both super oxide dismutase 1 (SOD1) mice and on patients suffering from ALS have found degeneration of neuromuscular junctions prior to the loss of motor neurons. This indicated that ALS is considered to be a distal axonopathy (Fischer, Culver et al. 2004).
The peripheral nervous system has the ability to regenerate axons in response to an injury. Axonal stumps possess the ability to regenerate and grow in response to Schwann cells and their basal lamina (Fischer, Culver et al. 2004). Macrophages and Schwann cells phagocytose the myelin debris (Fansa and Keilhoff 2003) that results from the injury. Fibroblasts and Schwann cells provide a matrix for axonal regrowth. They secrete neurotrophic factors that support and enhance neuron survival (Ide 1996). In Wallerian degeneration Schwann cells carry out the first step in myelin sheath evacuation by myelin fragmentation. The degraded myelin is phagocytosed by macrophages for full myelin clearance (Stoll, Griffin et al. 1989). This is an important step prior to nerve regeneration. Schwann cells in the region of the damaged neurons secrete a number of growth factors such as glial-cell derived neurotrophic factor (GDNF), brain derived neurotrophic factor (BDNF), insulin-like growth factor (IGF-1) and nerve growth factor (NGF) (Funakoshi, Frisen et al. 1993).

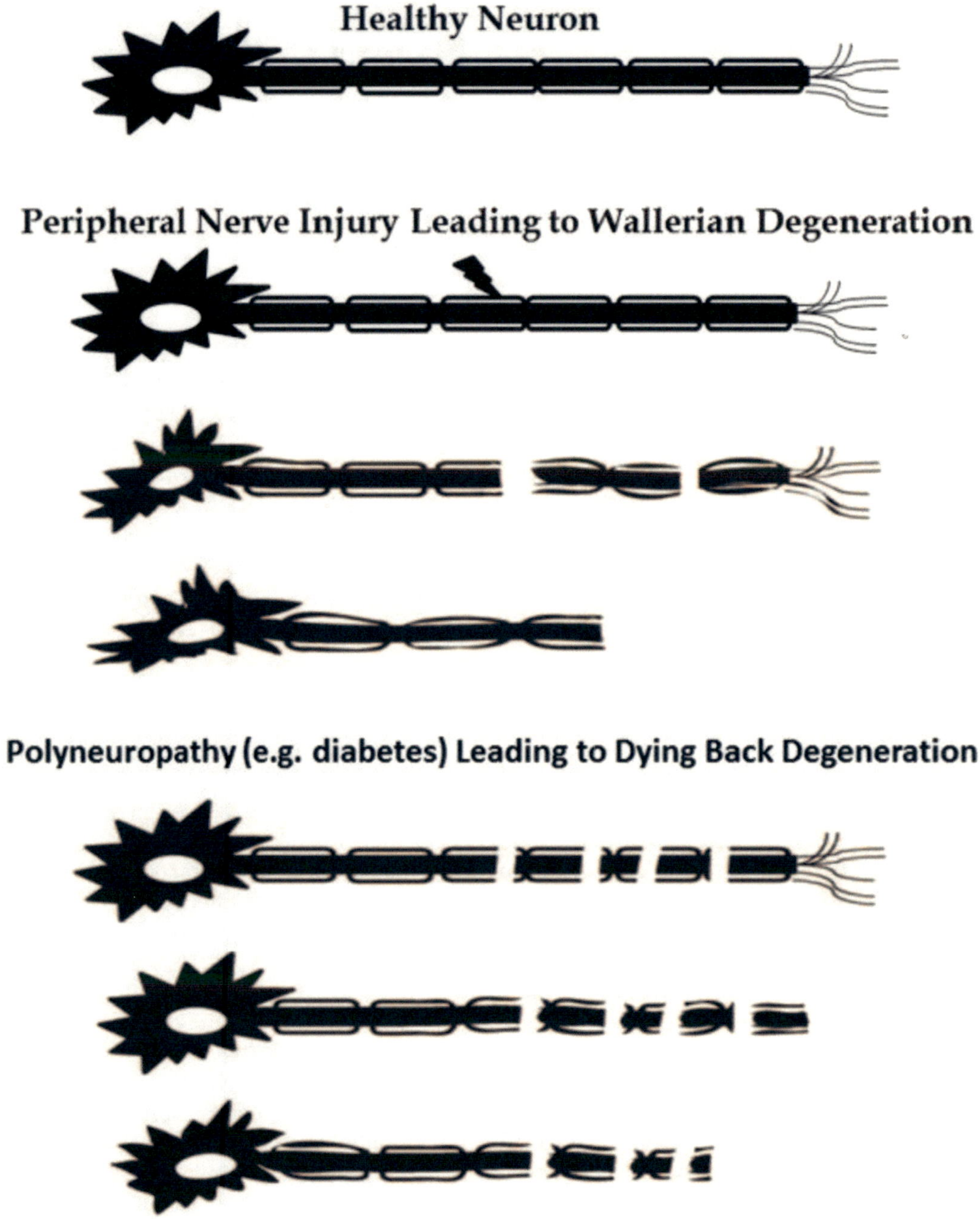

Fig. 1. Comparison of Wallerian and "Dying Back" degeneration in neurons.

Nerve regeneration starts at the node of Ranvier near the proximal stump. The basal lamina that remains post-injury, which surrounds the axon and the Schwann cells, acts as a conduit or tube for the regenerating axon. The damaged nerve stump distal to the injury supports regeneration by assisting regenerating sprouts to extend in the direction of the distal stump (Hoke 2006).
The next step in axonal regeneration occurs when the axons enter the distal stump. They have to grow over a long distance in an environment that is considerably different from the embryonic one originally encountered. The regenerating nerve also has to remyelinate. The last step to complete the regenerative process is for the axon to find and reinnervate their original targets be they muscle or sensory organs (Abrams and Widenfalk 2005).

1.1.1 Therapeutic targets

A damaged peripheral nerve can be divided into a number of parts. Each one needs to be considered individually as a therapeutic target (Figure 2).

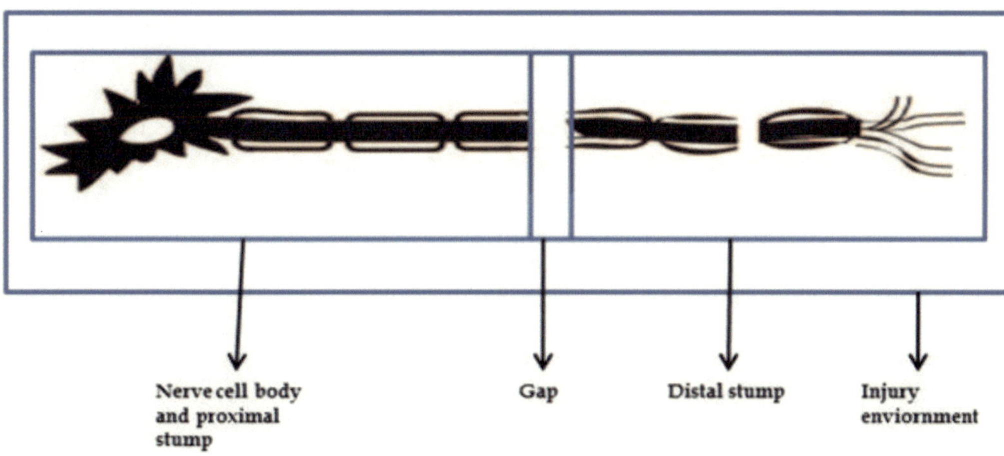

Fig. 2. Identification of the four different parts of a damaged neuron.

The first part is the nerve cell body and the proximal stump. The nerve cell body is necessary for providing the metabolic machinery to support axonal growth. Trauma and neurodegenerative processes affect the axon but can also damage the nerve cell body. Treatments that aim to protect nerve cell body health after injury have been aimed at neuroprotection and trying to minimise cell death. Neurotrophic factors mediate neuronal survival and factors such as nerve growth factor (NGF) (Levi-Montalich, 1987), glial derived neurotrophic factor (GDNF) (Lewis, Neff et al. 1993), IGF-1 (Henderson, Phillips et al. 1994) and vascular endothelial growth factor (VEGF) (Storkebaum, Lambrechts et al. 2004) have been employed for their neuroprotective effects. Other factors that are feasible in minimising nerve cell body death are anti-apoptotic factors. The X-linked inhibitor of apoptosis protein (XIAP) mediated protection of motor neurons as shown in *in vitro* models of ALS and in diabetic neuropathy (Garrity-Moses, Teng et al. 2004). Other anti-apoptotic factors such as Bcl-2 and Bcl-xL which prevent apoptosis both *in vitro* and *in vivo* (Yamashita, Mita et al. 2001; Matsuoka, Ishii et al. 2002; Yamashita, Mita et al. 2003; Garrity-Moses, Teng et al. 2005) are attractive for neuroprotection A problem associated with therapies that solely act on the proximal stump of a damaged nerve is the growth of axons into this milieu without being able to leave it. Excessive neuronal growth can lead to neuromas which prevent reinnervation of the distal stump and cause pain.

The second part of the injured peripheral nerve that needs to be considered is the gap. The success of the axon regrowth depends on the severity of the injury, the distance that needs to be bridged and how soon any intervention occurs post-injury (Midha, Munro et al. 2005; Weber and Mackinnon 2005). Nerve grafts assist in directing nerve regrowth. Grafting along with gene therapy has been used to assist in this process. The principle was proven by adenoviral transduction of nerve grafts (Blits, Dijkhuizen et al. 1999). In this experiment, sections of peripheral intercostal nerves were transduced with adenovirus expressing LacZ as a reporter gene. These nerves were then grafted into transacted sciatic nerves, avulsed neutral root, hemi-sected spinal cord and intact brain. Expression of LacZ could still be detected up to 7 days post-implantation.

The third part of the injured nerve is the distal stump and the neuromuscular junction. The distal stump of the damaged nerve provides support for neuronal regrowth via the release of stimulatory factors. These factors assist generating nerve sprouts to extend towards the target tissue (Abrams and Widenfalk 2005). One therapeutic strategy is to silence the expression of genes that inhibit nerve regrowth. Silencing the expression of the components of the inhibitory signalling cascade, using siRNAs, such as p75NTR, NgR and RhoA was shown to promote neurite outgrowth in cultured DRGs (Ahmed, Dent et al. 2005). This is a viable strategy for peripheral nerve injury therapy (Abrams and Widenfalk 2005).

The fourth and final part of a damaged peripheral nerve is the environment in which it is situated. The environment surrounding a damaged peripheral nerve is a target for *ex vivo* gene therapy. Stem cells that have been genetically engineered to enhance neurotrophic factors are a therapeutic option for injured peripheral nerves that has received considerable attention (Tohill and Terenghi 2004). Periaxonal grafts of nerve stem cells that secrete GDNF have been found to assist in providing a supportive environment for nerve regeneration (Deshpande, Kim et al. 2006).

2. Gene and cell therapy

Gene and cell therapies have the potential to be effective in peripheral neuropathy treatment. A number of factors need to be taken into account to allow this to happen. The correct vector (viral or non-viral) or cell type has to be chosen for the neuropathy based on vector or cell tropism. The vector tropism will help determine the method of delivery of the vector. Delivery will either be directly into the site of injury or degeneration, or remote from the site of injury. In the case of remote delivery the choice of therapeutic will depend on its' ability to cross the blood nerve barrier, in the case of AAV-9, or its' ability to be moved via retrograde transport from, for example, an intramuscular injection to the site of nerve injury. The therapeutic gene delivered using a vector has to be selected for optimum effect and if cell therapy is used whether the cells are engineered to secrete a neurotrophic factor.

2.1 Gene therapy vectors

Gene therapy vectors can be divided into viral and non-viral vectors based on their origin. The intent is to deliver a therapeutic gene to the affected area and affect a positive outcome. A variety of different viruses can be converted to viral vectors with different affinities for the peripheral nervous system. For example, herpes vectors have a natural tropism for the neurons of the Dorsal Root Ganglia (DRG) (Fink, Ramakrishnan et al. 1996). Similarly, a wide variety of methods exist for non-viral gene delivery. These can be engineered for enhanced gene delivery to the nerve.

2.1.1 Non-viral vectors

Non-viral vectors can include plasmid DNA containing the therapeutic gene of interest, cationic and polycationic polymers. The major advantage these have over viral vectors is their safety. The major disadvantage for gene transfer in the nervous system is they have a very low efficiency when compared to viral vectors (Costantini, Bakowska et al. 2000; Hsich, Sena-Esteves et al. 2002). The plasmid DNA vector can be delivered unmodified or with a targeting molecule attached to improve delivery. One such targeting molecule it the tet peptide developed by our research group (Liu, Teng et al. 2005). This peptide was identified based on its' homology to the tetanus toxin and it enhances neurotropism. This peptide was used by Park and colleagues to successfully target plasmid DNA the neural cells and DRG cells *in vitro* (Park, Lasiene *et al. 2007)* and *in vivo* via an injection into lateral ventricle of mice. The tet-1 complexed plasmid was found to target adult neural progenitor cells (NPCs) (Kwon, Lasiene et al. 2010).

2.1.2 Viral vectors

Viral vectors consist of viruses whose genome has been modified to carry the therapeutic gene. The genome is usually altered such that the vector is unable to replicate. In the peripheral nervous system there are a number of different viral vectors that have been used; Adenoviral vectors (Ad), Adeno associated vectors (AAV), Herpes simplex virus (HSV) type 1 and Lentiviral vectors.

2.1.2.1 Adenoviral vectors

Adenoviral vectors have been extensively used in gene therapy research. They have been shown to transduce post-mitotic dorsal root ganglions (DRGs), neurons (Glatzel, Flechsig et al. 2000) and Schwann cells (Shy, Tani et al. 1995; Dijkhuizen, Pasterkamp et al. 1998; Sorensen, Haase et al. 1998). They are non integrating vectors and therefore are limited to short-term expression which is a disadvantage. Ad vectors also have the drawback of eliciting an immune response which is an undesirable attribute in a therapeutic agent.

2.1.2.2 Adeno-associated vectors (AAV)

Adeno-associated vectors (AAV) are a very attractive vector for gene therapy. AAV vectors have long term and stable transgene expression and also efficiently transduce post-mitotic neurons. A disadvantage of AAV vectors is that there is a limit to the size of the transgene it can carry. This can make it unsuitable for larger transgenes. There are a number of AAV serotypes that have different tropisms for neural cells. AAV2 has been demonstrated to transduce DRGs, Schwann cells and fibroblasts (Fleming, Ginn et al. 2001). AAV9 has the ability to transduce a number of different neural cells types (Foust, Nurre et al. 2009). A study by our research group in mice showed that different AAV serotypes had different longitudinal spread within the spinal cord (Snyder, Gray et al. 2011) suggesting that similar differences in spread exist within the peripheral nervous system exist.

2.1.2.3 Herpes Simplex Virus (HSV) type 1

Herpes Simples Virus (HSV) type 1 is naturally neurotrophic. HSV-1 produces a lytic infection of skin cells and then migrates to the nerve processes. It is then transported in retrograde fashion to the sensory cell body of DRGs (Pradat and Mallet 2003). The ability of HSV type 1 to transduce sensory neurons makes it an ideal choice for neuropathies affecting sensory neurons (Glorioso and Fink 2004). The main disadvantage of HSV type 1 vectors is the immune response elicited against the virus proteins and the cell toxicity of the virions (Pradat and Mallet 2003).

2.1.2.4 Lentiviral vectors

Lentiviral vectors are also naturally neurotrophic (Fleming, Ginn et al. 2001). They integrate into the host genome which makes the expression of the carried transgene both stable and long-term (Blits, Boer et al. 2002; Hu, Leaver et al. 2005). Lentiviral vectors have limited immunogenicity and can accommodate a larger transgene than AAV (Federici and Boulis 2009). The modification of the lentiviral coat, which is termed pseudotyping, to enhance its transduction ability has been extensively studied. Pseudotyping of lentivirus with the rabies-G glycoprotein exploits the natural uptake of the rabies virus by axon terminals at neuromuscular junctions. This has been used to improve motor neuron gene delivery (Mazarakis, Azzouz et al. 2001; Cronin, Zhang et al. 2005)

Vector	Advantages	Disadvantages
Adenoviral	Easily transduces post-mitotic cells	Short expression time Immunogenic
HSV type 1	Naturally neurotrophic Retrogradely transported	Naturally immunogenic
AAV	Integrates and gives prolonged expression. A number of different serotypes available	Small cloning capacity
Lentiviral	Stable, integrated expression Retrogradely transported Large cloning capacity	Integration mutagenesis

Table 1. Comparison of different viral vectors.

2.1.3 Transport of vectors

The ability of vectors to be transported in a retrograde manner into the nervous system makes them more amenable for gene therapy of peripheral neuropathies. It allows the therapy to be administered at a site distant from and less invasive for the targeted area. Although Ad and AAV vectors are not naturally neurotrophic, they both have the ability to be transported in a retrograde manner and infect both sensory and motor neurons. A number of research groups have shown Ad vectors to be transported in a retrograde manner after intramuscular and intraneural injections (Finiels, Ribotta et al. 1995; Ghadge, Roos et al. 1995; Boulis, Bhatia et al. 1999). It is also possible to modify these vectors to enhance their affinity for neurons and as a consequence increase the rate of retrograde transport. Inoculation with botulinum toxin was found to enhance Ad vector transport and increase expression of the transgene in motor neurons (Millecamps, Mallet et al. 2002).

Different AAV serotypes have been shown to be transported in a retrograde fashion following both intramuscular and intraneural delivery (Boulis, Noordmans et al. 2003; Kaspar, Llado et al. 2003; Kaspar, Vich et al. 2004). A number of research groups have been working on improving the affinity AAV vectors have for neural cells. One means of achieving this is to modify the protein coat of the vector to incorporate neurotrophic peptides to enhance its' therapeutic effect. Peptides that mimic the binding capacity of the tetanus toxin, the NMDA receptor and peptides that mimic the activity of dynein have been inserted into the protein coat of AAV2 vectors to improve their neurotropism (Xu, Ma et al. 2005; Federici, Liu et al. 2007).

HSV-1 is a viral vector that is naturally neurotrophic. Recombinant HSV-1 has demonstrated the ability to transduce both motor and sensory neurons after intramuscular and subcutaneous delivery (Yamamura, Kageyama et al. 2000; Glorioso and Fink 2004). However, HSV mediated gene expression is transient. The lack of durability in expression impedes the application of HSV mediated gene delivery to chronic and ongoing neuropathies.

There is extensive research to show that lentiviral vectors have the ability to be transported in a retrograde manner. In a similar manner to AAV, the lentiviral vector can be engineered to enhance its' effect. The rabies virus is transported axonally via a neuromuscular junction. A lentiviral vector that is pseudotyped with the rabies G protein will have increased axonal transport and will reach the spinal cord motor neurons (Cronin, Zhang et al. 2005). Transduction of motor neurons in the lumbar spinal cord by a rabies-G pseudotyped lentiviral vector has been shown after peripheral administration intramuscularly (Mazarakis, Azzouz et al. 2001). Our research group has published data demonstrating that a pseudotyped human immunodeficiency virus type 1 (HIV-1) based lentiviral vector was capable of transducing specific cells types and increasing retrograde axonal transport (Federici, Kutner et al. 2007).

2.2 Cell therapy

The use of cell therapy in peripheral neuropathy especially peripheral nerve injury has been the focus of research. The peripheral nervous system has the ability to regenerate axons and reinnervate end organs. However, this can be problematic in the case of chronic denervation of distal nerves.

2.2.1 Schwann cells (SC)

Schwann cells (SC) have been shown to support peripheral nerve repair. They achieve this by changing their phenotype from myleinating to growth supporting (Shy, Shi et al. 1996; Mirsky and Jessen 1999). If the Schwann cells themselves are denervated for a prolonged period of time their ability to support peripheral nerve regrowth is impaired and inhibited (de Medinaceli and Rawlings 1987; Fu and Gordon 1995). One therapeutic option is to supplement or replace the deprived Schwann cells with healthy ones from another nerve. Infusion of healthy Schwann cells has been able to support regeneration and remyleination of both the spinal cord (Takami, Oudega et al. 2002; Pearse, Pereira et al. 2004) and in peripheral nerves (Guenard, Kleitman et al. 1992). The limiting factor in this is the number of Schwann cells obtainable from this source. There is also the fact that obtaining the Schwann cells from nerve tissue itself causes damage.

2.2.2 Neural stem cells (NSCs)

Neural stem cells (NSCs) have the ability to differentiate into neurons, astrocytes and oligodendrocytes (Parker, Anderson et al. 2005). They can also be induced to differentiate into Schwann cells (Blakemore 2005). NSCs secrete the growth factors that help support nerve regeneration (Heath 2000). They can be sourced from either fetal, adult or a non-neuronal tissue source. Implantation of NSCs has been shown to promote axonal regeneration and to form Schwann cell like peripheral myelin sheaths (Blakemore 2005). Therefore NSCs transplanted into a peripheral nerve injury site can help overcome the issue of limited sources of healthy Schwann cells and they can also promote peripheral nerve regeneration. The fact that NSCs can be grown and amplified *in vitro* is an added advantage. NSCs have been used in sciatic nerve injury repair.

2.2.3 Mesenchymal stem cells (MSC)

Mesenchymal stem cells (MSC) are adult derived stem cells that have the ability to differentiate down three lineages; adipogenic, chondrogenic and osteogenic. There have been a number of studies that show MSCs possess immunomodulatory properties *in vitro* on cell populations of both passive and adaptive immunity(Uccelli, Moretta et al. 2006). A study in a mouse model of experimental autoimmune encephalomyelitis (EAE), which is a model for human multiple sclerosis (MS), injected MSCs on one side of the brain and induced peripheral T cell tolerance to myelin proteins. This reduced the migration of pathogenic T cells to the CNS. On the other side of the brain the MSCs were found to preserve axons and reduce myelination (Bai, Lennon et al. 2009; Constantin, Marconi et al. 2009). Injection of MSCs into the spinal cord of transgenic SOD1 (G93A) mice, a model for ALS, was found to improve motor neuron survival, prolong life and improve motor performance (Vercelli, Mereuta et al. 2008). There have been a number of studies looking at the therapeutic effect of MSCs in peripheral nerve injury models. In a rat model of sciatic nerve injury MSCs were injected into the lumber DRG. The MSCs were found to have an analgesic effect affecting the expression of neuropetides galanin and neuropeptide Y (NPY) (Coronel, Musolino et al. 2009). Treatment of damaged nerves directly with MSCs has also been demonstrated to be effective. In a rat model of facial nerve injury MSCs were applied to a transected facial nerve after anastomosis. Results showed that the MSC treated nerve did better in terms of axonal organisation and myelin thickness when compared to nerves that had only been sutured (Satar, Karahatay et al. 2009) In another study MSCs were injected subepineurally one week after sciatic nerve injury in rabbits. Nerves that were grafted with MSCs showed better functional recovery, and improved nerve regeneration (Duan, Cheng et al. 2011)

Cell Type	Source	Advantages
Schwann Cells	Nerve tissue	Autologous source
NSC	Fetal or adult	Neural in origin
MSC	Adult tissues (bone marrow, adipocytes)	Ability to differentiate into different lineages Home to injury site

Table 2. Comparison of different cell types.

3. Peripheral nerve disorders

3.1 Diabetic neuropathy

Diabetic neuropathy is a complication of both insulin-dependent and insulin-independent diabetes mellitus. There are a number of possible contributing factors to the development of diabetic neuropathy such as oxidative stress, non-enzymatic glycation of nerve endings and mitochondrial damage (Mata, Chattopadhyay et al. 2006). A lack of or a reduction in neurotrophic factor levels is also considered a possible factor. Research has demonstrated that supplementation of neurotrophic factors can help delay the progression of diabetic neuropathy and other polyneuropathies.

Both nerve growth factor (NGF) and vascular endothelial growth factor (VEGF) have had therapeutic success in animal models of diabetic neuropathy. A HSV based vector expressing NGF was used to transduce dorsal root ganglion of diabetic mice. Results showed that it prevented loss of sensory nerve action potential (Goss, Goins et al. 2002). Subcutaneous delivery of VEGF in an HSV vector was transported in a retrograde manner to the DRGs and was found to preserve nerve fibres in diabetic mice (Chattopadhyay, Krisky et al. 2005). Placental growth factor (PlGF) is a member of the VEGF family. PlGF-2 has been found to display neurotrophic actions acting through neuropillin - 1 (NP-1) in DRGs *in vitro*. *In vivo*, PlGF-2 plasmid was injected with electroporation into the skeletal muscle of diabetic mice. Results showed a restoration of sensory deficits in these diabetic mice that was mediated via NP-1 (Murakami, Imada et al. 2011). Another study used a regulatable HSV vector to deliver erythropoietin (EPO) to diabetic mice. The HSV vector expression was controlled using the tet-on system which means EPO was expressed in response to presence of doxycycline (DOX). Mice were inoculated via their footpad and were administered DOX on a controlled basis. This regulated expression of EPO was found to be effective in protecting against the progression of neuropathy in these diabetic animals (Wu, Mata et al. 2011).

There is currently a clinical trial underway for diabetic neuropathy. VM202 which is human hepatocyte growth factor encoded in a plasmid. It is a Phase 1/2 open label trial examining safety and the effect of dose escalation with the gene therapy being administered via intramuscular injection into the calf muscle (www.clinicaltrials.gov , NCT01002235). A second phase 2 clinical trial is using zinc finger proteins in the treatment of diabetic neuropathy. Zinc finger proteins have the ability to increase expression of endogenous genes and can be designed to target specific genes (Davis and Stokoe 2010). In this trail the zinc finger protein is targeting VEGF and increasing its expression (www.clinicaltrials.gov, NCT01079325).

3.2 Peripheral nerve injury

A large number of the existing therapies for peripheral nerve diseases are concentrated on the proximal stump of the nerve (Federici and Boulis 2007). The ability of a number of viral vectors to be transported in a retrograde manner means they have been utilised to deliver neurotrophic factors (Romero, Rangappa et al. 2001; Natsume, Wolfe et al. 2003; Araki, Shiotani et al. 2006). In the case of peripheral nerve injury the site of the damaged nerve is first identified using current therapies. This has the advantage of exposing the damaged proximal stump of the nerve to allow the therapeutic vectors access. The viral vector can be engineered to enhance their uptake and retrograde transport. This can help improve their therapeutic effect and help prevent further nerve degeneration. Neuro-targeting peptides can be incorporated into the viral coat and into plasmids to enhance vector uptake as previously outlined (Federici, Liu et al. 2005; Park, Lasiene et al. 2007; Kwon, Lasiene et al. 2010).

An adenoviral vector was used to deliver glial derived neurotrophic factor (GDNF) intramuscularly in a chronic constricted nerve injury rat model of peripheral nerve injury. The injury to the limb was found to increase mechanical and thermal hypersensitivity. GDNF/Akt signalling was lost, particularly, in the distal stump of the sciatic nerve. Ad-GDNF therapy was found to restore GDNF/Akt signalling and this was associated with improved myelination and behavioural outcomes (Shi, Liu et al. 2011). An Ad vector was also used to deliver bone morphogenetic protein 7 (BMP-7) in a rat model of sciatic injury. BMPs promote neuronal differentiation and have been implicated in the survival of peripheral nerves (Beck, Drahushuk et al. 2001; Guha, Gomes et al. 2004; Schluesener, Meyermann et al. 1995) and in this study Ad-BMP-7 improved hind-limb recovery and reduced macrophage activation, nerve demyelination and axonal degeneration (Tsai, Pan et al. 2010).

Stem cells can also be utilised in peripheral nerve injury repair. One group used neural stem cells that had been engineered to secrete glial cell-line derived neurotrophic factor (GDNF). These cells were administered to the sciatic nerve of rats that had previously received spinal cord embryonic stem cell-derived motor neuron transplantation (Deshpande, Kim et al. 2006). The increased level of expression of GDNF in the sciatic nerve attracted embryonic stem cell- derived axons. Theses axons reached the muscle and formed physiologically active neuromuscular junctions.

3.3 Neuropathic pain

Neuropathic pain is caused by either dysfunction of the CNS, PNS or a primary lesion. This can manifest itself as hypersensitivity to pain (hyperalgesia) or as a painful response to a stimulus that would not normally cause pain (allodynia). Currently opiates are the mainstay of treatment for the majority of chronic pain states (Beutler and Reinhardt 2009). Their use has generally improved outcome (Portenoy 1995; Levy 1996) but due to side-effects opiates have not been effective in a significant number of patients (Caraceni and Portenoy 1999; Weiss, Emanuel et al. 2001). The possibility of delivering a therapeutic gene to alleviate the symptoms of pain has been studied in a number of animal models of neuropathic pain as well as the possibility of also of modulating both the excitatory and inhibitory pathways of pain has also been examined in these disease models (Cope and Lariviere 2006).

As previously discussed the HSV-1 vector is naturally neurotrophic and it has been utilised extensively in sensory neuropathies. Administration of a HSV-1 vector expressing glutamic acid decarboxylase (GAD) subcutaneously has been found to alleviate pain in a model of spinal nerve ligation. Increased expression of GAD in the DRGs resulted in attenuation of the symptoms of mechanical allodynia and thermal hyperalgesia (Hao, Mata et al. 2003). GDNF expressed by either a HSV-1 or lentiviral vector has also been found to be effective in reversing pain manifestations in spinal nerve ligation pain model. The HSV-GDNF was delivered subcutaneously and the lentiviral-GDNF was delivered via intraspinal injections (Hao, Mata et al. 2003; Pezet, Krzyzanowska et al. 2006). Treatment with both vectors was found to significantly alleviate both thermal and mechanical hyperalgesia symptoms.

Another focus has been on the opiate system. HSV-1 vectors encoding human proenkephalin A, which is an opiate peptide precursor, has been found to have anti-hyperalgesia effects in mice models of hyperalgesia (Wilson, Yeomans et al. 1999; Yeomans, Jones et al. 2004).

A further possibility is to knockdown expression of gene involved in pain pathways. Lentiviral vectors have been used to deliver short hairpin RNAs to knockdown expression of a voltage-gated sodium channel (NaV1.8). This ion channel is thought to be involved in the pathogenesis of neuropathic pain in DRGs. Delivery of the lentivirus expressing the shRNA to primary DRGs was found to knockdown protein and messenger RNA (mRNA) levels and to also decrease the NaV1.8 mediated current densities (Mikami and Yang 2005). Another study used an AAV vector to deliver a shRNA to knockdown expression of GTP cyclohydrolase I (GCHI). Activation of expression of GTPI cyclohydrolase in DRGs has been shown to be significantly involved in development and longevity of pain symptoms. The shRNA was delivered to the sciatic nerve and expression of the transgene was detected in the DRGs. Knockdown of GTP1 cyclohydrolase resulted in a sharp decline in pain symptoms in the animal model and also showed reduced microglial activation in the dorsal horn which inferred a link between pain relief and reduced inflammation (Kim, Lee et al. 2009).

3.4 Motor neuron disease

Motor neuron diseases, which include amyotrophic lateral sclerosis (ALS) and spinal muscular atrophy (SMA), are progressive neurodegenerative diseases that result in progressive loss of both upper and lower motor neurons. Both diseases are invariably fatal and current therapies are merely palliative. The possibility of gene or cell therapy as a therapeutic option for motor neuron disease is being extensively researched.

Successful gene transfer has been achieved in motor neuron disease by both intramuscular (Kahn, Haase et al. 1996, Wang, Lu et al. 2002, Lesbordes, Cifuentes-Diaz et al. 2003) and intraneural delivery(Boulis, Noordmans et al. 2003; Boulis, Willmarth et al. 2003). *Ex vivo* gene therapy involving genetic modification of cells that are then transplanted into the injured region has also been investigated in relation to motor neuron disease. This has involved grafting cells that have to ability to secrete neurotrophic factors. An example of this involved the implantation of myoblasts that had been retrovirally transduced with GDNF. These cells were implanted into the hindlimb of SOD1 mouse model of ALS. GDNF gene delivery was found to prevent motor neuron loss and disease progression (Mohajeri, Figlewicz et al. 1999). There is a Phase 2 clinical trial for an ALS therapy currently taking place in which neural stem cells are being injected to the spinal cord of ALS patients (www.clinicaltrials.gov NCT01348451).

4. Conclusion

Peripheral neuropathies in the form of diabetic neuropathy, peripheral nerve injury and neuropathic pain are painful and debilitating conditions. Amyotrophic lateral sclerosis (ALS) and spinal muscular atrophy (SMA) are not peripheral neuropathies in the strictest sense but they are related as disorders of the cells that form the peripheral nerves. Current best clinical practise offers drug treatment for pain relief and nerve grafting for damaged nerves. These treatments have some success but room for improvement exists.

Gene and cell therapies have the potential to improve treatment outcomes in these peripheral neuropathies. Gene therapy vectors potential to transduce neurons and be transported in a retrograde manner has been exploited in animal models of these diseases and has shown beneficial effects. Efforts to improve tropism of vectors by pseudotyping and by incorporating neurotrophic peptides into viral coats increase specificity of these vectors and reduce the problem of off-target effects. In a similar manner cell therapies can be used in these diseases. Cell therapies can be used in an unmodified state where they can effect change at the site of injury or can be engineered to secrete a specific factor that will support nerve regrowth and repair.

The movement of potential therapies into clinical trials is ongoing. In the meantime research continues to improve and refine understanding of peripheral neuropathies while working on therapy concepts to treat these conditions.

5. References

Abrams, M. and J. Widenfalk (2005). "Emerging strategies to promote improved functional outcome after peripheral nerve injury." Restor Neurol Neurosci 23(5-6): 367-382.

Ahmed, Z., R. G. Dent, et al. (2005). "Disinhibition of neurotrophin-induced dorsal root ganglion cell neurite outgrowth on CNS myelin by siRNA-mediated knockdown of NgR, p75NTR and Rho-A." Mol Cell Neurosci 28(3): 509-523.

Araki, K., A. Shiotani, et al. (2006). "Adenoviral GDNF gene transfer enhances neurofunctional recovery after recurrent laryngeal nerve injury." Gene Ther 13(4): 296-303.

Bai, L., D. P. Lennon, et al. (2009). "Human bone marrow-derived mesenchymal stem cells induce Th2-polarized immune response and promote endogenous repair in animal models of multiple sclerosis." Glia 57(11): 1192-1203.

Beck, H. N., K. Drahushuk, et al. (2001). "Bone morphogenetic protein-5 (BMP-5) promotes dendritic growth in cultured sympathetic neurons." BMC neuroscience 2: 12.

Beutler, A. S. and M. Reinhardt (2009). "AAV for pain: steps towards clinical translation." Gene therapy 16(4): 461-469.

Blakemore, W. F. (2005). "The case for a central nervous system (CNS) origin for the Schwann cells that remyelinate CNS axons following concurrent loss of oligodendrocytes and astrocytes." Neuropathology and applied neurobiology 31(1): 1-10.

Blits, B., G. J. Boer, et al. (2002). "Pharmacological, cell, and gene therapy strategies to promote spinal cord regeneration." Cell Transplant 11(6): 593-613.

Blits, B., P. Dijkhuizen, et al. (1999). "Adenoviral vector-mediated expression of a foreign gene in peripheral nerve tissue bridges implanted in the injured peripheral and the central nervous system." Exp Neurol 160: 256-267.

Boulis, N. M., V. Bhatia, et al. (1999). "Adenoviral nerve growth factor and beta-galactosidase transfer to spinal cord: a behavioral and histological analysis." J Neurosurg Spine 90(1): 99-108.

Boulis, N. M., A. J. Noordmans, et al. (2003). "Adeno-associated viral vector gene expression in the adult rat spinal cord following remote vector delivery." Neurobiol Dis 14(3): 535-541.

Boulis, N. M., N. E. Willmarth, et al. (2003). "Intraneural colchicine inhibition of adenoviral and adeno-associated viral vector remote spinal cord gene delivery." Neurosurgery 52(2): 381-387; discussion 387.

Caraceni, A. and R. K. Portenoy (1999). "An international survey of cancer pain characteristics and syndromes. IASP Task Force on Cancer Pain. International Association for the Study of Pain." Pain 82(3): 263-274.

Chattopadhyay, M., D. Krisky, et al. (2005). "HSV-mediated gene transfer of vascular endothelial growth factor to dorsal root ganglia prevents diabetic neuropathy." Gene Ther 12(18): 1377-1384.

Constantin, G., S. Marconi, et al. (2009). "Adipose-derived mesenchymal stem cells ameliorate chronic experimental autoimmune encephalomyelitis." Stem Cells 27(10): 2624-2635.

Cope, D. K. and W. R. Lariviere (2006). "Gene therapy and chronic pain." ScientificWorldJournal 6: 1066-1074.

Coronel, M. F., P. L. Musolino, et al. (2009). "Bone marrow stromal cells attenuate injury-induced changes in galanin, NPY and NPY Y1-receptor expression after a sciatic nerve constriction." Neuropeptides 43(2): 125-132.

Costantini, L. C., J. C. Bakowska, et al. (2000). "Gene therapy in the CNS." Gene therapy 7(2): 93-109.

Cronin, J., X. Y. Zhang, et al. (2005). "Altering the tropism of lentiviral vectors through pseudotyping." Curr Gene Ther 5(4): 387-398.

Davis, D. and D. Stokoe (2010). "Zinc finger nucleases as tools to understand and treat human diseases." BMC medicine 8: 42.

de Medinaceli, L. and R. R. Rawlings (1987). "Is it possible to predict the outcome of peripheral nerve injuries? A probability model based on prospects for regenerating neurites." Bio Systems 20(3): 243-258.

Deshpande, D. M., Y. S. Kim, et al. (2006). "Recovery from paralysis in adult rats using embryonic stem cells." Ann Neurol 60(1): 32-44.

Dijkhuizen, P. A., R. J. Pasterkamp, et al. (1998). "Adenoviral vector-mediated gene delivery to injured rat peripheral nerve." J Neurotrauma 15(6): 387-397.

Duan, X. H., L. N. Cheng, et al. (2011). "In vivo MRI monitoring nerve regeneration of acute peripheral nerve traction injury following mesenchymal stem cell transplantation." European journal of radiology.

Dubovy, P. (2011). "Wallerian degeneration and peripheral nerve conditions for both axonal regeneration and neuropathic pain induction." Annals of anatomy = Anatomischer Anzeiger : official organ of the Anatomische Gesellschaft 193(4): 267-275.

Fansa, H. and G. Keilhoff (2003). "[Factors influencing nerve regeneration]." Handchir Mikrochir Plast Chir 35(2): 72-82.

Federici, T. and N. Boulis (2007). "Gene therapy for peripheral nervous system diseases." Curr Gene Ther 7(4): 239-248.

Federici, T. and N. M. Boulis (2009). "Invited review: festschrift edition of neurosurgery peripheral nervous system as a conduit for delivering therapies for diabetic neuropathy, amyotrophic lateral sclerosis, and nerve regeneration." Neurosurgery 65(4 Suppl): A87-92.

Federici, T., R. Kutner, et al. (2007). "Cell targeting in the CNS using HIV-1-based lentiviral vectors bearing alternative glycoproteins and promoters." Mol Ther 15(Suppl 1).

Federici, T., J. Liu, et al. (2005). "In Vivo Spinal Cord Uptake and Neuronal Binding Properties of Tet1: A Potential Means for Enhanced Spinal Cord AAV Delivery." Mol Ther 11(Suppl. 1): S332.

Federici, T., J. Liu, et al. (2007). "A Means for Targeting Therapeutics to Peripheral Nervous System Neurons with Axonal Damage." Neurosurg 60(5): 911-918.

Finiels, F., M. G. y. Ribotta, et al. (1995). "Specific and efficient gene transfer strategy offers new potentialities for the treatment of motor neuron diseases." Neuroreport 7: 373-378.

Fink, D. J., R. Ramakrishnan, et al. (1996). "Advances in the Development of Herpes Simplex Virus-Based Gene Transfer Vectors for the Nervous System." Clin Neurosci 3(5): 284-291.

Fischer, L., D. Culver, et al. (2004). "Amyotrophic lateral sclerosis is a distal axonopathy: evidence in mice and man." Exp Neurol 185(2): 232-240.

Fleming, J., S. L. Ginn, et al. (2001). "Adeno-associated virus and lentivirus vectors mediate efficient and sustained transduction of cultured mouse and human dorsal root ganglia sensory neurons." Hum Gene Ther 12(1): 77-86.

Foust, K. D., E. Nurre, et al. (2009). "Intravascular AAV9 preferentially targets neonatal neurons and adult astrocytes." Nat Biotechnol 27(1): 59-65.

Fu, S. Y. and T. Gordon (1995). "Contributing factors to poor functional recovery after delayed nerve repair: prolonged denervation." The Journal of neuroscience : the official journal of the Society for Neuroscience 15(5 Pt 2): 3886-3895.

Funakoshi, H., J. Frisen, et al. (1993). "Differential expression of mRNAs for neurotrophins and their receptors after axotomy of the sciatic nerve." The Journal of cell biology 123(2): 455-465.

Garrity-Moses, M., Q. Teng, et al. (2004). "Adenoviral XIAP expression protects motor neurons in an in vivo model of ALS." Soc Neurosci Abstr: 312.310.

Garrity-Moses, M. E., Q. Teng, et al. (2005). "Neuroprotective adeno-associated virus Bcl-(x)L gene transfer in models of motor neuron disease." Muscle Nerve 32(6): 734-744.

Ghadge, G., R. Roos, et al. (1995). "CNS gene delivery by retrograde transport of recombinant replication-defective adenoviruses." Gene Ther 2(2): 132-137.

Glatzel, M., E. Flechsig, et al. (2000). "Adenoviral and adeno-associated viral transfer of genes to the peripheral nervous system." Proc Natl Acad Sci U S A 97(1): 442-447.

Glorioso, J. C. and D. J. Fink (2004). "Herpes vector-mediated gene transfer in treatment of diseases of the nervous system." Annu Rev Microbiol 58: 253-271.

Goss, J. R., W. F. Goins, et al. (2002). "Herpes simplex-mediated gene transfer of nerve growth factor protects against peripheral neuropathy in streptozotocin-induced diabetes in the mouse." Diabetes 51(7): 2227-2232.

Guenard, V., N. Kleitman, et al. (1992). "Syngeneic Schwann cells derived from adult nerves seeded in semipermeable guidance channels enhance peripheral nerve regeneration." The Journal of neuroscience : the official journal of the Society for Neuroscience 12(9): 3310-3320.

Guha, U., W. A. Gomes, et al. (2004). "Target-derived BMP signaling limits sensory neuron number and the extent of peripheral innervation in vivo." Development 131(5): 1175-1186.

Hao, S., M. Mata, et al. (2003). "HSV-mediated gene transfer of the glial cell-derived neurotrophic factor provides an antiallodynic effect on neuropathic pain." Mol Ther 8(3): 367-375.

Heath, C. A. (2000). "Cells for tissue engineering." Trends in biotechnology 18(1): 17-19.

Henderson, C. E., H. S. Phillips, et al. (1994). "GDNF: a potent survival factor for motoneurons present in peripheral nerve and muscle." Science 266(5187): 1062-1064.

Hoke, A. (2006). "Mechanisms of Disease: what factors limit the success of peripheral nerve regeneration in humans?" Nat Clin Pract Neurol 2(8): 448-454.

Hsich, G., M. Sena-Esteves, et al. (2002). "Critical issues in gene therapy for neurologic disease." Human gene therapy 13(5): 579-604.

Hu, Y., S. G. Leaver, et al. (2005). "Lentiviral-mediated transfer of CNTF to schwann cells within reconstructed peripheral nerve grafts enhances adult retinal ganglion cell survival and axonal regeneration." Mol Ther 11(6): 906-915.

Ide, C. (1996). "Peripheral nerve regeneration." Neurosci Res 25(2): 101-121.

Kahn, A., G. Haase, et al. (1996). "Gene therapy of neurological diseases." C R Seances Soc Biol Fil 190(1): 9-11.

Kaspar, B. K., J. Llado, et al. (2003). "Retrograde viral delivery of IGF-1 prolongs survival in a mouse ALS model." Science 301(5634): 839-842.

Kaspar, B. K., V. Vich, et al. (2004). "AAV Retrograde Transport Potential and Therapeutic Approaches for ALS." Molecular Therapy 9(Suppl 1): S18.

Kim, S. J., W. I. Lee, et al. (2009). "Effective relief of neuropathic pain by adeno-associated virus-mediated expression of a small hairpin RNA against GTP cyclohydrolase 1." Molecular pain 5: 67.

Kwon, E. J., J. Lasiene, et al. (2010). "Targeted nonviral delivery vehicles to neural progenitor cells in the mouse subventricular zone." Biomaterials 31(8): 2417-2424.

Lesbordes, J. C., C. Cifuentes-Diaz, et al. (2003). "Therapeutic benefits of cardiotrophin-1 gene transfer in a mouse model of spinal muscular atrophy." Hum Mol Genet 12(11): 1233-1239.

Levy, M. H. (1996). "Pharmacologic treatment of cancer pain." The New England journal of medicine 335(15): 1124-1132.

Lewis, M. E., N. T. Neff, et al. (1993). "Insulin-like growth factor-I: potential for treatment of motor neuronal disorders." Exp Neurol 124(1): 73-88.

Liu, J. K., Q. Teng, et al. (2005). "A novel peptide defined through phage display for therapeutic protein and vector neuronal targeting." Neurobiol Dis 19(3): 407-418.

Mata, M., M. Chattopadhyay, et al. (2006). "Gene therapy for the treatment of sensory neuropathy." Expert Opin Biol Ther 6(5): 499-507.

Matsuoka, N., K. Ishii, et al. (2002). "Overexpression of basic fibroblast growth factor and Bcl-xL with adenoviral vectors protects primarily cultured neurons against glutamate insult." Neurosurgery 50(4): 857-862; discussion 862-853.

Mazarakis, N. D., M. Azzouz, et al. (2001). "Rabies virus glycoprotein pseudotyping of lentiviral vectors enables retrograde axonal transport and access to the nervous system after peripheral delivery." Hum Mol Genet 10(19): 2109-2121.

Midha, R., C. A. Munro, et al. (2005). "Regeneration into protected and chronically denervated peripheral nerve stumps." Neurosurgery 57(6): 1289-1299; discussion 1289-1299.

Mikami, M. and J. Yang (2005). "Short hairpin RNA-mediated selective knockdown of NaV1.8 tetrodotoxin-resistant voltage-gated sodium channel in dorsal root ganglion neurons." Anesthesiology 103(4): 828-836.

Millecamps, S., J. Mallet, et al. (2002). "Adenoviral retrograde gene transfer in motoneurons is greatly enhanced by prior intramuscular inoculation with botulinum toxin." Hum Gene Ther 13(2): 225-232.

Mirsky, R. and K. R. Jessen (1999). "The neurobiology of Schwann cells." Brain pathology 9(2): 293-311.

Mohajeri, M., D. Figlewicz, et al. (1999). "Intramuscular grafts of myoblasts genetically modified to secrete glial cell line-derived neurotrophic factor prevent motoneuron loss and disease progression in a mouse model of familial amyotrophic lateral sclerosis." Hum Gene Ther 10(11): 1853-1866.

Murakami, T., Y. Imada, et al. (2011). "Placental growth factor-2 gene transfer by electroporation restores diabetic sensory neuropathy in mice." Experimental neurology 227(1): 195-202.

Natsume, A., D. Wolfe, et al. (2003). "Enhanced functional recovery after proximal nerve root injury by vector-mediated gene transfer." Exp Neurol 184(2): 878-886.

Park, I. K., J. Lasiene, et al. (2007). "Neuron-specific delivery of nucleic acids mediated by Tet1-modified poly(ethylenimine)." J Gene Med 9(8): 691-702.

Parker, M. A., J. K. Anderson, et al. (2005). "Expression profile of an operationally-defined neural stem cell clone." Experimental neurology 194(2): 320-332.

Pearse, D. D., F. C. Pereira, et al. (2004). "cAMP and Schwann cells promote axonal growth and functional recovery after spinal cord injury." Nature medicine 10(6): 610-616.

Pezet, S., A. Krzyzanowska, et al. (2006). "Reversal of neurochemical changes and pain-related behavior in a model of neuropathic pain using modified lentiviral vectors expressing GDNF." Mol Ther 13(6): 1101-1109.

Portenoy, R. K. (1995). "Pharmacologic management of cancer pain." Seminars in oncology 22(2 Suppl 3): 112-120.

Pradat, P. F. and J. Mallet (2003). "Gene transfer into the central and peripheral nervous system: applications for the treatment of neurodegenerative diseases and peripheral neuropathies." Biotechnol Genet Eng Rev 20: 49-76.

Romero, M., N. Rangappa, et al. (2001). "Functional regeneration of chronically injured sensory afferents into adult spinal cord after neurotrophin gene therapy." J Neurosci 21(21): 8408-8416.

Satar, B., S. Karahatay, et al. (2009). "Repair of transected facial nerve with mesenchymal stromal cells: histopathologic evidence of superior outcome." The Laryngoscope 119(11): 2221-2225.

Schluesener, H. J., R. Meyermann, et al. (1995). "Immunolocalization of vgr (BMP-6, DVR-6), a TGF-beta related cytokine, to Schwann cells of the rat peripheral nervous system: expression patterns are not modulated by autoimmune disease." Glia 13(1): 75-78.

Shi, J. Y., G. S. Liu, et al. (2011). "Glial cell line-derived neurotrophic factor gene transfer exerts protective effect on axons in sciatic nerve following constriction-induced peripheral nerve injury." Human gene therapy 22(6): 721-731.

Shy, M. E., Y. Shi, et al. (1996). "Axon-Schwann cell interactions regulate the expression of c-jun in Schwann cells." Journal of Neuroscience Research 43(5): 511-525.

Shy, M. E., M. Tani, et al. (1995). "An adenoviral vector can transfer lacZ expression into Schwann cells in culture and in sciatic nerve." Ann Neurol 38(3): 429-436.

Snyder, B. R., S. J. Gray, et al. (2011). "Comparison of Adeno-Associated Viral Vector Serotypes for Spinal Cord and Motor Neuron Gene Delivery." Hum Gene Ther.

Sorensen, J., G. Haase, et al. (1998). "Gene transfer to Schwann cells after peripheral nerve injury: a delivery system for therapeutic agents." Ann Neurol 43(2): 205-211.

Stoll, G., J. W. Griffin, et al. (1989). "Wallerian degeneration in the peripheral nervous system: participation of both Schwann cells and macrophages in myelin degradation." Journal of neurocytology 18(5): 671-683.

Storkebaum, E., D. Lambrechts, et al. (2004). "VEGF: once regarded as a specific angiogenic factor, now implicated in neuroprotection." Bioessays 26(9): 943-954.

Takami, T., M. Oudega, et al. (2002). "Schwann cell but not olfactory ensheathing glia transplants improve hindlimb locomotor performance in the moderately contused adult rat thoracic spinal cord." The Journal of neuroscience : the official journal of the Society for Neuroscience 22(15): 6670-6681.

Tohill, M. and G. Terenghi (2004). "Stem-cell plasticity and therapy for injuries of the peripheral nervous system." Biotechnol Appl Biochem 40(Pt 1): 17-24.

Tsai, M. J., H. A. Pan, et al. (2010). "Adenoviral gene transfer of bone morphogenetic protein-7 enhances functional recovery after sciatic nerve injury in rats." Gene therapy 17(10): 1214-1224.

Uccelli, A., L. Moretta, et al. (2006). "Immunoregulatory function of mesenchymal stem cells." European journal of immunology 36(10): 2566-2573.

Vercelli, A., O. M. Mereuta, et al. (2008). "Human mesenchymal stem cell transplantation extends survival, improves motor performance and decreases neuroinflammation in mouse model of amyotrophic lateral sclerosis." Neurobiology of disease 31(3): 395-405.

Wang, L. J., Y. Y. Lu, et al. (2002). "Neuroprotective effects of glial cell line-derived neurotrophic factor mediated by an adeno-associated virus vector in a transgenic animal model of amyotrophic lateral sclerosis." J Neurosci 22(16): 6920-6928.

Weber, R. V. and S. E. Mackinnon (2005). "Bridging the neural gap." Clin Plast Surg 32(4): 605-616, viii.

Weiss, S. C., L. L. Emanuel, et al. (2001). "Understanding the experience of pain in terminally ill patients." Lancet 357(9265): 1311-1315.

Wilson, S. P., D. C. Yeomans, et al. (1999). "Antihyperalgesic effects of infection with a preproenkephalin-encoding herpes virus." Proc Natl Acad Sci U S A 96(6): 3211-3216.

Wu, Z., M. Mata, et al. (2011). "Prevention of diabetic neuropathy by regulatable expression of HSV-mediated erythropoietin." Molecular therapy : the journal of the American Society of Gene Therapy 19(2): 310-317.

Xu, J., C. Ma, et al. (2005). "A combination of mutations enhances the neurotropism of AAV-2." Virology 341(2): 203-214.

Yamamura, J., S. Kageyama, et al. (2000). "Long-term gene expression in the anterior horn motor neurons after intramuscular inoculation of a live herpes simplex virus vector." Gene Ther 7(11): 934-941.

Yamashita, S., S. Mita, et al. (2001). "Bcl-2 expression by retrograde transport of adenoviral vectors with Cre-loxP recombination system in motor neurons of mutant SOD1 transgenic mice." Gene Ther 8(13): 977-986.

Yamashita, S., S. Mita, et al. (2003). "Bcl-2 expression using retrograde transport of adenoviral vectors inhibits cytochrome c-release and caspase-1 activation in motor neurons of mutant superoxide dismutase 1 (G93A) transgenic mice." Neurosci Lett 350(1): 17-20.

Yeomans, D. C., T. Jones, et al. (2004). "Reversal of ongoing thermal hyperalgesia in mice by a recombinant herpesvirus that encodes human preproenkephalin." Mol Ther 9(1): 24-29.